KT-553-996

Fundamentals of Skeletal Radiology

FIFTH EDITION

CLYDE A. HELMS, MD
Professor of Radiology and Orthopedic Surgery
Department of Radiology
Duke University School of Medicine
Durham, North Carolina

BMA LIBRARY
BRITISH MEDICAL ASSOCIATION

ELSEVIER

ELSEVIER

1600 John F. Kennedy Blvd.
Ste 1600
Philadelphia, PA 19103-2899

FUNDAMENTALS OF SKELETAL RADIOLOGY, FIFTH EDITION ISBN: 978-0-323-61165-7

Copyright © 2020 by Elsevier, Inc. All rights reserved.
Previous editions copyrighted 1995, 2005, 2014

No part of this publication may be reproduced or transmitted in any form or by any means, electronic or mechanical, including photocopying, recording, or any information storage and retrieval system, without permission in writing from the publisher. Details on how to seek permission, further information about the Publisher's permissions policies and our arrangements with organizations such as the Copyright Clearance Center and the Copyright Licensing Agency, can be found at our website: www.elsevier.com/permissions.

This book and the individual contributions contained in it are protected under copyright by the Publisher (other than as may be noted herein).

Notices

Practitioners and researchers must always rely on their own experience and knowledge in evaluating and using any information, methods, compounds or experiments described herein. Because of rapid advances in the medical sciences, in particular, independent verification of diagnoses and drug dosages should be made. To the fullest extent of the law, no responsibility is assumed by Elsevier, authors, editors or contributors for any injury and/or damage to persons or property as a matter of products liability, negligence or otherwise, or from any use or operation of any methods, products, instructions, or ideas contained in the material herein.

Library of Congress Cataloging-in-Publication Data or Control Number: 2018955733

Content Strategist: Russell Gabbedy
Content Development Specialist: Angie Breckon
Publishing Services Manager: Shereen Jameel
Project Manager: Rukmani Krishnan
Design Direction: Bridget Hoette

Printed in China

Last digit is the print number: 9 8 7 6 5 4 3 2 1

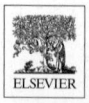

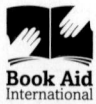

Working together to grow libraries in developing countries

www.elsevier.com • www.bookaid.org

To Hideyo Minagi – the finest teacher I have ever known.

Foreword to the Second Edition

Clyde Helms, as a radiologist in training during the mid-1970s, was, in many ways, the ideal radiology resident. Able, perceptive, informed, and responsible, he progressed through the various stages of residency training in superb fashion. On the other hand, he was different. Whereas the traditional "best resident" always had at hand exhaustive lists of differential diagnoses, Dr. Helms quietly ignored the trivial, the esoteric, and the information that was not likely to serve him in his work as a radiologist in the "real world," sometimes to the discomfiture of the radiology faculty of the University of California, San Francisco (of which I was then a junior member). Whereas the traditional "best resident" was suitably in awe of the faculty (many of whom were truly awesome), Dr. Helms fearlessly challenged what he perceived as unsupportable dogma. Not one to sit still for pretension, he poked gentle (and sometimes not so gentle) fun at the faculty. Occasional pranks were perpetrated, sometimes at the expense of members of the faculty. No one was immune, no matter how lofty his status. Dr. Helms, as the Sinatra song goes, did it his way. Irreverent, witty, occasionally outrageous, and a superb radiologist, he completed his residency and went on to fulfill his military commitment.

He returned to UCSF 3 years later as a faculty member in the skeletal radiology section. That he had not changed was immediately apparent. Faculty meetings were disrupted by his irreverent remarks, frequently hilarious. Now a mentor, his teaching reflects the same realistic, nontraditional approach he used as a resident. He emphasizes not the exotic or esoteric but the practical, the information that is critical in the day-to-day practice of radiology. Incorporated into his teaching method are mnemonics, one or two of which might not be recommended for family viewing. On the other hand, if they work, why not use them? An increasingly large number of young radiologists (his residents and former residents) will attest that, indeed, they do work. The teaching may be unorthodox, but the learning is real and substantial.

This volume is also unorthodox. Several excellent, superbly researched and crafted treatises on skeletal radiology are available to the radiology resident and practicing radiologist. This volume is not intended as an exhaustive compendium of skeletal radiology. Rather it is, as indicated by the title, an exposition of the *basics* of skeletal radiology. In keeping with his personalized, unusual approach to teaching, he begins with a discussion of radiologic examinations that should *not* be performed. The remainder of the book deals with skeletal conditions that radiologists are likely to encounter any day of the week. The reader who wishes to become familiar with Scheie syndrome or trichorhinophalangeal dysplasia type II must look elsewhere.

Rather than the usual, formal language found in other radiology texts, the reader will encounter the vernacular used by all radiologists when they discuss their work with other radiologists. The text is much like Dr. Helms himself—witty, irreverent, unpretentious, and fast-paced. The reader will find the book refreshing, eminently readable, and highly informative.

The ideal condition
Would be, I admit, that men should be right by instinct;
But since we are all likely to go astray,
The reasonable thing is to learn from those who can teach.

—SOPHOCLES

Clyde Helms can teach!

Hideyo Minagi, MD

Preface

When I was a resident at University of California, San Francisco (UCSF) in the 1970s, the teacher we all tried to emulate was Hideyo Minagi. He not only taught us radiology, he taught us how to behave, how to treat people, and how to be professionals. He told me that you shouldn't tell an audience everything you know – that was an effort to impress them; instead, you should tell them what they need to know – that was an effort to teach them. I hope this book follows that advice. This book is much the same in this fifth edition as it was 30 years ago. The fundamentals don't change that much. I have cleaned it up a bit and added better illustrations here and there, but essentially it's the same book.

When the first edition came out, I was concerned about what others might think of me for being somewhat irreverent and flippant in a supposedly scholarly work. As I got older and more mature I didn't really care what other people thought about me. As I have gotten even older, I now realize others were never thinking about me at all. The hard part about condensing a huge topic like musculoskeletal radiology into a small book is deciding what to omit. To paraphrase Mark Twain, "I would have written a shorter book if I had more time."

Table of Contents

1 **Unnecessary Examinations,** *1*

2 **Benign Lytic Lesions,** *7*

3 **Malignant Tumors,** *35*

4 **"Don't Touch" Lesions,** *59*

5 **Trauma,** *83*

6 **Arthritis,** *119*

7 **Metabolic Bone Disease,** *151*

8 **Miscellaneous Conditions,** *167*

9 **Magnetic Resonance Imaging of the Knee,** *181*

10 **Magnetic Resonance Imaging of the Shoulder,** *199*

11 **Lumbar Spine: Disc Disease and Stenosis,** *211*

12 **Magnetic Resonance Imaging of the Foot and Ankle,** *225*

13 **Miscellaneous Magnetic Resonance Imaging,** *239*

INDEX, *247*

APPENDIX, AVAILABLE ONLINE IN EXPERTCONSULT

CHAPTER 1

Unnecessary Examinations

Before beginning to learn how to interpret pathologic skeletal films, it is important to briefly consider unnecessary skeletal radiographic examinations. Dr. Ferris Hall from Boston first brought to my attention the idea that just because we *could* x-ray something didn't mean that we *should*. His article entitled "Overutilization of Radiologic Examinations" in the August 1976 issue of *Radiology*[1] details many examples of overuse and misuse of radiologic examinations. This article, even though it is over 35 years old, and a similar one by Dr. Herbert Abrams in the *New England Journal of Medicine*,[2] should be mandatory reading for every intern before he or she begins to order examinations.

There are many reasons why it is undesirable to have unnecessary radiologic examinations: excess cost, excess radiation, waste of patient's time, waste of technician's and radiologist's time, false hopes and expectations based on the outcome of the examination, and, not least of all, they indicate a breakdown in the logical thought pattern concerning the patient's workup.

Many examinations are ordered because of so-called medicolegal considerations. It is believed that if a certain finding is not documented (e.g., a broken rib), the doctor could be sued. In fact, few, if any, examples of medicolegal "covering yourself" types of examinations are valid. With the move toward greater consumer awareness, lawsuits in the future are more likely to result from unnecessary radiation exposure because of needless examinations rather than from too few examinations.

EXAMPLES OF UNNECESSARY EXAMINATIONS

Skull Series

Except for a depressed skull fracture or the presence of intracranial metallic fragments, there is no reason to order a skull series for trauma. This was once one of the most abused examinations in radiology, costing millions of dollars per year unnecessarily. Although the number of unnecessary skull films has decreased, they remain a costly burden in many emergency departments. There is virtually no finding on a skull series that will alter the next step in the patient's workup. Presence or absence of a fracture should not influence whether or not the patient receives a computed tomography (CT) scan or a magnetic resonance imaging (MRI) exam. A CT scan or an MRI exam are obtained for other reasons: continued unconsciousness or focal neurologic signs. The plain films only delay the eventual diagnosis, and in a patient with a subdural or an epidural hematoma, that delay could be fatal.[3] The mortality from intracranial bleeds is significantly increased as the time to surgical decompression is increased; therefore any delay caused by obtaining unnecessary examinations (skull films) is potentially harmful. There are no findings on a plain skull series to indicate (or not indicate) subdural or epidural hematoma (Fig. 1.1). Fewer than 10% of patients with fractures have subdural or epidural hematomas, and up to 60% of patients with subdural or epidural bleeds have no fractures.[4] Therefore why order the examinations? Medicolegal reasons? On the contrary! It is well documented that delays in diagnosis in this setting can be fatal, so ordering unnecessary examinations might in fact be asking for a lawsuit! The American College of Radiology has published appropriateness criteria for when to order particular exams, and has endorsed head CT as the initial study of choice in trauma.[5]

In spite of much documentation in the radiology and emergency room literature showing the lack of utility of skull films in trauma, they still are frequently routinely ordered in many emergency rooms throughout North America. A survey performed in 1991 by Hackney and published in *Radiology*[6] showed that over 50% of the hospitals in the study "often or always" obtained skull films for trauma. Every hospital had CT available. What were they thinking? Obviously they are not thinking about what a skull film will show them that might affect their treatment, because it won't change a thing, whether it's positive or negative.

Sinus Series

It is true that an opaque sinus and/or an air–fluid level can be seen with sinusitis. But often the patient with these findings is asymptomatic, and just as often in another patient, the sinus series can be normal when the patient has typical clinical findings of sinusitis. Both of these patients are treated based on their clinical, not radiographic, presentation, which is appropriate. Therefore the information from the sinus series is ignored. If that is the way you practice—and many

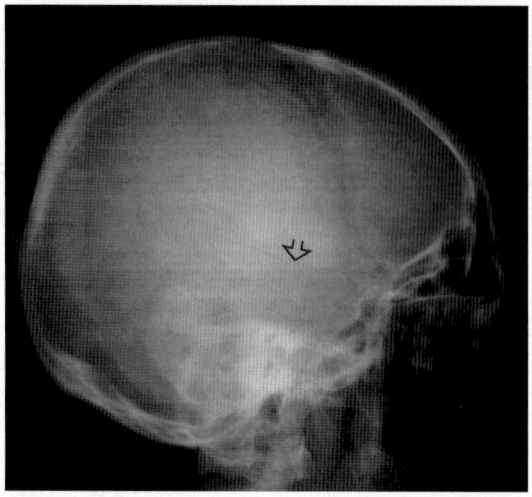

FIG. 1.1 **Skull Fracture.** A thin radiolucent line characteristic of a skull fracture is noted *(arrow)* extending obliquely across the temporal bone. A fracture in this area is often associated with an epidural hematoma because the middle meningeal artery lies here. This finding by itself, however, has little or no significance and must be correlated with clinical findings.

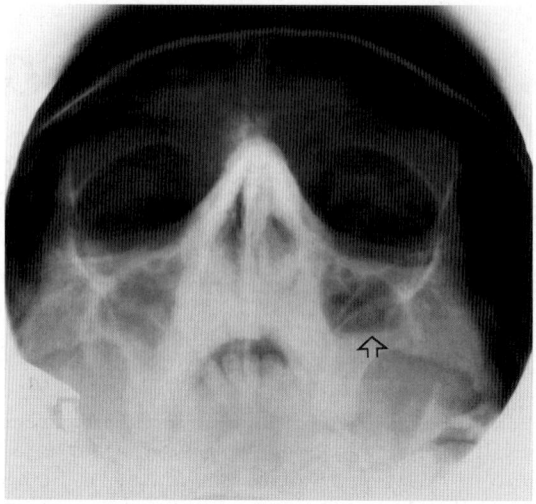

FIG. 1.2 **Waters' View of the Sinuses.** This film is obtained with the patient's head slightly tilted upward (as if he were drinking water—apologies to Dr. Waters). It is an excellent film to obtain when the maxillary sinuses need to be seen. When done in an upright position, air–fluid levels can be seen *(arrow)*.

recommend that as being proper—don't order the sinus series; treat the patient. Reserve the sinus series for the patient who doesn't respond to treatment or has an unusual presentation. Also, if it is only sinusitis you are concerned with, most times, a simple upright Waters' view (Fig. 1.2) to examine the maxillary and frontal sinuses, rather than a full sinus series, will suffice, saving money and decreasing patient exposure.[7]

Nasal Bone

A nasal series is often requested to see if a patient has suffered a broken nose after trauma to the face. So what if the nasal bone is fractured? It won't be casted. It won't be reduced. In other words, no treatment will be given regardless of what the x-ray shows. Therefore don't order the films in the first place. Occasionally a nasal bone is badly enough displaced to warrant intervention, but even then an acute, posttraumatic x-ray adds nothing for the patient except expense and radiation exposure. A facial series or a CT to search for additional fractures might be in order, but not a nasal series.

Rib Series

Fractured ribs are commonly seen in any radiologic practice. The significance of the finding of a fractured rib or ribs is not well appreciated by most physicians. If the truth be known, the finding of a rib fracture after trauma has almost no clinical significance and does not alter treatment. One must rule out a pneumothorax and even a lung contusion, both of which are uncommon and are best done on chest films, not a rib series. In older patients with chest wall pain and rib fractures from undetermined causes, it is extremely difficult and often impossible to differentiate a pathologic rib fracture through a metastatic focus from a posttraumatic rib fracture. Hence, x-raying a patient with focal rib pain to find a fracture serves little purpose other than to find a cause for the pain. Most rib series can be eliminated without changing the way the patient is treated.

Coccyx

Although not a common x-ray examination, we have occasional requests to x-ray the coccyx to rule out a fracture. As with the nasal bone and ribs, a fracture in this location will not be casted or reduced. Also, this examination has significantly more gonadal radiation dose than a rib or nasal series. Because no treatment is predicated on the x-ray results, don't order the x-ray for routine trauma to the coccyx.

Lumbar Spine

Plain films of the lumbar spine are probably the most abused examinations in radiology. They give the highest gonadal radiation dose of any plain film examination, and in most cases, they offer no diagnostic information that will be acted on by the physician. A significant number of lumbar spine films are done in a population under the age of 40 with acute onset of back pain after lifting or straining. There is virtually no plain-film x-ray finding in this patient subgroup that can be responsible for the acute problem or that can be treated with intervention. Even the severest spondylolisthesis cannot unequivocally be said to be the origin of the symptoms. Disc herniation cannot be identified. Tumors and infections are not clinical considerations in this setting. Treatment invariably consists of rest, nonsteroidal antiinflammatory drugs, generally relaxing the muscle groups, and then flexion and extension exercises to strengthen the muscles. Radiographs have nothing to offer unless the pain is very atypical or the clinical picture is clouded by other considerations (such as intravenous drug use, in which case infection must be ruled out).

The gonadal radiation dose from a lumbar spine film is the same as that from a daily chest x-ray for 6,[8] 16,[9] or 98 years,[10] depending on which study you choose to believe. These studies were based on a three-view lumbosacral spine series and do not include the oblique views routinely obtained in many practices. Subtle osseous changes found on oblique views are thought by many orthopedists to be insignificant in most cases anyway.

So when should a lumbosacral spine series be ordered? In cases of severe trauma, possible primary or metastatic tumor, and possible infection. Acute low back pain with radicular signs is no indication for a spine series. An MRI exam will show disc herniation and would be the preferred examination over plain films, if clinically warranted. Generally a lumbar spine MRI exam is performed only after a failed course of conservative therapy if disc disease is clinically suspected.

Metabolic Bone Survey

Many institutions routinely order metabolic bone surveys in patients with hyperparathyroidism or renal osteodystrophy to look for Looser's fractures, brown tumors, and subperiosteal bone resorption. Most institutions have replaced the bone survey with hand films, which are preferable in regard to patient expense and radiation dose. Subperiosteal bone resorption is seen earliest and easiest on the middle phalanges and radial sides (Fig. 1.3) and is virtually pathognomonic for hyperparathyroidism. Looser's fractures are rare and not treated anyway. Brown tumors are uncommon and also are not treated. Therefore if no treatment is based on the x-ray findings, the survey only satisfies curiosity and is not worth the patient's money or radiation exposure.

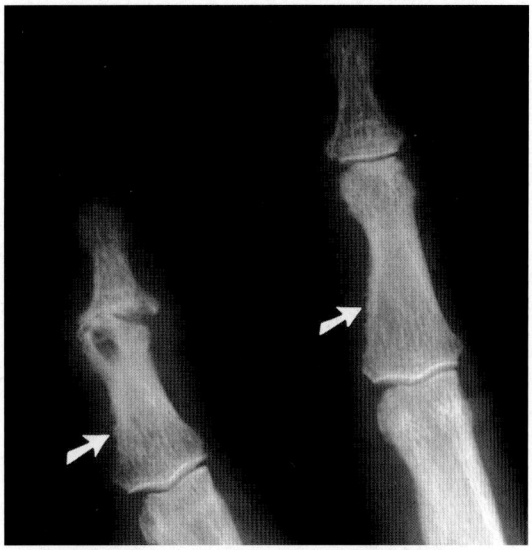

FIG. 1.3 **Phalanges with Subperiosteal Bone Resorption.** Subperiosteal bone resorption is seen as a subtle irregularity or interruption of the cortex. It is best seen on the radial aspect of the middle phalanges *(arrows)* and is pathognomonic for hyperparathyroidism.

Metastatic Bone Survey

Little useful information is obtained from the majority of metastatic bone surveys. Occult lesions that are not found on radionuclide bone scans are seldom encountered. Radionuclide scans are more effective at picking up most metastatic lesions and could be substituted for bone surveys with less cost and better diagnostic yield.[11] Many investigators believe that searching for bone metastases is not warranted in every patient with a primary tumor unless finding metastatic disease will obviate surgery or otherwise change the patient's therapy. Radionuclide bone scans with x-rays of questionable or clinically suspicious areas makes more sense than a complete metastatic bone survey. An exception to this is in patients with multiple myeloma. Radionuclide bone scans are often negative in multiple myeloma even with marked skeletal involvement; hence a plain film bone survey is warranted in these patients.

Ankle Series

The most common cause for presentation to emergency rooms in North America is an ankle sprain, with over 30,000 ankle sprains/day reported.[12] Ligamentous injuries can easily be clinically differentiated from significant fractures. One study showed a 50% reduction of ankle films with no fractures missed if the radiology resident would simply examine the patient.[13] Another

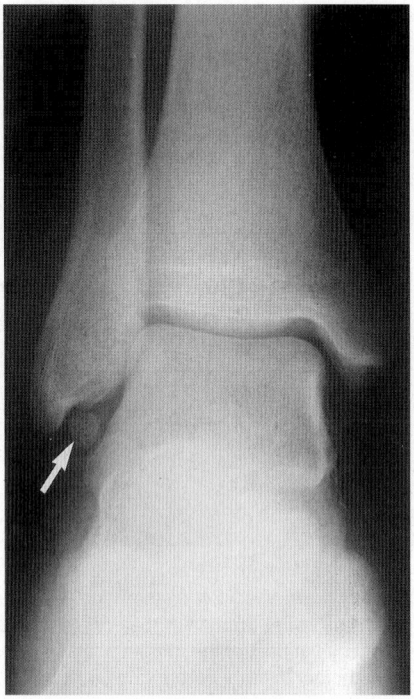

FIG. 1.4 **Ankle After Trauma.** Calcific densities around the ankle that can be mistaken for avulsions are often seen *(arrow)*. When rounded and smoothly corticated, as in this example, they are either accessory ossicles or old avulsions. An acute avulsion is best diagnosed clinically by noting point tenderness at ligament insertion sites. Because a ligament can avulse with or without a fragment of bone being attached, the x-ray finding will not influence the patient's treatment.

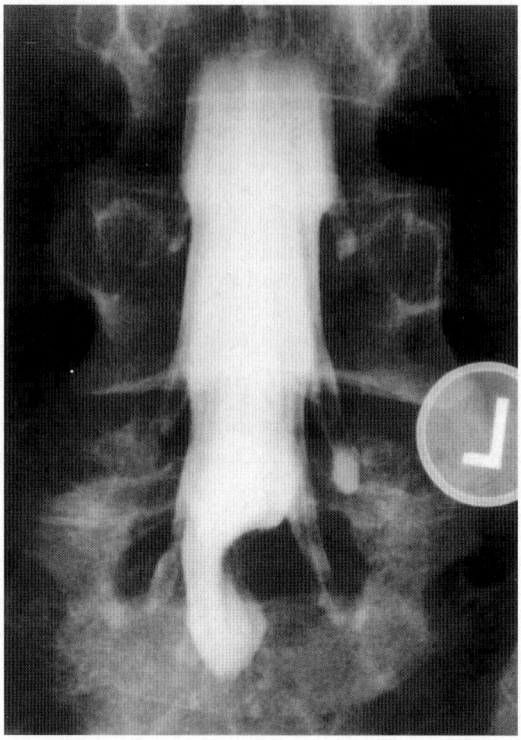

FIG. 1.5 **Lumbar Myelogram.** An iodinated contrast material has been injected into the subarachnoid space by way of a spinal needle. A large extradural defect is seen that is caused by a disc protrusion. A tumor could have a similar appearance. This examination can be quite painful, has occasional long-lasting complications, and gives no information that could not be obtained with an magnetic resonance imaging (MRI) examination. In some institutions, it requires an overnight stay in the hospital as well. For these reasons, the standard of practice today is an MRI exam.

study revealed that if the patient were able to walk three steps immediately after the injury or during the examination in the ER, there was almost zero chance of a fracture.[14] This study was one of several to utilize what has been called the "Ottawa Rules" for when to obtain ankle x-rays. They are so-named after the hometown of the first authors to implement them and are in widespread use today in the majority of emergency departments in North America. Small bony avulsions receive the same treatment as ligament tears, and are often difficult to differentiate from accessory ossicles (Fig. 1.4). Therefore in most cases, the x-ray is not a factor in determining the patient's treatment and should be skipped.

Lumbar Myelograms

One of the most painful radiologic examinations extant is the lumbar myelogram, in which a spinal needle is placed into the subarachnoid space of the lumbar spine and contrast material is injected (Fig. 1.5). Although this is done for tumors, it is most commonly performed in the workup of lumbar disc disease. Many studies show that CT or MRI of the lumbar spine is more accurate than myelography in diagnosing disc disease, and they emphasize that CT or MRI should be the study of choice. Many surgeons, however, still request myelograms in addition to the CT or MRI study when only the CT or MRI need be performed. In addition to being painful, the myelogram produces side effects in some people that can be pronounced and debilitating; the myelogram occasionally necessitates overnight hospitalization; the radiation dose from the myelogram is higher overall than with CT; and, most important perhaps, the myelogram is not as accurate and does not give as complete a picture of additional

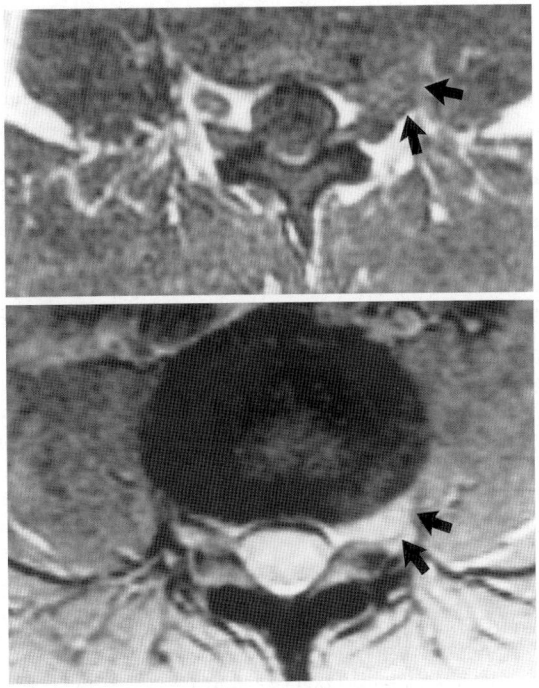

FIG. 1.6 **Lumbar Magnetic Resonance Imaging (MRI).** Axial T1-weighted (top) and T2-weighted (bottom) images through the L4-5 disc space show a focal lateral disc protrusion *(arrows)*, which is encroaching on the left neuroforamen. This type of disc protrusion would likely not be seen with a myelogram.

back structures as the CT or MRI examination (Fig. 1.6). We can hope that the myelogram will go the way of the pneumoencephalogram and the epidural venogram.

So far as choosing between a CT and an MRI of the lumbar spine for disc disease and spinal stenosis, an MRI exam will give much more diagnostic information and is considered the state-of-the-art imaging exam for the spine. Although, as the next section shows, MRI of the lumbar spine is one of the most overutilized imaging tests in the country.

Magnetic Resonance Imaging Lumbar Spine

A lot has been written in the lay press in the past few years concerning the overutilization of medical testing at a time when our economy is reeling from skyrocketing medical costs. One of the imaging tests mentioned near the top of every list is MRI of the lumbar spine. Multiple studies have shown that as many as one-third of asymptomatic individuals over the age of 50 will have one or more focal disc protrusions.[15] Oftentimes the patient's pain is from some other source rather than from the disc, yet it coincidentally corresponds to the location of the disc protrusion resulting in unnecessary surgery. More times than not, the MRI shows abnormalities that have no clinical correlation whatsoever, resulting in diagnostic confusion. In most cases, an MRI of the lumbar spine should not be performed unless 6–8 weeks of conservative care have been afforded, and, even then, if surgery is not being considered, why pay for an expensive imaging study? Certainly an MRI would be a reasonable imaging study if the clinical presentation were atypical or if trauma, tumor, or infection were clinically suspected. Several studies have shown that surgeons and other medical specialists who own their own MRI units order many more exams than when the MRI is not self-owned. Lumbar spine MRIs tend to be the most overutilized exam I see on a daily basis.

Cervical Spine

Many emergency rooms routinely order cervical spine (C-spine) films on all trauma patients, primarily because of the horrible consequences of not stabilizing a fractured neck. This is ridiculous. It has been demonstrated in numerous publications that patients who are alert and have no C-spine pain have almost zero chance of having a fracture.[16] If the patient is unconscious, obtunded for whatever reason, not able to communicate, or has a significant fracture elsewhere, all bets are off. But if the patient is alert and has no pain with motion on clinical exam of the neck, no posterior midline tenderness, and no neurologic deficits, no C-spine film need be performed.[17]

As for plain films of the C-spine in trauma, a case should be made for skipping a plain-film C-spine series and going straight to a CT scan. The obvious reason for this is that a negative plain film will not exclude a fracture; therefore a CT scan will be performed regardless of what the plain film shows (a CT is always obtained when a fracture is found). One caveat is that if the CT shows no fracture, the patient could still have ligamentous disruption, which would not be seen on a CT unless there is malalignment. To diagnose ligamentous disruption, a flexion–extension plain film or an MRI needs to be done. Some say performing a CT on every patient that now gets only a plain film would inundate most scanners with unnecessary exams, since the majority of plain films of the C-spine aren't really needed. Hello! If they aren't really needed, then don't get them!

TECHNICAL CONSIDERATIONS

Avoiding unnecessary examinations constitutes only one way to decrease unnecessary radiation exposure in the general population. Another way to significantly diminish exposure is to collimate the x-ray beam tighter. One study reported that if collimation were limited just to the size of the film, radiation dose could be reduced by one-third.[18] Exposure could be further reduced by having proper filtration, fast screen–film combination, and adequate gonadal shielding. Digital radiography, which is now widely used, will further help decrease radiation dose. Certainly, having properly trained technicians and properly functioning equipment will diminish the number of retakes. These should be high-priority goals for all radiologists to make our specialty more cost-effective and to provide better service to both the referring clinician and the patient. It should be part of every radiologist's responsibility to help educate and guide the unknowing clinician in obtaining the appropriate imaging exams while eliminating those that are unnecessary.

REFERENCES

1. Hall F. Overutilization of radiological examinations. *Radiology*. 1976;120:443–448.
2. Abrams HL. The "overutilization" of x-rays: sounding board. *N Engl J Med*. 1979;300:1213–1216.
3. Seelig JM, Becker DP, Miller JD, et al. Traumatic acute subdural hematoma. *N Engl J Med*. 1981;304:1511–1518.
4. Masters JS, McClean PM, Arcarese JS, et al. Skull x-ray examinations after head trauma. *N Engl J Med*. 1987;316:84–91.
5. American College of Radiology. ACR appropriateness criteria head trauma. 2001. Available at: http: //www.acr.org.
6. Hackney DB. Skull radiography in the evaluation of acute head trauma: a survey of current practice. *Radiology*. 1991;181:711–714.
7. Williams JJ, Roberts L, Distell B, Simel D. Diagnosing sinusitis by x-ray: comparing a single Waters' view to 4-view paranasal sinus radiographs. *J Gen Intern Med*. 1992;7:481–485.
8. Webster EW, Merrill OE. Radiation hazards: II. Measurements of gonadal dose in radiologic examinations. *N Engl J Med*. 1957;257:811–819.
9. Antoku S, Russell WJ. Dose to the active bone marrow, gonads, and skin from roentgenography and fluoroscopy. *Radiology*. 1957;101:669–678.
10. Andron GM, Crooks HE. Gonad radiation dose from diagnostic procedures. *Br J Radiol*. 1957;30:295–297.
11. Mall JC, Bekerman C, Hoffer PB, et al. A unified radiological approach to the detection of skeletal metastases. *Radiology*. 1976;118:323–329.
12. Cheung Y, Rosenberg ZS. MR imaging of ligamentous abnormalities of the ankle and foot. *Magn Reson Imaging Clin N Am*. 2001;9:507–531.
13. Auletta A, Conway W, Hayes C, Guisto D, Gervin A. Indications for radiography in patients with acute ankle injuries: role of the physical examination. *Am J Roentgenol*. 1991;157:789–791.
14. Stiell I, Greenberg G, McKnight R, et al. Decision rules for the use of radiography in acute ankle injuries. *JAMA*. 1993;269:1127–1132.
15. Jarvik JJ, Hollingworth W, Hoagerty P, Haynor DR, Deyo RA. The Longitudinal Assessment of Imaging and Disability of the Back (LAIDBACK) study: baseline data. *Spine*. 2001;26:1158–1166.
16. Mirvis S, Diaconis J, Chirico P, Reiner B, Joslyn J, Militello P. Protocol-driven radiologic evaluation of suspected cervical spine injury: efficacy study. *Radiology*. 1989;170:831–834.
17. Hoffman JR, Mower WR, Wolfson AB, Todd KH, Zucker MI. Validity of a set of clinical criteria to rule out injury to the cervical spine in patients with blunt trauma. *N Engl J Med*. 2000;343:94–99.
18. Morgan RH, Hearings before the Committee on Commerce, Science and Transportation. *U.S. Senate, An Oversight of Radiation Health and Safety*. 95th Congress, 1st session; 1977:241–266.

CHAPTER 2

Benign Lytic Lesions

A benign, bubbly lytic lesion of bone is probably one of the most common skeletal findings a radiologist encounters. The differential diagnosis can be quite lengthy and is usually given on an "Aunt Minnie" basis (I know that's Aunt Minnie because she *looks* like Aunt Minnie); in other words, the differential diagnosis is structured on how the lesion looks to the radiologist, using his or her experience as a guide. This method, called "pattern identification," certainly has merit, but it can lead to many erroneous conclusions if not tempered with some logic. For instance, most radiologists would justifiably miss the diagnosis of a rare presentation of a primary malignant neoplasm that initially looks benign. Many of these radiologists would subsequently insist on including primary malignant neoplasms in their benign lytic differential, even though the rare malignancy is "one in a million." If every differential is geared to cover even the long shots, there would be a lot of extremely long differentials, and the clinicians wouldn't get much useful information from us. We might as well give the clinician the index to a multivolume bone book as give a differential that will never miss anything.

Then again, you don't want a differential diagnosis list that is wrong half the time. You could almost do better with a coin flip. I'm willing to accept a differential that is accurate (that is, one that contains the correct diagnosis) 95% of the time. This is acceptable to me for most skeletal entities; however, I would be remiss if I were willing to accept a 1 out of 20 miss rate for fractures and dislocations. Nevertheless, for most of the entities in this book, I will accept a 95% accuracy differential and would expect most radiologists to concur. If you want to be more accurate than that, you simply add more diagnoses to the list of differential possibilities.

The shorter the differential diagnosis list, the handier it is to remember and apply. As the differential list gets longer, it generally gets more accurate, but it can be difficult to remember and often falls into disuse. Mnemonics are helpful in recalling long lists of information, and I will pass on many that I use; many people, however, do not like to use mnemonics (for no good reason that I've been able to ascertain) and will just have to use whatever method that works for them to remember the differentials. The list of entities that cause benign lytic lesions is quite long, and therefore a mnemonic is helpful in recalling them.

I was a flight surgeon in the air force before my radiology residency, and I would spend a half day a week or so with the radiologist, trying to pick up some pearls. This radiologist was Ivan Barrett, and he did me a great favor. He taught me the mnemonic FEGNOMASHIC, which is made up from the first letter of each of the entities in the differential of benign lytic lesions of bone. For instance, the *F* stands for fibrous dysplasia, the *E* for enchondroma, and so on, as I will show. I diligently learned what each letter stood for, even though I had no idea what most of the processes were or looked like on an x-ray. Before I could learn another mnemonic from Ivan (I was a slow learner), I moved away to begin residency.

Sure enough, the first week of residency, in a formal conference with 15 to 20 residents present, I was chosen as the sacrificial lamb among the first-year residents to take an unknown case. It happened to be a benign lytic lesion, which I proceeded to expound on with a list of 12 to 15 differential possibilities. The conference room got quiet, I was thanked cordially but a little frostily, and the conference was adjourned. One of the first-year residents, whom I barely knew at the time, asked how I knew so many of the possibilities on that case, since the staff man showing the case (who was a chest radiologist) didn't even know that many. I explained, with a straight face, that those just seemed like the logical things to mention. I was trying to be matter-of-fact and not come off as too much of a show-off, but I couldn't help laughing. I then told the resident how I had learned a single mnemonic, and by getting lucky, it made me seem to know a lot more than I really did. He and the rest of my fellow residents were relieved that I really wasn't any smarter or more advanced than them and quickly learned the mnemonic themselves. I became hopelessly addicted to mnemonics from that day on.

FEGNOMASHIC

FEGNOMASHIC is defined in "Funk and Wagner's" unabridged dictionary, 13th edition, as "one who uses mnemonics." It serves as a nice starting point for discussing possibilities that appear as benign lytic lesions in bone. That mnemonic has been in general use for many years, but I have never heard a claim as to who first coined it. The first mention of it that I saw in print was in 1972 in a radiology article by Gold, Ross, and Margulis.[1] By itself, it is merely a long list—about 14 entities—and needs to be coupled with other criteria to shorten the list into manageable form for each particular case. For instance, if the lesion is epiphyseal, only three to five entities, depending on how accurate you care to be, need to be mentioned. If multiple lesions are present, only half a dozen entities need to be discussed. Ways of narrowing the differential are discussed later in this chapter.

The next step after learning the names of all the lesions is getting some idea of what each one looks like. This is where experience becomes a factor. For the medical student or first-year resident, it's difficult to go beyond saying that they all look lytic or bubbly and benign. However, the fourth-year resident should have no trouble differentiating between a unicameral bone cyst and a giant cell tumor because he or she has seen examples of each many times before and knows what each looks like. The fourth-year resident may have a hard time verbalizing the differences but should be able to tell them apart.

A novice can quickly gain experience by looking at the examples of each of these lesions in a major skeletal radiology text. In fact, I highly recommend that you compare my description and differential points on each lesion with multiple examples in other books. Some of these lesions can only be diagnosed radiologically on a "pattern identification" or "Aunt Minnie" basis. In other words, there are no hard and fast criteria to differentiate some of the lesions from the others.

After getting a feel for what each lesion looks like radiographically and overcoming the frustration that builds when you realize that many of them look alike, you should try to learn ways to differentiate each lesion from the others. I have developed a number of keys that I call "discriminators" that will help to differentiate each lesion. These discriminators are 90% to 95% useful (I will mention when they are more or less accurate, in my experience) and are by no means meant to be absolutes or dogma. They are guidelines but have a high confidence rate.

Textbooks rarely tell you that a finding "always" or "never" occurs. They temper their descriptions with "virtually always," "invariably," "usually," or "characteristically." I have tried to pick out findings that come as close to "always" as I can, realizing that I will often only be 95% accurate. That's good enough for me. If it's not good enough for you, you'll have to get your own differential criteria or discriminators. Try these and see if they work for you. If they don't, modify them as necessary. But whatever you do, develop *reasons* for including things in your differential. Have concrete criteria of some kind for including or excluding each entity.

I will give a brief description of each entity, as complete descriptions are readily available in any skeletal radiology text. What I will dwell on, however, are the points that are unique for each entity, thereby enabling differentiation from the others. Table 2.1 is a synopsis of these discriminators.

FIBROUS DYSPLASIA

It is unfortunate that this differential starts with fibrous dysplasia because fibrous dysplasia can look like almost anything. It can be wild looking, a discrete lucency, patchy, sclerotic, expansile, multiple, and a host of other descriptions. Unless it is a classic example, it can be difficult to look at a bubbly lytic lesion and unequivocally say it is or is not fibrous dysplasia. When assessing such a lesion, radiology residents usually say, "I suppose it *could* be fibrous dysplasia, but I'm not sure." The resident is feeling insecure and becomes defensive right off, setting the tone for the entire differential diagnosis. It would be better if the differential started on a positive note, say, with giant cell tumor or chondroblastoma, where there are some hard and definite criteria. That way the resident would set the tone of self-assurance and decisiveness rather than appear wishy-washy. Then, when mentioning fibrous dysplasia and using the same words, "I suppose it *could* be fibrous dysplasia, but I'm not sure," it's looked upon as thoughtful deliberation rather than insecurity or ignorance. It's pure gamesmanship, but it makes a difference in how you are perceived.

How do you know whether to include or exclude fibrous dysplasia if it can look like almost anything? Experience is the best guideline. In other words, look in a few texts and find as many different examples as you can; get a feeling for what fibrous dysplasia looks like. A few examples are shown here (Figs. 2.1 to 2.6), but poring over another text for 10 to 15 minutes will be time well spent.

Fibrous dysplasia will not have periostitis associated with it; therefore if periostitis is present, you can safely exclude fibrous dysplasia. It would be possible to have a pathologic fracture through an area of fibrous dysplasia, which then had periostitis, but I have never seen this occur. Fibrous dysplasia virtually never undergoes malignant degeneration and should not be a painful lesion in the long bones unless there is a fracture.

TABLE 2.1
Differential criteria for benign lytic bone lesions

MNEMONIC: FEGNOMASHIC			
F	*Fibrous Dysplasia* = No pain or periosteal reaction; if in tibia, mention adamantinoma		
E	*Enchondroma* = Must have calcification, except in phalanges; no pain or periostitis		
	Eosinophilic Granuloma (EG) = Must be under 30		
G	*Giant Cell Tumor (GCT)* = (1) Epiphyses must be closed; (2) must be epiphyseal *and* abut the articular surface; (3) eccentric; (4) well-defined but nonsclerotic border		
N	*Nonossifying fibroma (NOF)* = Must be under 30; no pain or periostitis		
O	*Osteoblastoma* = Mentioned whenever ABC is mentioned, even if over 30		
M	*Mets and Myeloma* = Must be over 40		
A	*Aneurysmal Bone Cyst (ABC)* = Must be under 30; expansile		
S	*Solitary Bone Cyst* = Must be centrally located; under age 30; no pain or periostitis		
H	*Hyperparathyroidism (Brown Tumor)* = Must have other evidence of hyperparathyroidism; *Hemangiomas*		
I	*Infection* = If adjacent to a joint, must involve the joint (weak)		
C	*Chondroblastoma* = Must be under 30; epiphyseal		
	Chondromyxoid Fibroma = Mention when considering nonossifying fibroma		
Less Than 30	No periostitis or pain	Epiphyseal	Multiple
EG	Fibrous dysplasia	Chondroblastoma	(Mnemonic: FEEMHI)
ABC	Enchondroma	Infection	Fibrous dysplasia
NOF	NOF	GCT	EG
Chondroblastoma	Solitary bone cyst	Geode	Enchondroma
Solitary bone cyst		(EG and ABC are optional)	Mets and Myeloma
			Hyperparathyroidism Hemangiomas
			Infection

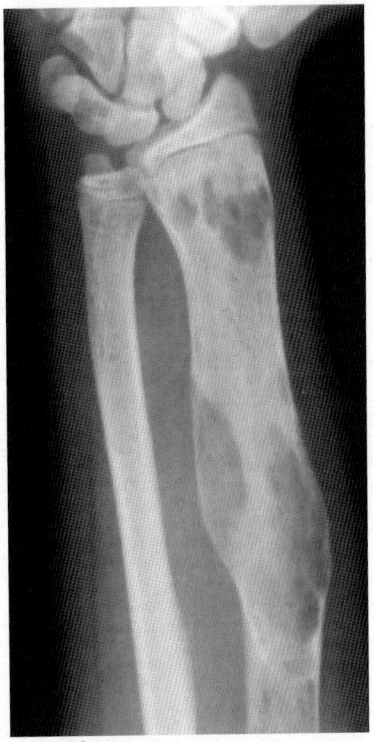

FIG. 2.1 **Fibrous Dysplasia.** A predominantly lytic lesion with some sclerosis and expansion is seen in the distal half of the radius in a child. A long lesion in a long bone typifies fibrous dysplasia. Although parts of this lesion indeed have a ground-glass appearance, most of it does not. Expansion and bone deformity like this is commonly seen in fibrous dysplasia.

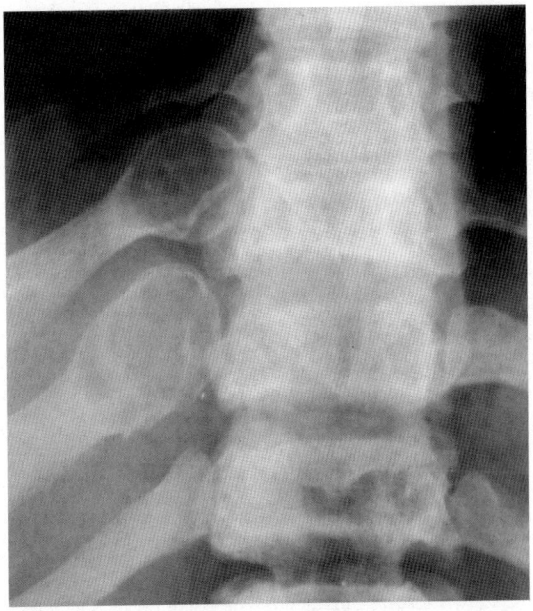

FIG. 2.2 **Fibrous Dysplasia.** The ribs are often involved with fibrous dysplasia, as in this example. When the posterior ribs are involved, the process is often a lytic expansile lesion, whereas when the anterior ribs are involved, it is commonly a sclerotic process.

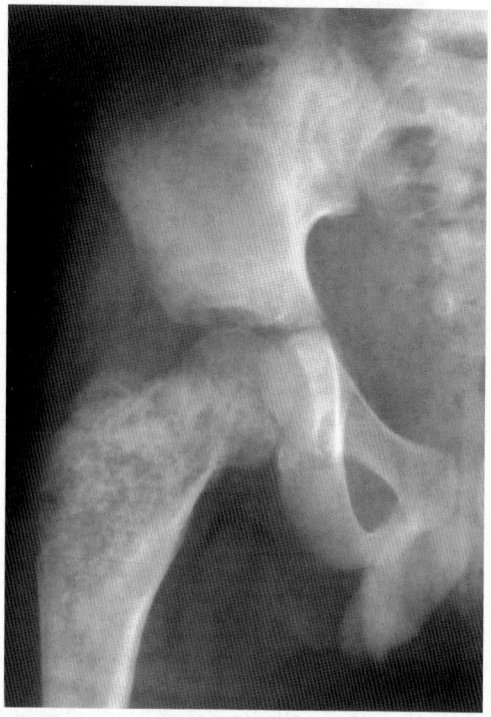

FIG. 2.3 **Fibrous Dysplasia.** An expansile mixed lytic/sclerotic process in the proximal femur is a common pattern for fibrous dysplasia. Note that the supra-acetabular region is also involved. The ipsilateral proximal femur is invariably affected when the pelvis is involved with fibrous dysplasia.

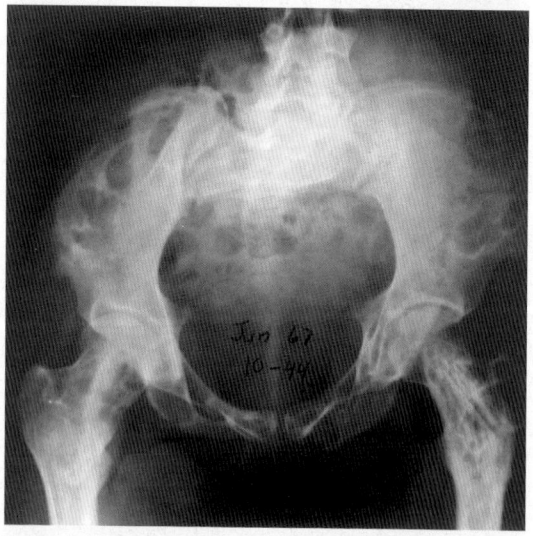

FIG. 2.4 **Fibrous Dysplasia.** The entire pelvis and proximal femurs are diffusely involved with polyostotic fibrous dysplasia. The pelvis is severely deformed with predominantly lytic lesions. The proximal femurs are involved with both lytic and sclerotic lesions.

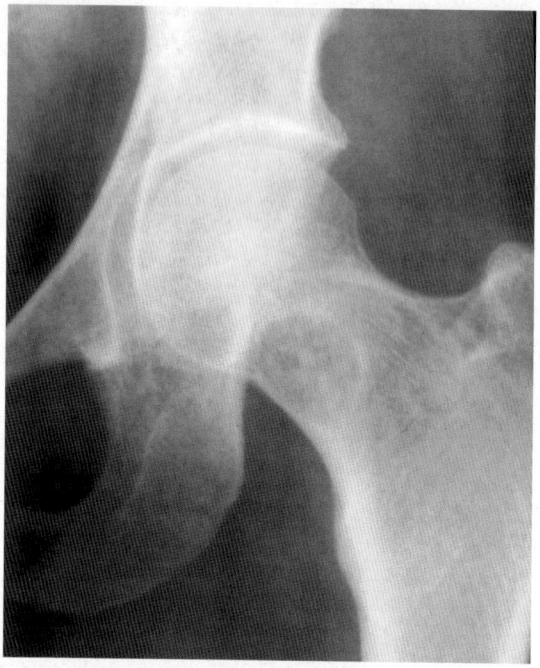

FIG. 2.5 **Monostotic Fibrous Dysplasia.** The proximal femur is a common place for monostotic fibrous dysplasia. This presentation is typical and should not be confused with an infection. Some speckled calcification is noted within the lesion that should not be misconstrued as chondroid calcification in an enchondroma.

Fibrous dysplasia can be either monostotic (most commonly) or polyostotic and has a predilection for the pelvis, proximal femur, ribs, and skull. When it is present in the pelvis, it is invariably present in the ipsilateral proximal femur (Figs. 2.3 and 2.4). I have seen only one case in which the pelvis was involved with fibrous dysplasia and the proximal femur was spared. The proximal femur, however, may be affected alone, without involvement in the pelvis (Figs. 2.5 and 2.6).

The classic description of fibrous dysplasia is that it has a ground-glass or smoky-appearing matrix. This description confuses people rather than helps them, and I do not recommend using "ground-glass appearance" as a buzz word for fibrous dysplasia. Fibrous dysplasia is often purely lytic and becomes hazy or takes on a ground-glass look as the matrix calcifies. It can go on to calcify quite a bit, and then it presents as a sclerotic lesion. Also, I often see other lytic lesions that have a distinct ground-glass appearance; therefore the ground-glass quality can be misleading.

When a lesion in the tibia that has fibrous dysplasia in the differential diagnosis is encountered, an adamantinoma should also be mentioned (Fig. 2.7). An adamantinoma is

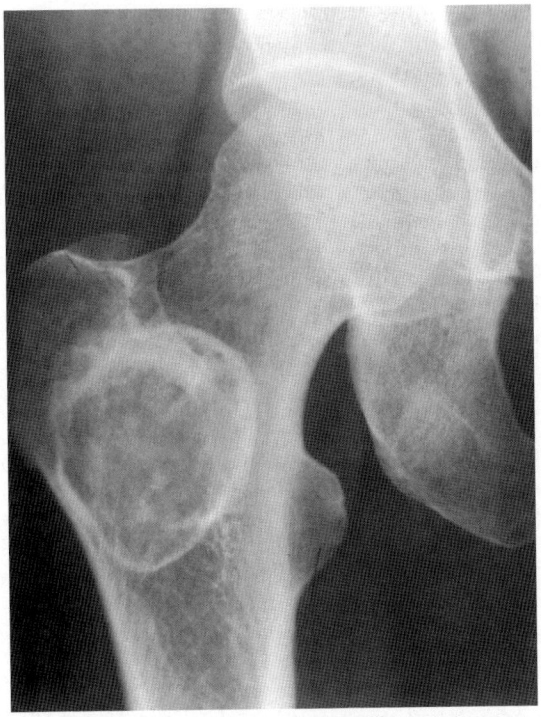

FIG. 2.6 **Monostotic Fibrous Dysplasia.** Another example of proximal femur involvement that shows a lytic lesion with a thick sclerotic border reminiscent of a chronic infection. This is characteristic of fibrous dysplasia in the hip.

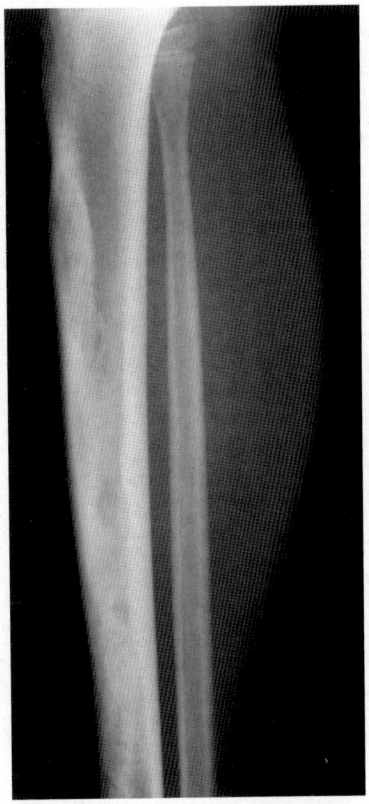

FIG. 2.7 **Adamantinoma.** A wild-looking mixed lytic and sclerotic lesion in the tibia that resembles fibrous dysplasia is classic for an adamantinoma. This lesion occurs almost exclusively in the tibia and has some malignant potential. An adamantinoma should always be considered when a lesion resembling fibrous dysplasia is seen in the tibia.

a malignant tumor that radiographically and histologically resembles fibrous dysplasia. It occurs almost exclusively in the tibia (for unknown reasons) and is rare. Because it is rare, you may choose not to include it in your memory bank—you won't miss more than one or two in your life, even if you're a busy radiologist.

Polyostotic fibrous dysplasia occasionally occurs in association with café au lait spots on the skin (dark-pigmented, freckle-like lesions) and precocious puberty. This complex is called McCune–Albright syndrome. The bony lesions in this syndrome, and even in the simple polyostotic form, often occur unilaterally (that is, in one-half of the body). This doesn't happen often enough to be of any diagnostic use in differentiating fibrous dysplasia from other lesions. The presence of multiple lesions in the jaw has been termed "cherubism," which relates to the physical appearance of the affected child. Such children present with puffed-out cheeks, producing an "angelic" look. The jaw lesions in cherubism regress in adulthood.

Fibrous dysplasia often has areas of chondroid matrix which, when biopsied, can resmble chondrosarcoma (as can any chondral tissue). I have seen sampling errors result in inappropriate radical surgery when the diagnosis should have been made on the plain films with no biopsy performed.

Discriminator:

No periosteal reaction.

ENCHONDROMA AND EOSINOPHILIC GRANULOMA

Enchondroma

The most common benign cystic lesion of the phalanges is an enchondroma (Fig. 2.8). Enchondromas occur in any bone formed from cartilage and may be central, eccentric, expansile, or nonexpansile. They invariably contain calcified chondroid matrix (Fig. 2.9A) except when in the phalanges. If a cystic lesion is present without calcified chondroid matrix anywhere except in the phalanges, I will not include enchondroma in my differential.

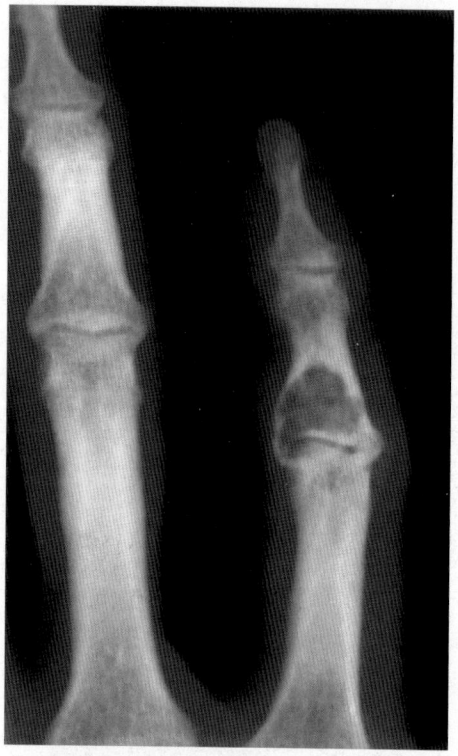

FIG. 2.8 **Enchondroma.** A benign lytic lesion in the hand is an enchondroma until proven otherwise. This is a common presentation of an enchondroma. Enchondromas in any other part of the body should contain some calcified chondroid matrix before they are included in the differential. However, calcified chondroid matrix is unusual in the phalanges.

Occasionally it can be difficult to differentiate between an enchondroma and a bone infarct. Although some of the following criteria are helpful in separating an infarct from an enchondroma, they are not foolproof. An infarct usually has a well-defined, densely sclerotic, serpiginous border, whereas an enchondroma does not (Fig. 2.9B). An enchondroma often causes endosteal scalloping, whereas a bone infarct will not.

It is difficult, if not impossible, to differentiate an enchondroma from a chondrosarcoma. Clinical findings (primarily pain) serve as a better indicator than radiographic findings, and indeed pain in an apparent enchondroma should warrant further investigation. Periostitis should not be seen in an enchondroma either. Trying to differentiate an enchondroma from a chondrosarcoma histologically is also difficult, if not impossible, at times. Therefore biopsy of an apparent enchondroma should not be performed routinely for histologic differentiation.[2] Magnetic resonance imaging (MRI) criteria for benign versus malignant includes lack of a soft tissue mass and no surrounding T2 high-signal edema in benign enchondromas.

Because an enchondroma can histologically mimic a chondrosarcoma, painless chondroid lesions of all types should not be routinely biopsied. Most tumor surgeons prefer to watch them with serial imaging (every 6 months to a year) and close clinical supervision. Radiologists should refrain from putting in a formal report "cannot exclude chondrosarcoma" when looking at a benign appearing chondroid lesion, even though that is technically correct. The problem is there are few surgeons who will not biopsy a lesion if the dictation mentions chondrosarcoma as a possibility. I have seen multiple examples of radical surgery for benign cartilaginous lesions because a biopsy was incorrectly interpreted as chondrosarcoma (including a forequarter shoulder amputation). The correct dictation for an enchondroma should simply say "benign appearing chondroid lesion with no aggressive features noted"—no differential diagnosis should be given.

Multiple enchondromas occur on occasion, and this condition has been termed Ollier disease (Fig. 2.10A). It is not hereditary and does not have an increased rate of malignant degeneration. Older books say that Ollier disease has a high rate of malignant degeneration; that is because any chondroid lesion can look "malignant" when biopsied and needs to be correlated radiographically and clinically. The presence of multiple enchondromas associated with soft tissue hemangiomas is known as Maffucci syndrome (Fig. 2.10B). This syndrome also is not hereditary; however, it is characterized by an increased incidence of malignant degeneration of the enchondromas. Mafucci syndrome is quite rare, whereas Ollier disease is not.

Discriminators:

1. Must have calcification (except in phalanges).
2. No periostitis.

Eosinophilic Granuloma

Eosinophilic granuloma (EG) is a form of histiocytosis X, the other forms being Letterer–Siwe disease and Hand–Schüller–Christian disease. Although these forms may be merely different phases of the same disease, most investigators categorize them separately. The bony manifestations of all three disorders are similar and are discussed in this text simply as eosinophilic granuloma, or EG.

EG, unfortunately for radiologists, has many appearances. It can be lytic or blastic, it may be well-defined

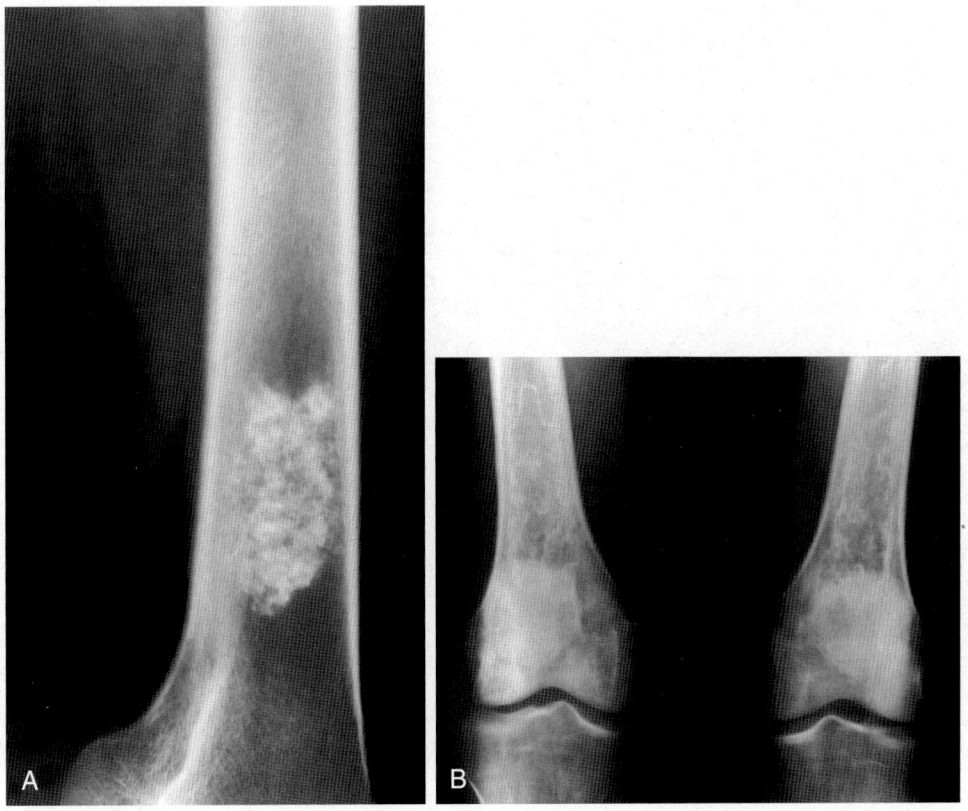

FIG. 2.9 (A) **Enchondroma.** A lesion in the distal femur is seen with irregular speckled calcification typical of chondroid matrix. This is virtually pathognomonic of an enchondroma. A chondrosarcoma could have an identical appearance but should be painful for consideration in the differential diagnosis. A bone infarct can be similar in appearance to an enchondroma. (B) **Bone infarcts.** Bilateral lytic lesions in the femurs are noted with a densely calcified serpiginous border characteristic of bone infarcts. Compare these lesions with (A), which does not have a well-defined serpiginous border. Often the differentiation between bone infarcts, as in this example, and an enchondroma (A) is not so clear-cut. (Case courtesy of Dr. Hideyo Minagi.)

or ill-defined (Figs. 2.11 and 2.12), it may or may not have a sclerotic border, and it may or may not elicit a periosteal response.[3] The periostitis, when present, is typically benign in appearance (thick, uniform, wavy) but can be lamellated or amorphous. EG can mimic Ewing sarcoma and present as a permeative (multiple small holes) lesion.

How, then, can one distinguish EG from any of the other lytic lesions in this differential? Let me say right out that it is difficult to exclude EG from almost any differential of a bony lesion. Although some authorities say that up to 20% of EG occurs in patients over the age of 30, others claim that it is rare in older age groups. I have seen only one or two cases of EG in someone over the age of 30 and have seen at least 100 cases in children and young adults. Therefore I find the 30-year cutoff point quite useful and am willing to exclude the diagnosis of EG in anyone over the age of 30. (I accept the fact that I will miss the diagnosis in older age groups, but I hate to clutter up *every* differential with EG.)

EG is most often monostotic, but it can be polyostotic and thus has to be included whenever multiple lesions are present.

EG may or may not have a soft tissue mass associated with it, so the presence or absence of a soft tissue mass will not help in the differential diagnosis. In fact, I know of no entity in which presence or absence of an associated soft tissue mass will warrant inclusion or exclusion of a processs from a differential. It is important to note the presence of a soft tissue mass (or its absence), but it will do little to narrow your differential diagnosis.

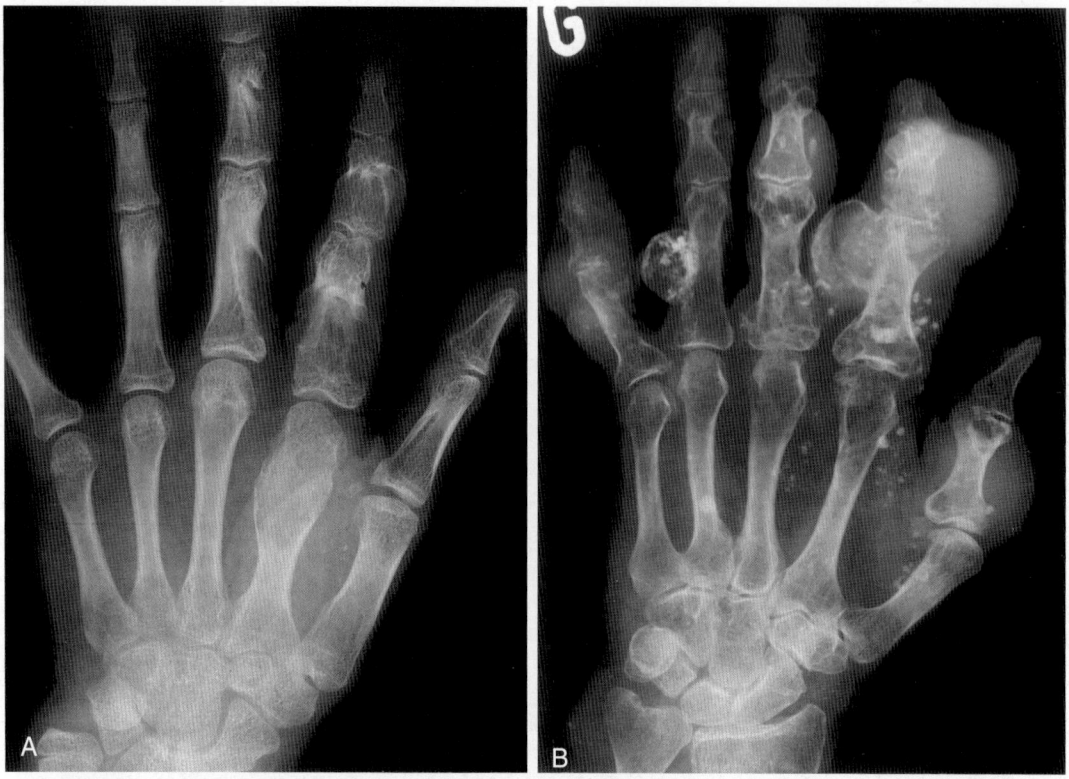

FIG. 2.10 (A) **Ollier.** Multiple lytic lesions in the hand are seen in this patient, which are multiple enchondromas. This is known as Ollier disease. (B) **Maffucci.** Multiple enchondromas associated with soft tissue hemangiomas are seen in the hand in this patient. This is Maffucci syndrome. Note the multiple rounded calcifications in the soft tissues, which are phleboliths in the hemangiomas.

EG occasionally has a bony sequestrum (Fig. 2.13). Only three other entities have been described that, on occasion, have bone sequestra: osteomyelitis, lymphoma, and fibrosarcoma. Therefore when a sequestrum is identified, these four entities should be considered (Table 2.2). (Another entity, osteoid osteoma, can sometimes have an appearance that mimics a sequestrum—this is discussed in Chapter 8, Miscellaneous Conditions.)

Clinically, EG may or may not be associated with pain; therefore clinical history is noncontributory for the most part.

Discriminator:

Must be under age 30.

GIANT CELL TUMOR

Giant cell tumor (GCT) is an uncommon tumor found almost exclusively in adults in the ends of long bones and in flat bones.[4]

It is important to realize that one is unable to tell, regardless of its radiographic appearance, if a GCT is benign or malignant. In fact, histologically, a GCT cannot be reliably divided into either a benign or a malignant category. Most surgeons curettage and pack the lesions and consider them benign unless they recur. Even then, they can still be benign and recur a second or third time. About 15% of GCTs are said to be malignant based on their recurrence rate. Only rarely will GCTs metastasize. They metastasize to the lungs and then should be characterized as malignant.

I use four radiographic criteria for diagnosing GCTs (Figs. 2.14 and 2.15). If any of these criteria are not met when looking at a lesion, I discard GCT from my differential diagnosis.

Number one: GCT occurs only in patients with closed epiphyses; this is valid at least 98% to 99% of the time and is extremely useful. I will not entertain the diagnosis of GCT in a patient with open epiphyses.

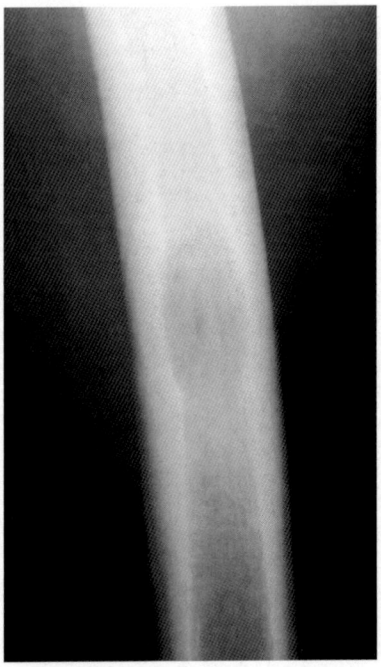

FIG. 2.11 **Eosinophilic granuloma.** A well-defined lytic lesion in the midshaft of a femur in a child. At biopsy this was shown to be eosinophilic granuloma. This is an entirely nonspecific pattern that could easily represent a focus of infection or one of several other processes. Because the lesion is present in a child, eosinophilic granuloma must be included in the differential diagnosis.

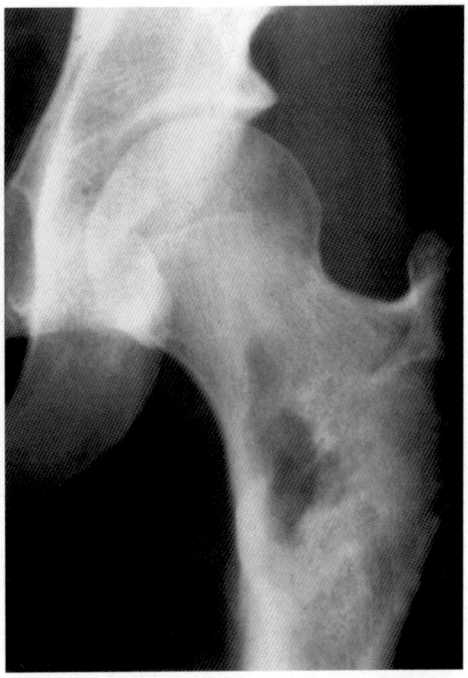

FIG. 2.12 **Eosinophilic granuloma.** A predominantly lytic process with some sclerosis is seen in the proximal femur in a child. Again, this case would have a long differential diagnosis. Eosinophilic granuloma must be mentioned because the patient is under the age of 30. In this example, the zone of transition is narrow and the lesion appears benign, but eosinophilic granuloma can have an aggressive appearance and mimic a sarcoma.

Number two: The lesion must be epiphyseal and abut the articular surface. There is disagreement over whether GCTs begin in the epiphysis or metaphysis, or from the physeal plate itself; however, except for rare cases, when radiologists see the lesions, they are epiphyseal and are flush against the articular surface. The metaphysis also has some of the tumor in it because the lesions are generally very large. I'm not terribly interested in the embryogenesis of a lesion when I'm looking at it as an unknown and a handful of surgeons are breathing down my neck wanting a differential diagnosis. I (and they) want to be able to intelligently say what it is or is not. Therefore I don't get caught up in the argument of where the lesion began. When you see a GCT, it will be epiphyseal. Perhaps more important, it should be flush against the articular surface of the joint. This occurs in 98% to 99% of GCTs;[4] therefore if I have a lesion that is separated from the articular surface by a definite margin of bone, I will not include GCT in the diagnosis.

Number three: These lesions are said to be eccentrically located in the bone, as opposed to being centrally placed in the medullary cavity. I don't find this to be a terribly helpful description, but it is one of the classic "rules" of a GCT. It is accurate; however, occasionally the lesion is so large that it's difficult to tell whether or not it is really eccentric.

Number four: The lesion must have a sharply defined zone of transition (border) that is not sclerotic. This is a very helpful finding in GCT. The only places this does not apply is in flat bones, such as the pelvis, and the calcaneus.

Using these four "rules" will allow one to eliminate GCT from a list of differential possibilities with accuracy and assurance when otherwise it would have to be included. Unwarranted inclusion of a lesion in a differential tends to clutter up the list and make it unnecessarily long.

It is important to realize that the four criteria for a GCT apply only to GCTs and to no other lesion. For instance, I know of no other lesion that is dependent on whether the epiphyses are open or closed. No other

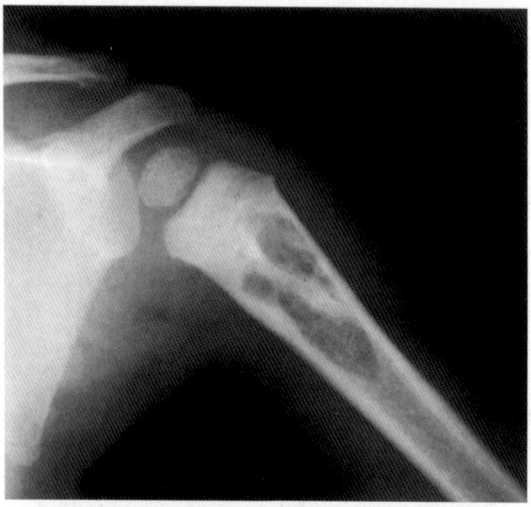

FIG. 2.13 **Eosinophilic Granuloma.** A well-defined lytic lesion with a dense bony sequestrum in the proximal humerus of a child should conjure up the diagnosis of an infection. Eosinophilic granuloma also occasionally has a bony sequestrum (as in this example) and must be considered.

TABLE 2.2 Entities that can present with a sequestration
Osteomyelitis
Eosinophilic granuloma
Malignant fibrous histiocytoma (includes fibrosarcoma and desmoids)
Lymphoma
(Osteoid osteoma can mimic a sequestration)

lesion in any of my lists can be defined by whether or not the zone of transition is sclerotic (many lesions, such as nonossifying fibromas, will usually have a sclerotic margin, but it doesn't occur enough to include as a differential point). No other lesion must always abut the articular surface, and no other lesion has the classic description of always being eccentrically placed (although several lesions, including nonossifying fibroma and chondromyxoid fibroma, are, in fact, eccentric in greater than 98% of cases).

So although these four criteria work nicely for GCT, they don't work at all for any other lesions. Residents have a tendency to apply these criteria to every lytic lesion encountered for the simple reason that they've learned the four criteria. Once one of the criteria is violated, the remainder don't even have to be used to eliminate a

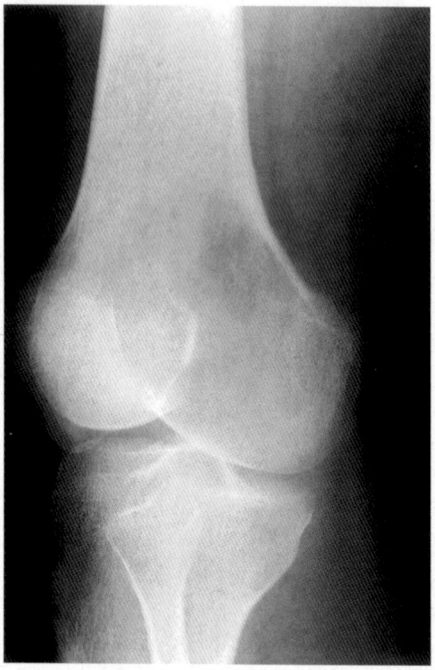

FIG. 2.14 **Giant Cell Tumor.** A well-defined lytic lesion in the distal femur that has all four criteria typical for a giant cell tumor: a well-defined but nonsclerotic zone of transition, the epiphyses are closed, the lesion is eccentrically placed in the bone, and the lesion is epiphyseal and abuts the articular surface. If any one of these criteria were *not* adhered to, I would not include giant cell tumor in my differential.

GCT. For instance, if a lytic lesion is found in the middiaphysis of a bone, GCT can be excluded. There's no need to check further to see if it's eccentric, if it has a nonsclerotic margin, or if the epiphyses are closed.

Again, these "rules" will be greater than 95% effective and, in my experience, close to 99% effective, but only in long bones. Flat bones such as the pelvis and the calcaneus are exceptions. If one or two cases are found that don't fit the criteria, another pathologist should probably review the slides. Many pathologists refer to aneurysmal bone cysts (ABCs) as GCTs; hence they have "GCTs" that don't obey *any* of the criteria. These pathologists may be correct, but they are not in the mainstream of what most people use for GCT criteria, both radiographically and histologically.

Discriminators: (long bones only)

1. Epiphyses must be closed.
2. Must abut the articular surface.
3. Must be well defined with a nonsclerotic margin.
4. Must be eccentric.

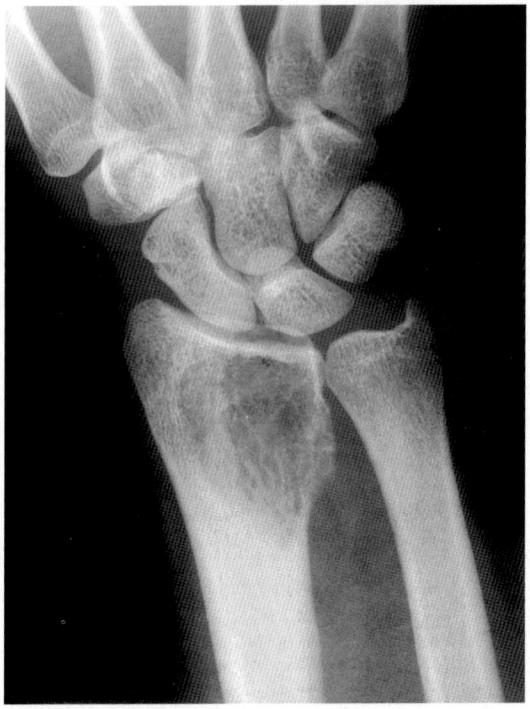

FIG. 2.15 **Giant Cell Tumor.** A typical example in the distal radius, which is a common location for giant cell tumor.

NONOSSIFYING FIBROMA

A nonossifying fibroma (NOF) (also called a fibroxanthoma) is probably the most common bone lesion encountered by radiologists. It reportedly occurs in up to 20% of children and spontaneously regresses so as to be seen only rarely after the age of 30. "Fibrous cortical defect" is a common synonym, although some people divide the two lesions on the basis of size, with fibrous cortical defect being smaller than 2 cm in length and NOF being larger than 2 cm. Histologically, these lesions are identical; therefore it seems illogical to subdivide the lesion by its size.

NOFs are benign, asymptomatic lesions that typically occur in the metaphysis of a long bone emanating from the cortex (Figs. 2.16 to 2.18). They classically have a thin, sclerotic border that is scalloped and slightly expansile; however, this is a general description that probably applies to only 75% of the lesions. They do not have to have expansion or a scalloped or sclerotic border, and they are not limited to the metaphyses. Then how will you recognize them? The best way is, again, familiarize yourself with their general appearance by looking at examples in textbooks. That can be done in 15 minutes. It's important to

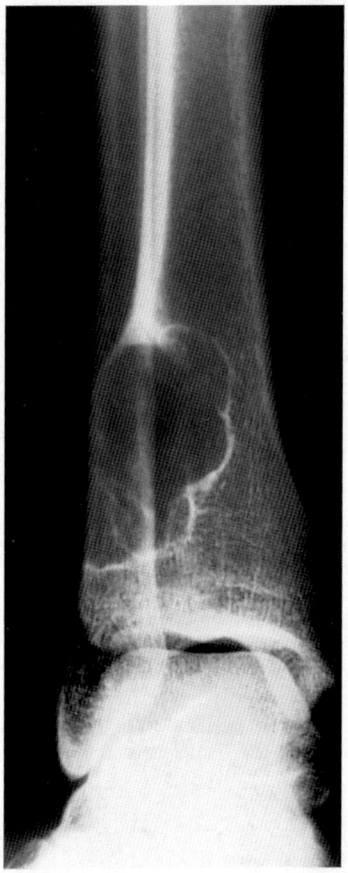

FIG. 2.16 **Nonossifying Fibroma.** A classic example of a nonossifying fibroma that is slightly expansile and lytic and has a scalloped, well-defined sclerotic border. The location in the metaphysis is characteristic. The fact that the cortex is not well seen should not imply cortical destruction, but rather that the cortex has been replaced with benign fibrous tissue. This was an incidental finding in a patient who was asymptomatic.

recognize these lesions because they are what I call "don't touch" lesions; that is, the radiologist's diagnosis should be the final word and thereby supplant a biopsy (see Chapter 4, "Don't Touch" Lesions). These lesions are so characteristic that no logical differential diagnosis should be entertained, although a few entities can indeed occasionally simulate them.

I use age 30 as a cutoff point for NOFs. If the patient is over 30 years of age, I will not include NOF in the differential diagnosis. The lesions must be asymptomatic and exhibit no periostitis, unless there is an antecedent history of trauma. NOFs routinely "heal" with sclerosis and eventually disappear (Figs. 2.19 and 2.20). During

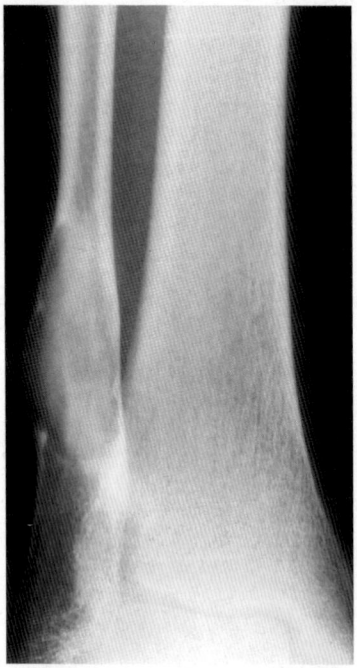

FIG. 2.17 **Nonossifying Fibroma.** A well-defined expansile lytic lesion in the distal fibula is noted, which is characteristic for a nonossifying fibroma. The patient was asymptomatic, and the lesion was an incidental finding. The faint sclerosis seen in the lesion is secondary to the partial calcification or ossification of the matrix, which, in a few years' time, will be complete as the lesion disappears.

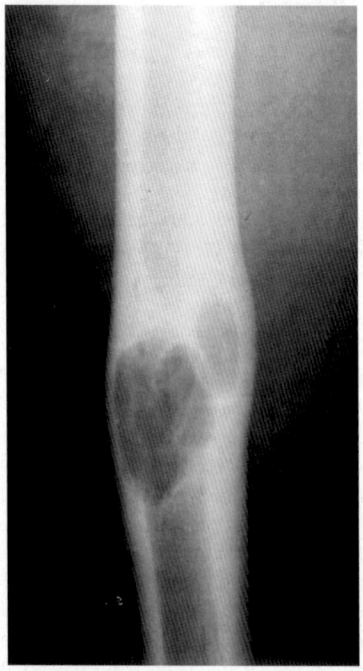

FIG. 2.18 **Nonossifying Fibroma.** A multilocular, expansile, well-defined lytic lesion in a long bone of a child who is asymptomatic. There is no need to do a biopsy for diagnosis because this is an obviously benign lesion and characteristic of a nonossifying fibroma.

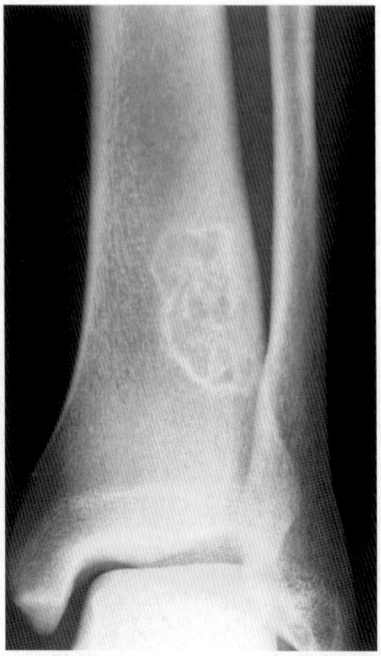

FIG. 2.19 **Healing Nonossifying Fibroma.** A lesion in a young adult, characteristic of a nonossifying fibroma that is beginning to disappear or "heal." As these lesions are typically not seen in patients over the age of 30, it is thought that they ossify and then blend into the normal bone.

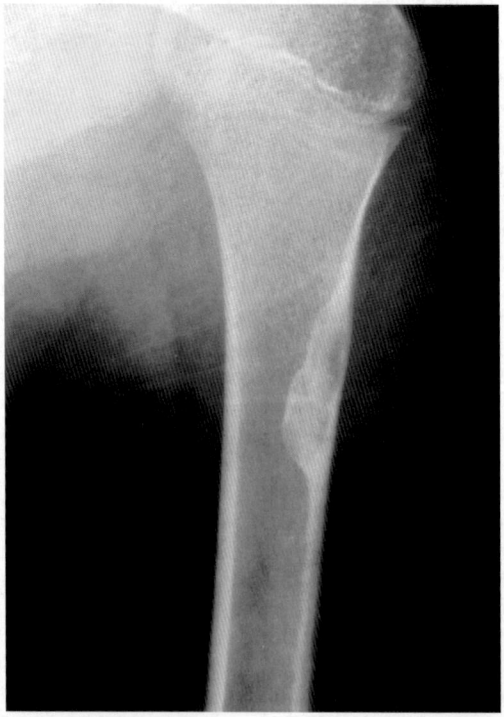

FIG. 2.20 **Healing Nonossifying Fibroma.** A typical nonossifying fibroma in the proximal humerus of a child that is beginning to ossify. In a few years' time, this lesion will essentially be nonexistent.

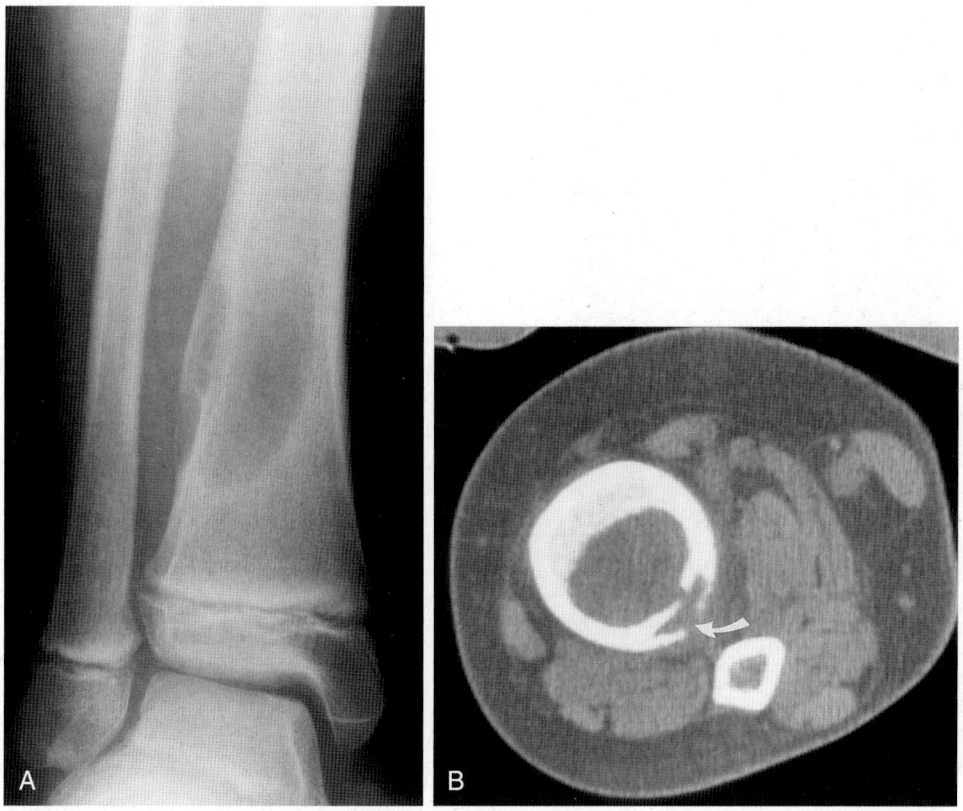

FIG. 2.21 **Computed Tomography (CT) of Nonossifying Fibroma.** An anteroposterior (AP) plain film (A) shows an expansile lytic lesion that was seen when this child had x-rays obtained for a sprained ankle. This is typical for a nonossifying fibroma. A CT scan was obtained through this lesion (for no good reason) (B); it shows some disruption of the cortex *(arrow)*, which was felt to represent "cortical destruction." The lesion was therefore biopsied and found to be a nonossifying fibroma. This cortex is not destroyed but rather replaced with benign fibrous tissue.

this "healing" period, they can appear hot on a radionuclide bone scan because there is osteoblastic activity. Computed tomography scan can show apparent cortical breakthrough, which is really only fibrous tissue replacing cortex (Fig. 2.21). These lesions can occasionally get quite large (Fig. 2.22); therefore growth or change in size should not alter the diagnosis. They are most commonly seen about the knee but can occur in any long bone.

The MR imaging appearance of an NOF is somewhat variable. Although they are essentially always low signal on T1WI, they can have high or low signal on T2WI (Fig. 2.23).

Discriminators:

1. Must be under age 30.
2. No periostitis or pain.

OSTEOBLASTOMA

Osteoblastomas are rare lesions that could justifiably be excluded from this differential without the fear of missing a diagnosis more than once in your lifetime. Why, then, include them? The mnemonic FEGNOMASHIC would not have nearly the same ring without the extra vowel, so osteoblastoma remains.

Osteoblastomas have two appearances:[1] They can look like large osteoid osteomas and are often called giant osteoid osteomas. Because osteoid osteomas are sclerotic lesions and do not resemble bubbly lytic lesions, this is not the type of osteoblastoma we are concerned with in this differential.[2] They can simulate ABCs. They are expansile, often having a soap bubble

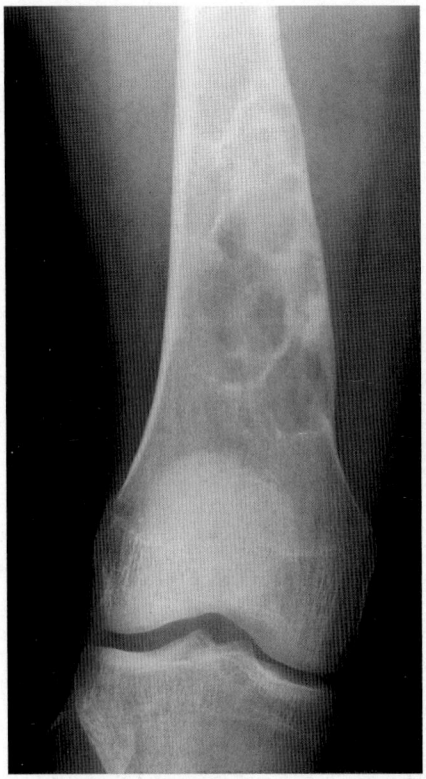

FIG. 2.22 **Large Nonossifying Fibroma.** This large, expansile, well-defined lytic lesion was noted in an asymptomatic 16 year old and biopsied because it had grown over a several-year follow-up. It was found to be a nonossifying fibroma. There is little justification for biopsying this lesion, even though it is larger than most nonossifying fibromas.

appearance (Fig. 2.24). If an ABC is being considered, so should an osteoblastoma. They most commonly occur in the posterior elements of the vertebral bodies, and about half of the cases demonstrate speckled calcifications. A classic radiology differential is that of an expansile lytic lesion of the posterior elements of the spine, and it includes osteoblastoma, ABC, and tuberculosis (Table 2.3).

Discriminator:

Mentioned when ABC is mentioned.

METASTATIC DISEASE AND MYELOMA

Metastatic disease (mets) should be considered for any lytic lesion—benign or aggressive in appearance—in a patient over the age of 40. Mets can appear perfectly benign radiographically (Fig. 2.25), so it is not valid to say, "Since this lesion looks benign, it should not be a met." Most mets have an aggressive appearance and won't be in the FEGNOMASHIC differential, but a significant number appear benign.

For statistical purposes, I will not mention mets in a patient under the age of 40. I'll be correct more than 99% of the time using 40 as a cutoff age. Otherwise, mets would have to be mentioned in every single case of a lytic lesion, and I'm trying to find ways to limit the list of differential possibilities. I'm not saying that mets don't occur in patients under the age of 40, only that I'm willing to miss them (unless I'm given a history of a known primary neoplasm). It is very uncommon for a person under age 40 to present with bone pain due to metastatic disease, whereas, over age 40, this is not uncommon.

Myeloma can present as either solitary or multiple lytic lesions, which are more correctly called plasmacytomas (Fig. 2.26). I try to mention plasmacytoma separately from metastatic disease because it can occur in a slightly younger population (35 years is my cutoff) and can precede clinical or hematologic evidence of myeloma by 3 to 5 years. In general, there is no harm in lumping all metastatic disease, including myeloma, into one group and using greater than age 40 as the limiting factor.

Virtually any metastatic process can present as a lytic, benign-appearing lesion; therefore it serves no purpose to try to guess the source of the met from its appearance. In general, lytic expansile mets tend to come from thyroid and renal tumors (Fig. 2.27). The only metastatic lesion that is said to always be lytic is renal cell carcinoma.

Discriminator:

Must be over age 40.

ANEURYSMAL BONE CYST

ABCs are the only lesions I know of that are named for their radiographic appearance. They are virtually always aneurysmal or expansile (Figs. 2.28 and 2.29). Rarely an ABC will present before it is expansile, but that is unusual enough to not worry about. ABCs primarily occur in patients who are under the age of 30, although occasionally one will be encountered in older patients. I use expansion and below the age of 30 as fairly rigid guidelines and seldom miss the diagnosis of ABC.

ABCs have a characteristic appearance on MRI exams with multiple fluid–fluid levels (Fig. 2.30).

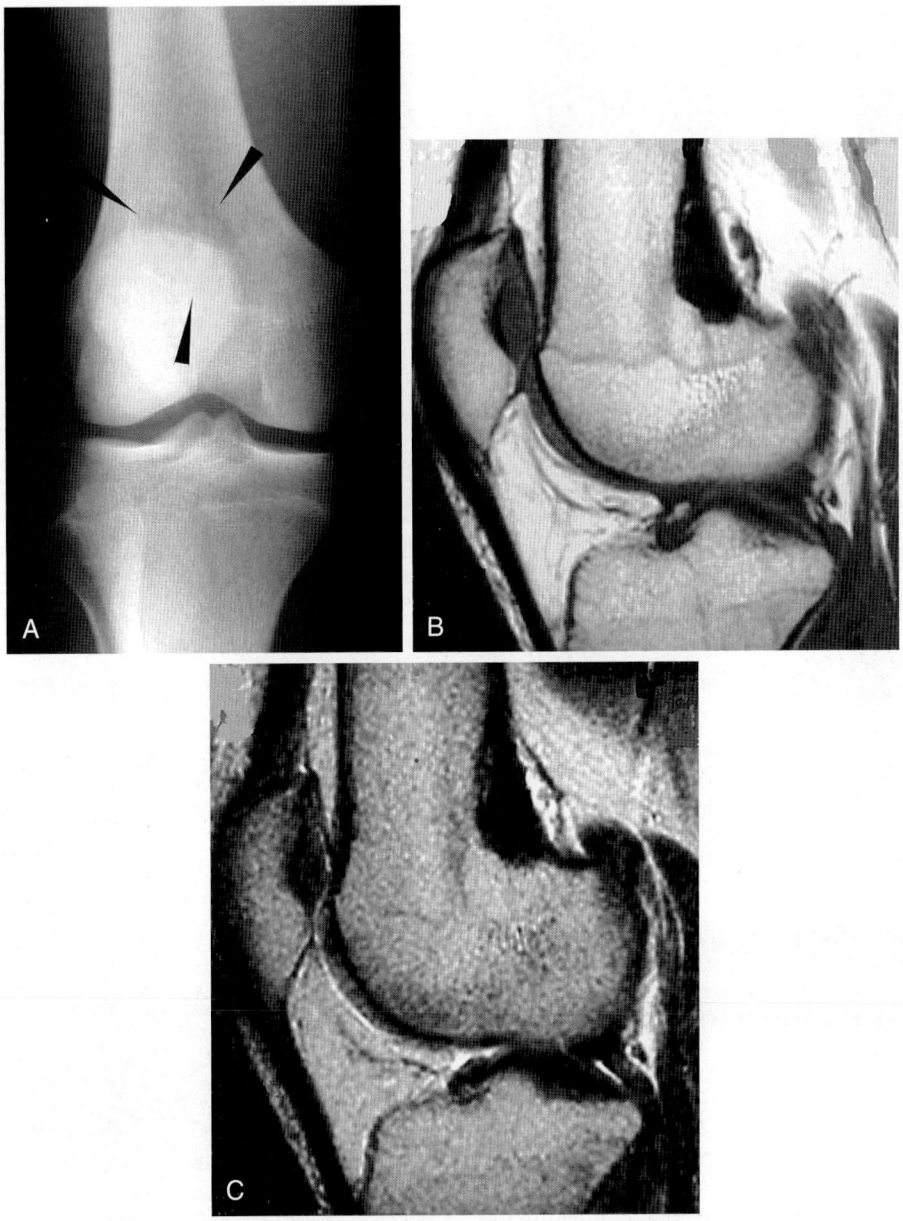

FIG. 2.23 **Magnetic Resonance Imaging (MRI) of Nonossifying Fibroma.** An anteroposterior (AP) plain film (A) of a knee in a 16-year-old girl shows a benign appearing lytic lesion *(arrows)*, which is consistent with an nonossifying fibroma (NOF). Sagittal T1- (B) and T2- (C) weighted images show a cortically based low signal lesion on both the T1 and the T2 sequences. This is characteristic for an NOF.

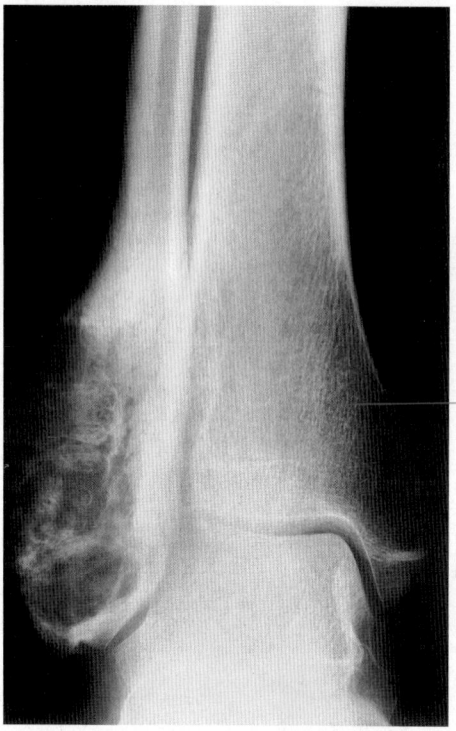

FIG. 2.24 **Osteoblastoma.** A well-defined, expansile, lytic lesion in a 35-year-old patient that looks like an aneurysmal bone cyst. This is only one appearance of this very rare lesion (the other appearance being a sclerotic lesion similar to an osteoid osteoma, although considerably larger).

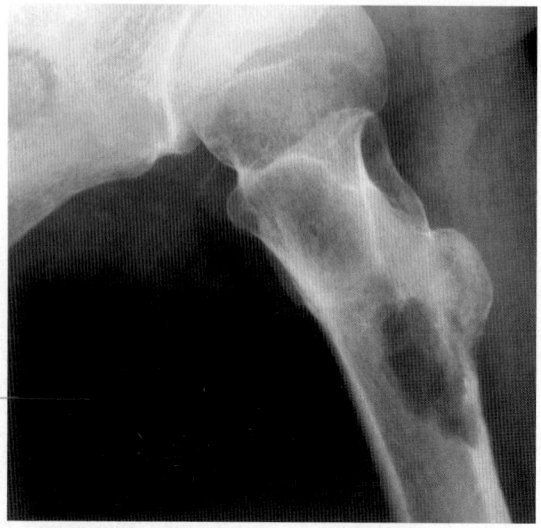

FIG. 2.25 **Metastatic Disease.** A typical renal metastasis is seen as a benign lytic lesion in the proximal femur in this patient.

TABLE 2.3 Differential diagnosis of expansile, lytic lesion in posterior elements of spine
Aneurysmal bone cyst
Osteoblastoma
Tuberculosis

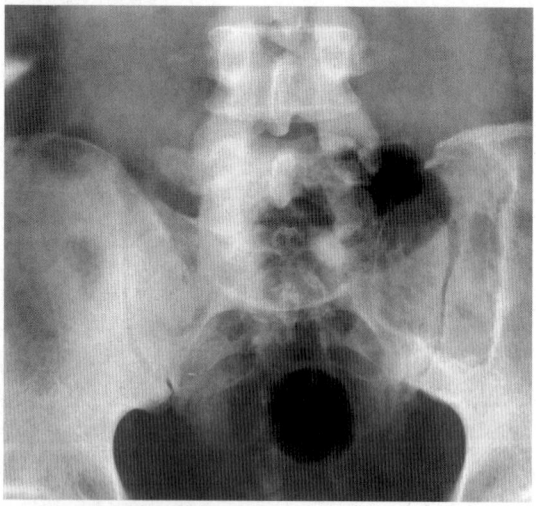

FIG. 2.26 **Plasmacytoma.** A large lytic lesion with a well-defined sclerotic border is seen in the left ilium in a patient with multiple myeloma. The ilium and sacrum are common sites for plasmacytomas.

Although other entities can have fluid–fluid levels and ABCs don't always have them, the appearance is nevertheless so characteristic for an ABC that it is almost pathognomonic.

There are two types of ABCs: a primary type and a secondary type. The secondary type occurs in conjunction with another lesion or from trauma, whereas a primary ABC has no known cause or association with other lesions. Secondary ABCs have been described to occur with GCTs, osteosarcomas, and almost any other lesion you can name; however, in my experience, this does not happen very often. As to occurring after trauma, I don't understand why they would be age-limited if trauma were the cause. Also, malignant tumors were once thought to occur after trauma because of the

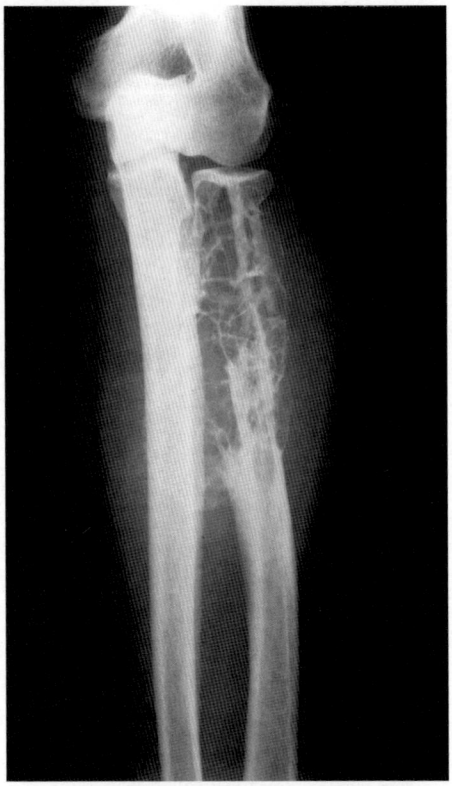

FIG. 2.27 **Metastatic Renal Cell Carcinoma.** A bubbly expansile lesion of the proximal radius is noted that is typical for renal cell carcinoma metastasis. It is similar in appearance to an aneurysmal bone cyst.

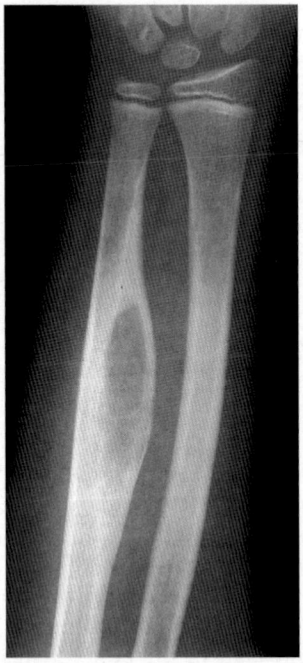

FIG. 2.28 **Aneurysmal Bone Cyst.** An expansile lesion in the diaphysis of the ulna in a young child that is typical for an aneurysmal bone cyst.

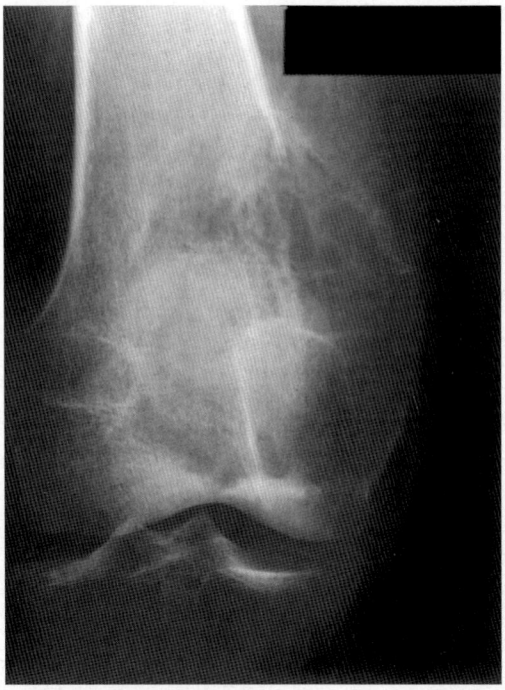

FIG. 2.29 **Aneurysmal Bone Cyst.** An expansile lytic lesion in a 25-year-old that is typical for an aneurysmal bone cyst. At first glance, one might consider this typical for a giant cell tumor. However, note the sclerotic margins and the fact that it does not abut the articular surface.

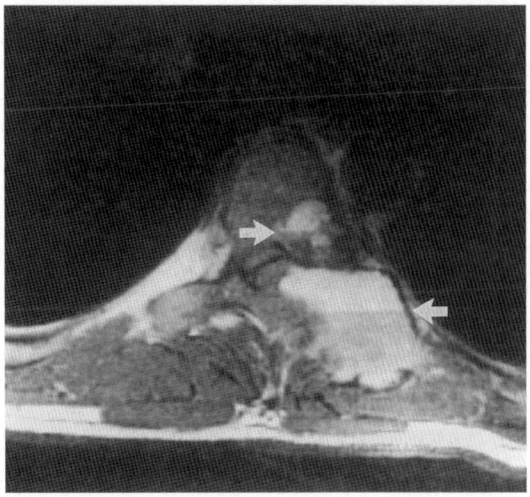

FIG. 2.30 **Aneurysmal Bone Cyst (Magnetic Resonance Imaging; MRI).** An axial proton-density magnetic resonance image through an expansile lytic lesion involving the posterior elements of a thoracic vertebral body reveals several fluid–fluid levels *(arrows)*. This appearance is classic for an aneurysmal bone cyst.

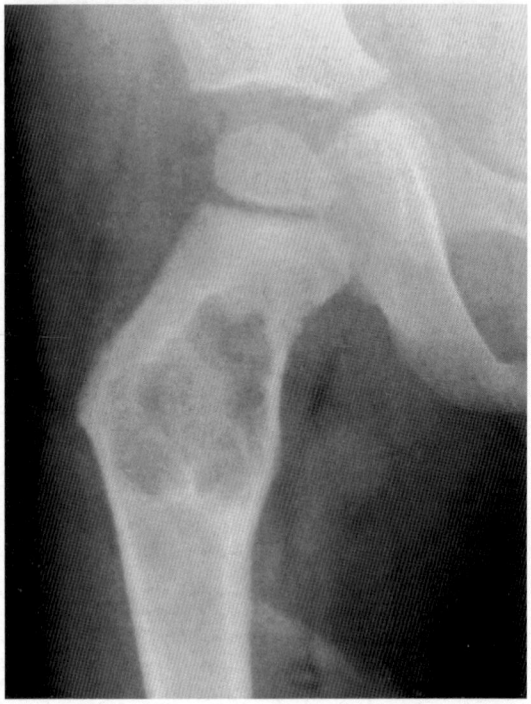

FIG. 2.31 **Solitary Bone Cyst.** A centrally placed lesion in the proximal femur that is classic for a solitary bone cyst.

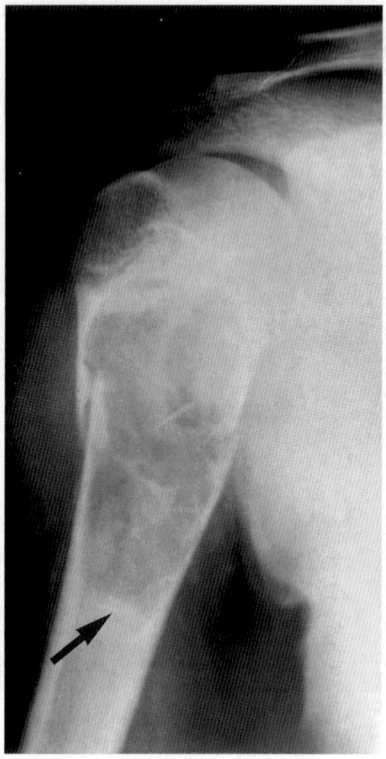

FIG. 2.32 **Solitary Bone Cyst.** A pathologic fracture has occurred through this lesion in the proximal humerus. Its location and appearance are typical for a solitary bone cyst. Note the cortical fragments *(arrow)* produced from the fracture that have sunk to the bottom of this fluid-filled lesion. This is termed a "fallen fragment sign." No other lesion has been reported to have a fallen fragment sign; therefore this is virtually pathognomonic.

frequent antecedent history of trauma with malignant bone tumors. This is not seriously considered today and is thought to be coincidental. I suspect that ABCs and trauma are also coincidental, but this is mere speculation.

ABCs typically present because of pain. They occasionally can occur in the epiphyses, but there is no location in which they should be given more weight in the differential. As with osteoblastoma, they often occur in the posterior elements of the spine.

Discriminators:

1. Must be expansile.
2. Must be under age 30.

SOLITARY BONE CYST

Solitary bone cysts are also called simple bone cysts or unicameral bone cysts. They are not necessarily unicameral (one compartment), however. This is the only lesion in FEGNOMASHIC that is always central in location (Fig. 2.31). Many of the other lesions may be central, but a solitary bone cyst can be excluded if it is not. It is one of the few lesions that doesn't occur most commonly around the knees. Two-thirds to three-fourths of these lesions occur in the proximal humerus and proximal femur. By itself this fact isn't that helpful, or one-third to one-fourth of the lesions would be missed.

Solitary bone cysts are usually asymptomatic unless fractured—a common occurrence (Fig. 2.32). Even when pathologic fractures occur, they rarely form periostitis. They usually occur in young patients, and it is unusual to see one in a patient over the age of 30. Although long bones are most commonly involved, solitary bone cysts have been described in almost every bone in the body. They begin at the physeal plate in long bones and grow into the shaft of the bone; therefore they are

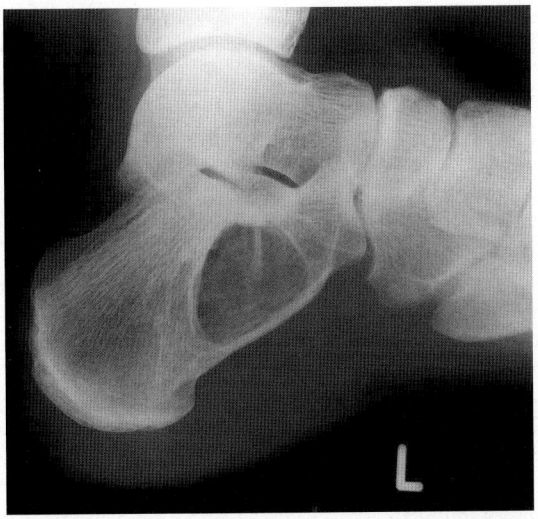

FIG. 2.33 **Solitary Bone Cyst.** A classic appearance of a solitary bone cyst in the calcaneus. This lesion in the calcaneus occurs only in this position (anterior to the midportion of the calcaneus and on the inferior border). Although other lesions could occur in this location, a solitary bone cyst of the calcaneus virtually never occurs away from this spot.

not epiphyseal lesions. They can, however, extend up into an epiphysis after the plate closes, but this is unusual. A fairly common location is in the calcaneus, where they have a characteristic triangular appearance (Fig. 2.33).

Discriminators:

1. Must be central.
2. Must be under age 30.

HYPERPARATHYROIDISM (BROWN TUMORS)

Brown tumors of hyperparathyroidism (HPT) can have almost any appearance, from a purely lytic lesion to a sclerotic process (Fig. 2.34). Generally, when the patient's HPT is treated, the brown tumor undergoes sclerosis and will eventually disappear. If a brown tumor is going to be considered in the differential, additional radiographic findings of HPT should be seen. Subperiosteal bone resorption is pathognomonic for HPT and should be searched for in the phalanges (particularly the radial aspect of the middle phalanges), distal clavicles (resorption), medial aspect of the proximal tibias, and sacroiliac joints (it has the appearance of bilateral sacroiliac joint erosive disease). Osteoporosis or osteosclerosis might

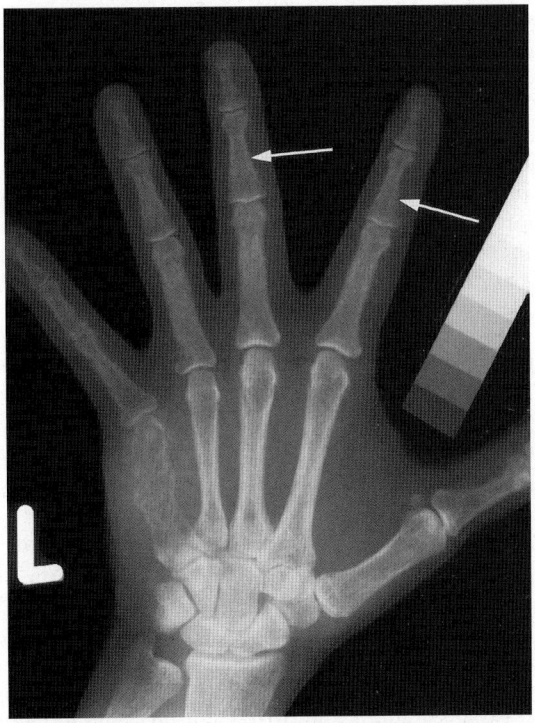

FIG. 2.34 **Brown Tumor.** An expansile lytic lesion in the fifth metacarpal that would have an extremely long differential diagnosis. Barely discernible is subperiosteal bone resorption on the radial aspect of the middle phalanges *(arrows)*. A second, smaller lytic lesion is seen at the proximal portion of the fourth proximal phalanx. It has a different appearance than the other lytic lesion, emphasizing how brown tumors can have almost any appearance. The multiplicity is typical for a brown tumor and limits the differential diagnosis. However, the finding of subperiosteal bone resorption makes any other diagnosis unlikely.

suggest that renal osteodystrophy with secondary HPT is present, but subperiosteal resorption must be present; otherwise brown tumor can be excluded from the differential.

We rarely see brown tumors today, likely due to the more aggressive treatment of renal disease with resulting fewer cases of HPT.

Discriminator:

Must have other evidence of HPT.

HEMANGIOMAS

Multiple hemangiomas, also known as cystic angiomatosis or cystic lymphangiomatosis, while uncommon, are seen more frequently than brown tumors and should probably replace them as the *H* in FEGNOMASHIC. Cystic angiomatosis usually is an incidental finding of multiple lytic lesions throughout the skeleton (Fig 2.35). Although they are incidental, some feel they are in a similar category to Goham's disease (massive osteolysis or disappearing bone disease), but without the destructive potential. Cystic angiomatosis should be considered when multiple lytic lesions are encountered that are asymptomatic.

INFECTION

Unfortunately there is no reliable way to radiographically exclude a focus of osteomyelitis (Fig. 2.36). It has a protean radiographic appearance and can occur at any location and in a patient of any age. It may or may not be expansile, have a sclerotic or nonsclerotic border, or have periostitis associated with it. Soft tissue findings such as obliteration of adjacent fat planes are notoriously unreliable and even misleading, as tumors and EG can do the same thing.

When osteomyelitis occurs near a joint, if the articular surface is abutted, invariably the adjacent joint will be involved and show either cartilage loss or an effusion, or both (Fig. 2.37). This finding is not particularly helpful, since any lesion can cause an effusion, but it's the best I can come up with.

When a sclerotic margin is present, infection usually causes the sclerotic margin to be thick and ill-defined or fuzzy on its outermost portion, but these findings are by no means always present and are only of limited usefulness.

If a bony sequestrum is present, osteomyelitis should be strongly considered. As previously mentioned, the only lesions described that demonstrate sequestra are infection, EG, lymphoma, and fibrosarcoma. Most cases of osteomyelitis, however, do not have sequestra, so this feature is also of limited use. Therefore infection will be in almost every differential diagnosis of a lytic lesion, which is all right, since it is one of the most common lesions encountered.

Discriminators:

None.

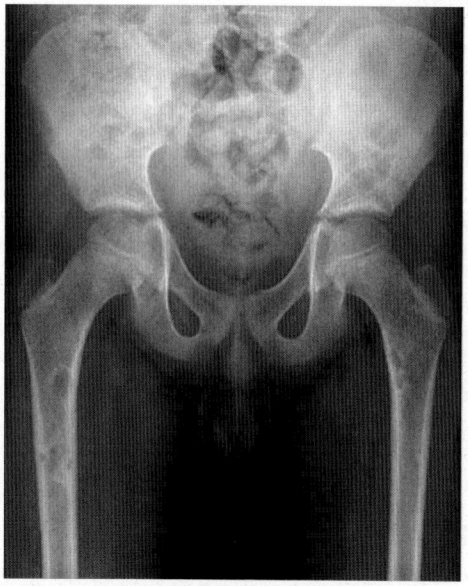

FIG. 2.35 **Cystic Angiomatosis.** Multiple lytic lesions are seen in the femurs and pelvis in this asymptomatic young woman, which were found to be hemangiomas.

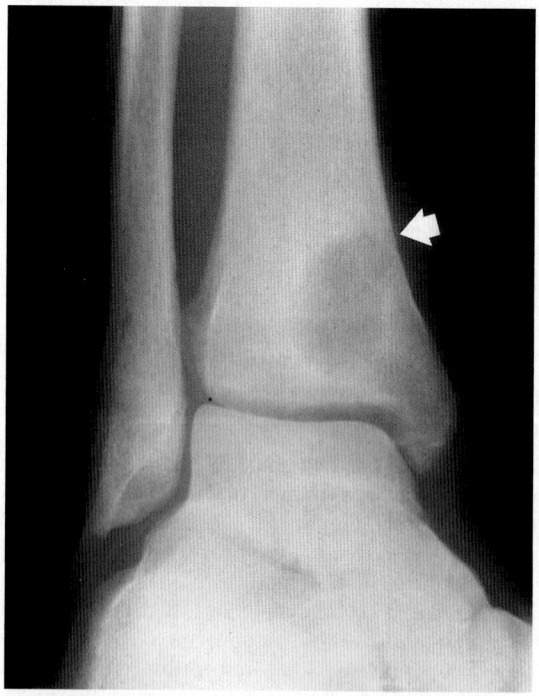

FIG. 2.36 **Brodie Abscess.** A focus of infection that was chronic in this patient is seen in the distal tibia. The differential diagnosis for this lesion would be quite long if the subtle periostitis *(arrow)* and the clinical history of pain were not noted. Although this is a typical appearance for a chronic osteomyelitis (Brodie abscess), infection can resemble almost anything.

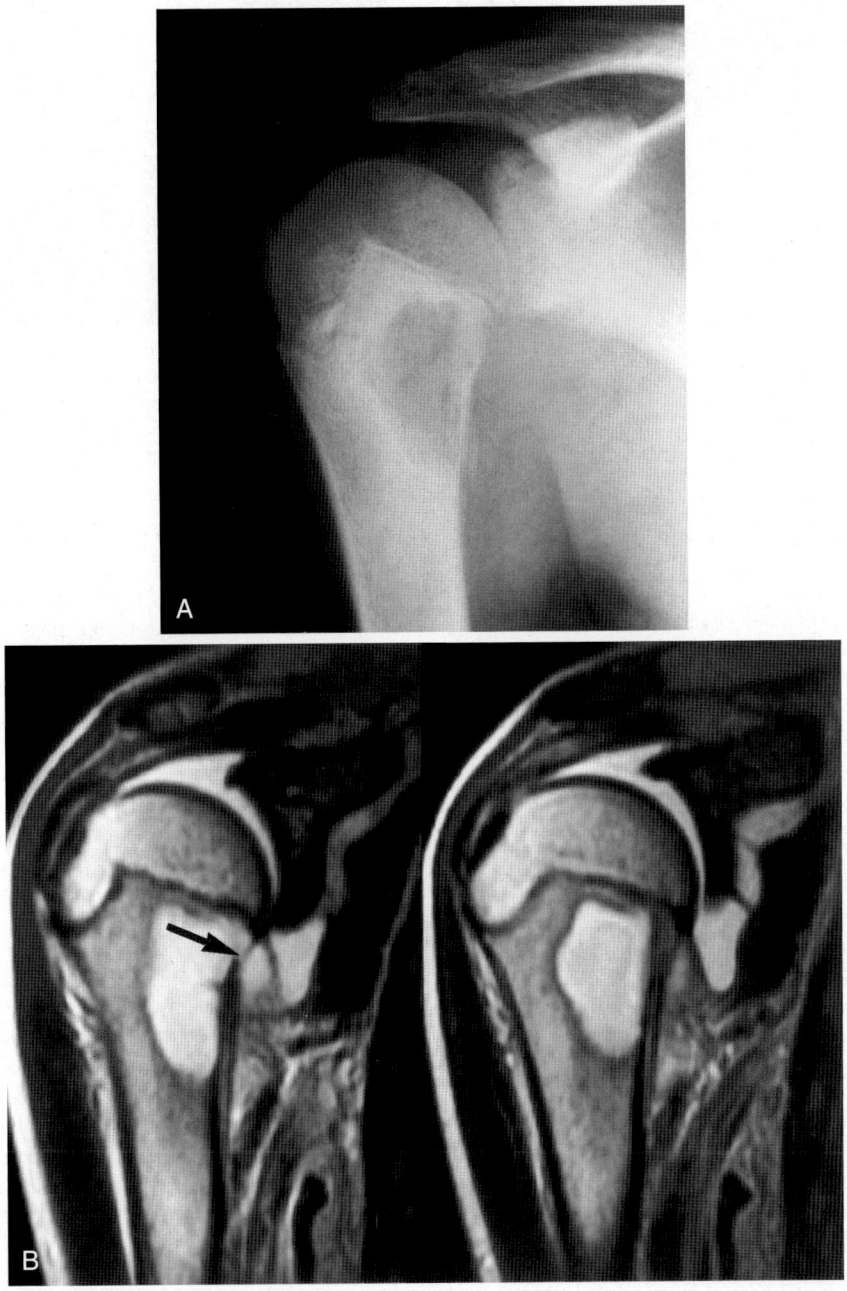

FIG. 2.37 **Osteomyelitis with Pyoarthritis.** A plain film of the shoulder (A) in this child with shoulder pain shows a well-defined lytic lesion. Coronal T2-weighted magnetic resonance imaging (MRI) (B) shows high signal throughout the lesion, which extends through the cortex *(arrow)* into the joint. This is a typical appearance for osteomyelitis with extension into the joint.

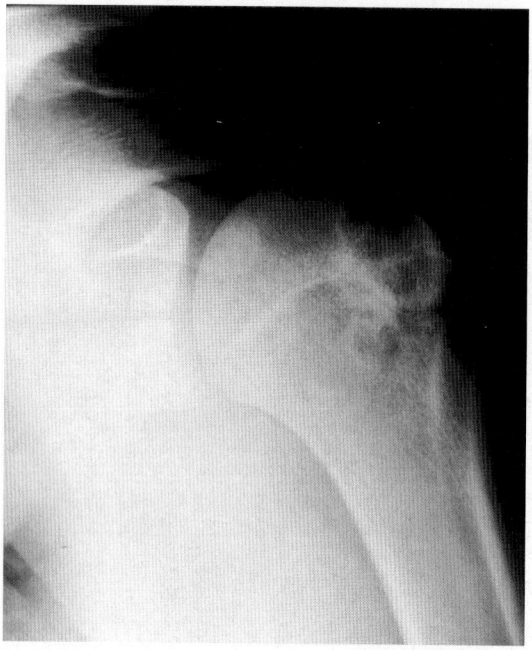

FIG. 2.38 **Chondroblastoma.** A lytic lesion with a well-defined sclerotic margin in the proximal humeral epiphysis extending slightly across the epiphyseal plate. This is a typical appearance of a chondroblastoma. Almost half of all chondroblastomas have a small portion of the lesion extending across the physeal plate.

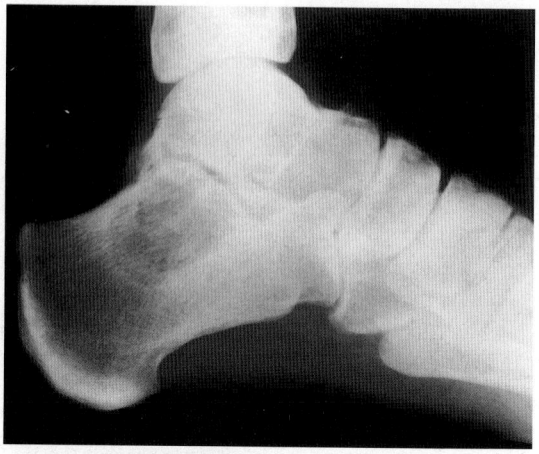

FIG. 2.39 **Chondroblastoma.** A lytic lesion in the calcaneus that abuts the superior portion of the calcaneus has a fairly short differential diagnosis. The differential is essentially the same as in an epiphysis. On biopsy, this lesion was found to be a chondroblastoma.

CHONDROBLASTOMA

Chondroblastomas are among the easiest lesions to deal with because they occur only in the epiphyses (a handful of cases have been reported in the metaphyses—they're rare), and they occur almost exclusively in patients under the age of 30 (Fig. 2.38). What could be easier? Anywhere from 40% to 60% demonstrate calcification, so absence of calcification is not helpful. Presence of calcification is helpful so long as you can be sure that it's not detritus or sequestra from infection or EG (both of which can occur in the epiphyses). Because I can never be certain about the calcification, I don't worry about it.

The differential diagnosis of a lytic lesion in the epiphysis of a patient under the age of 30 is short and simple:[1] infection (most common), chondroblastoma, and GCT (it has its own diagnostic criteria, so it can usually be definitely ruled out or in). This is an old, classic differential and probably takes care of 98% of epiphyseal lesions. If you want to be 99% certain, you must add two more lesions—ABC (be certain it is expansile) and EG—and add mets and myeloma if the age is over 40. I no longer recommend using the longer differential as it just seems to cause confusion. Residents remember that there are three entities in the epiphyseal differential and then pick from the longer list of five entities, often leaving out the main things while including EG and ABC. Most of you have too much to commit to memory already without trying to stuff in a few rare presentations that will not be seen very often.

A caveat on epiphyseal lesions is to always consider the possibility of a subchondral cyst or geode, which has been described in anything that can result in degenerative joint disease (DJD). Be certain no joint pathology that might cause DJD is present, or an unnecessary biopsy of a geode might be performed based on your differential of an epiphyseal lesion (see Chapter 4, "Don't Touch" Lesions).

The carpal bones, the tarsal bones, and the patella have a tendency to behave like epiphyses as far as their differential diagnosis of lesions is concerned. Therefore a lytic lesion in these areas has a similar differential as an epiphyseal lesion (Fig. 2.39); although in my experience, while this differential diagnosis in the epiphyses is close to 99% inclusive, in these other locations, it is only about 50% inclusive—still, a good differential to begin with.

Discriminators:

1. Must be under age 30.
2. Must be epiphyseal.

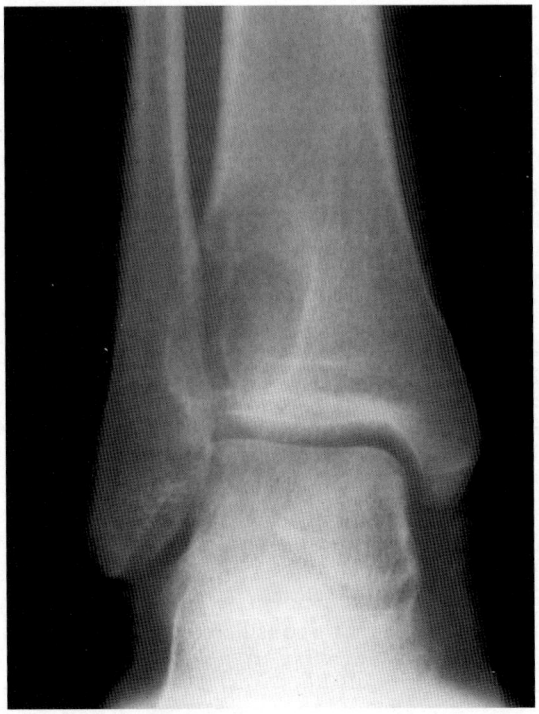

FIG. 2.40 **Chondromyxoid Fibroma.** This lytic lesion in the distal tibia with a well-defined sclerotic margin should have been a nonossifying fibroma. The differential diagnosis for this lesion would include several other entities, all of which are benign. Although a biopsy of this lesion probably should not have been done in this asymptomatic patient, it was performed, and the lesion was found to be a chondromyxoid fibroma.

CHONDROMYXOID FIBROMA

Like osteoblastoma, the chondromyxoid fibroma is such a rare lesion that failure to mention it is probably not going to result in missing more than one in your lifetime. Why include it then? I recommend not including it, but it's part of the classic differential. If you do mention it, at least know what it looks like. Basically, chondromyxoid fibromas resemble NOFs (Fig. 2.40). Unlike NOFs, however, they can be seen in patients of any age. They can present with pain also, which will not occur with an NOF.

Discriminator:

Mention when an NOF is mentioned.

ADDITIONAL POINTS

That, in essence, is my differential for a benign lytic lesion of bone. It is probably 98% accurate, which is good enough for me. To increase the accuracy to 99%, it would be necessary to add a host of uncommon or rare lesions, and the whole process would become too confusing for most residents to learn and would not be as helpful to clinicians. If you have a favorite lesion that is not in this list, by all means, add it. Likewise, if the list is already too cumbersome, forget about osteoblastoma, brown tumors, hemangiomas, and chondromyxoid fibroma. I'm unable to make it much simpler than that and still be reasonably accurate.

Some of the lesions I have purposefully omitted are intraosseous ganglion, pseudotumor of hemophilia, hemangioendothelioma, ossifying fibroma, intraosseous lipoma, glomus tumor, neurofibroma, plasma cell granuloma, and schwannoma. Others could be added to this list, of course, but are best left to the pathologist—not the radiologist—for the diagnosis.

There are several features that are somewhat useful in separating out the various lesions in FEGNOMASHIC (Table 2.1). For instance, if the patient is under the age of 30, be sure to consider EG, chondroblastoma, NOF, ABC, and solitary bone cyst. This is not a differential diagnosis to list when faced with a lytic lesion in a patient less than 30; several other lesions should be included in that differential. This means don't mention those five lesions in a patient over 30. If the patient is over 30, those five lesions can probably be excluded.

If periostitis or pain is present (assuming no trauma, which can be a foolhardy assumption), you can exclude fibrous dysplasia, solitary bone cyst, NOF, and enchondroma. If the lesion is epiphyseal, the classic differential is infection, GCT, and chondroblastoma. ABC and EG could be added to that differential too, but are not mandatory. If the patient is over 40 years of age, add mets and myeloma and remove ABC, chondroblastoma, and EG from the epiphyseal list. Don't forget to consider a subchondral cyst or geode in epiphyseal lesions.

The epiphyseal differential tends to work also for the tarsal bones (especially the calcaneus), the carpal bones, and the patella. In the calcaneus, a unicameral bone cyst should also be considered and has a characteristic appearance and location (Fig. 2.33). Apophyses are "epiphyseal equivalents" and have the same differential as epiphyses. The difference between an epiphysis and an apophysis is that epiphyses contribute to the length of a bone, whereas apophyses serve as ligamentous attachments.

A few findings that just don't seem to narrow the differential diagnosis are presence or absence of a soft tissue mass, expansion of the bone (except must be present in an

ABC), a sclerotic or nonsclerotic border (except must be nonsclerotic in GCT), presence or absence of bony struts or compartments in the lesion, and size of the lesion.

There are a few lesions that I call "automatics" (Box 2.1). That is, they need to be included automatically in almost every case. In patients less than 30, EG and infection must be included in every differential of a lytic bone lesion. In fact, they should be mentioned in any case except for trauma or arthritis because they can have virtually *any* appearance—lytic, sclerotic, mixed, benign, aggressive, etc. Hence they can mimic almost any bone lesion. I recommend mentioning EG and infection for every bone lesion in patients under the age of 30. Make sure you give a thoughtful pause after inspecting the film—as if you really considered the pros and cons of mentioning them. This is gamesmanship, but it adds to your credibility. In patients over the age of 40, mets and infection are "automatics." No consideration for the lesion's appearance or location needs to be made when using the automatics—simply find a lesion.

BOX 2.1
"Automatics"

UNDER AGE 30:
Eosinophilic granuloma
Infection

OVER AGE 40:
Mets
Infection

DIFFERENTIAL DIAGNOSIS OF A SCLEROTIC LESION

Many lytic lesions spontaneously regress and are not usually seen in patients over the age of 30. When these lesions regress, they often fill in with new bone and have a sclerotic or blastic appearance. Therefore when a sclerotic focus is identified in a 20- to 40-year-old patient, especially if it is an asymptomatic, incidental finding, the following lesions should be considered: NOF (Fig. 2.41),

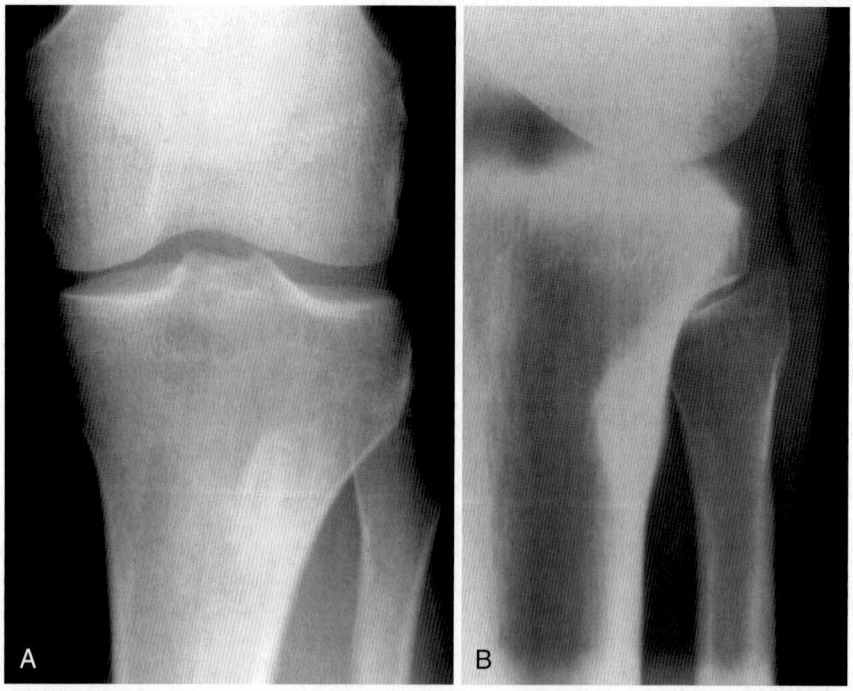

FIG. 2.41 (A) **Healing Nonossifying Fibroma.** This faintly sclerotic lesion in the proximal tibia of a 30-year-old asymptomatic patient is characteristic for a healing or disappearing nonossifying fibroma. Prior films showed a typical lytic nonossifying fibroma. (B) **Healing Nonossifying Fibroma.** This densely sclerotic lesion in the posterior proximal tibia in a young asymptomatic patient was thought to represent an osteoid osteoma or osteomyelitis. Even though the patient was asymptomatic, a biopsy was performed. It revealed a nonossifying fibroma that had ossified. In a patient over the age of 40, metastatic disease would need to be considered.

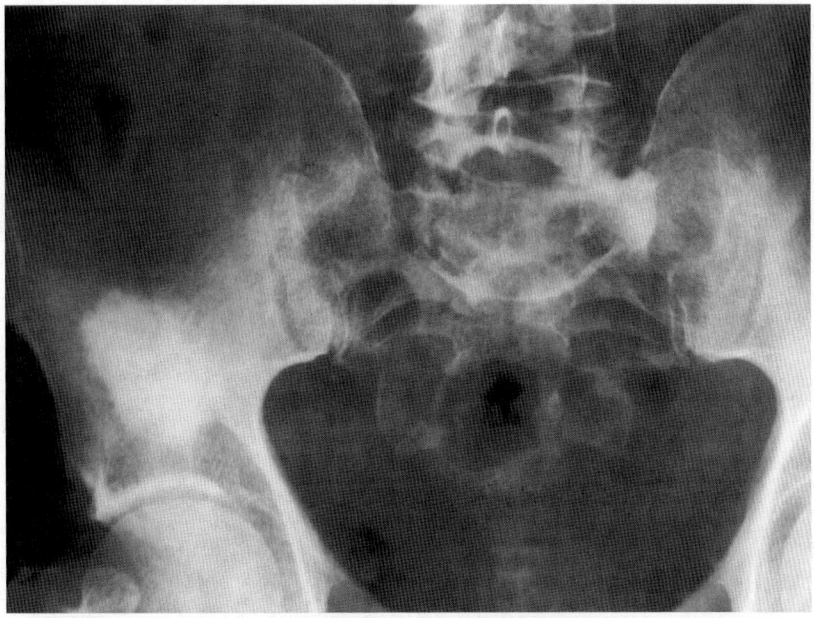

FIG. 2.42 **Giant Bone Island.** A large sclerotic lesion is seen in the right iliac bone, which could easily be mistaken for a focus of metastatic disease in a patient over the age of 40. This is a giant bone island and has the typical pattern of irregular "feathered" margins with the trabecula blending into the normal bone. The axis of the lesion is in the long axis of the bone or in the direction of the primary weight-bearing trabecula.

EG, solitary bone cyst, ABC, chondroblastoma. Several other lesions should be included that can also appear sclerotic: fibrous dysplasia, osteoid osteoma, infection, brown tumor (healing), and perhaps a giant bone island (Fig. 2.42). As these lesions continue to resolve, they often will be seen to have varying amounts of normal fatty marrow (Fig. 2.43). They should not be mistakenly called intraosseous lipomas just because they contain fat, although no harm would come from that misdiagnosis—it's still benign, and in most cases an incidental finding.

In any patient over the age of 40, the number one possibility for a sclerotic lesion should be metastatic disease (now that I've passed 40, I'm seriously considering moving the age to 50).

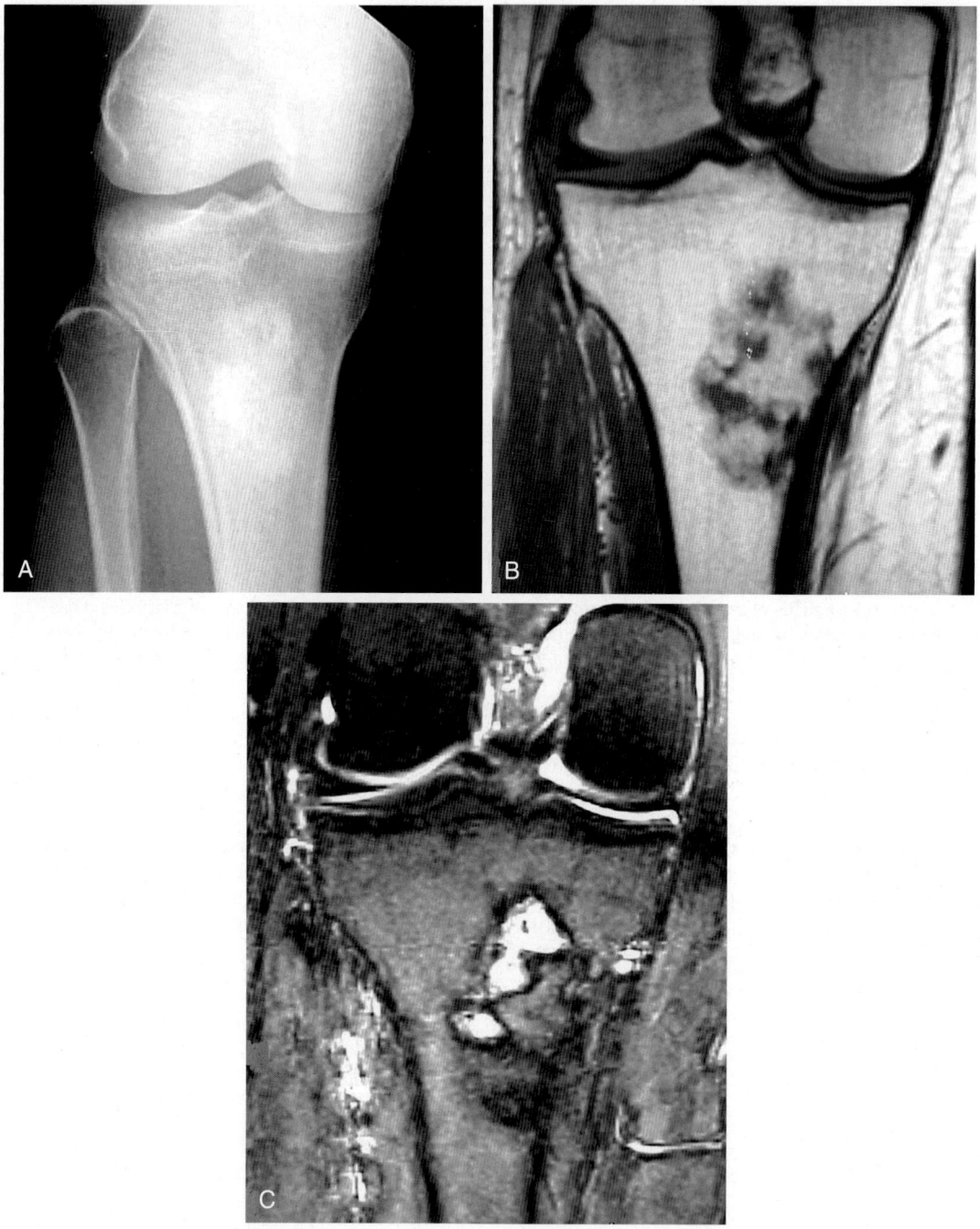

FIG. 2.43 **Resolving Nonossifying Fibroma (NOF).** An anteroposterior (AP) plain film of a knee (A) in a 28-year-old man shows a sclerotic lesion in the metaphysis of the tibia. Coronal T1 (B) and T2 (C) weighted images of the knee reveal a lesion that on T1WI has mixed high and low signal, consistent with fatty tissue in some areas, which is mixed high and low signal on the T2WI. This is typical for a resolving NOF.

REFERENCES

1. Gold RH, Ross SE, et al. The radiologic learning file. An introduction to diagnostic radiology. *Radiology*. 1972;104(1): 27–31.
2. Skeletal Lesions Interobserver Correlation among Expert Diagnosticians (SLICED) study group. Reliability of histopathologic and radiologic grading of cartilaginous neoplasms in long bones. *JBJS*. 2007;89:2113–2123.
3. David R, Oria R, Kumar R, et al. Radiologic features of eosinophilic granuloma of bone. Pictorial essay. *AJR*. 1989;153:1021–1026.
4. Dahlin D. Giant cell tumor of bone: highlights of 407 cases. *AJR*. 1985;144:955–960.

CHAPTER 3

Malignant Tumors

Radiology residents have difficulty dealing with malignant bone tumors, and the difficulty gets worse in the years after residency. This is simply because malignant bone tumors, thankfully, are not very common. Nevertheless, every radiologist will encounter one or two a year in most practices and should be able to recognize them and give a good differential diagnosis.

First, how do you recognize a malignant tumor and differentiate it from a benign process? This can be difficult, and oftentimes it is impossible. Recognizing that it is *aggressive* is usually easy, but saying that it is *malignant* is another matter altogether. Processes such as infection and eosinophilic granuloma can mimic malignant tumors and are, of course, benign. They will often be included in the differential diagnosis of an aggressive lesion along with malignant tumors.

DIFFERENTIATION OF MALIGNANT FROM BENIGN

What radiologic criteria are useful for determining malignant versus benign? Standard textbooks and the literature give four aspects of a lesion to be examined: (1) cortical destruction, (2) periostitis, (3) orientation or axis of the lesion, and (4) zone of transition.

Let me expound on each of these criteria and show why only the last one—the zone of transition—is the most reliable, being accurate to a 90% plus rate.

Cortical Destruction

Often cortical bone is replaced by part of the noncalcified matrix (fibrous matrix or chondroid matrix) of benign fibro-osseous lesions and cartilaginous lesions. This can give the false impression of cortical destruction on plain films (Fig. 3.1) or computed tomography (CT). Also, benign processes such as infection and eosinophilic granuloma can cause extensive cortical destruction and mimic a malignant tumor. Aneurysmal bone cysts are known to cause such thinning of the cortex as to make it radiographically undetectable (Fig. 3.2). For these reasons, I find cortical destruction to occasionally be misleading. Cortical destruction makes one think of a malignant lesion when using the Gestalt approach, but the lesion must also have other criteria for a malignant process, such as a wide zone of transition.

Periostitis

Periosteal reaction occurs in a nonspecific manner whenever the periosteum is irritated, whether it is irritated by a malignant tumor, a benign tumor, infection, or trauma. Callus formation in a fracture is actually just periosteal reaction of the most benign type. Periosteal reaction occurs in two types: benign (Fig. 3.3A and B) and aggressive (Fig. 3.3C and D). The difference between the two is based more on the timing of the growth of the irritation than on whether the process causing the periostitis is malignant or benign. For example, a slow-growing benign tumor will cause thick, wavy, uniform, or dense periostitis because it is a low-grade chronic irritation that gives the periosteum time to lay down thick new bone and remodel into more normal cortex. A malignant tumor causes a periosteal reaction that is high grade and more acute; hence the periosteum does not have time to consolidate. It appears lamellated (onion-skinned) or amorphous, or even sunburst. If the irritation stops or diminishes, the aggressive periostitis will solidify and appear benign. Therefore when periostitis is seen, the radiologist should try to characterize it into either a benign (thick, dense, wavy) type or an aggressive (lamellated, amorphous, sunburst) type.

Unfortunately, judging the lesion by its periostitis can be misleading. First, it takes considerable experience to accurately characterize periostitis because many times the reaction is not clearly benign or aggressive. Second, many benign lesions cause aggressive periostitis, such as infection, eosinophilic granuloma, aneurysmal bone cysts, osteoid osteomas, and even trauma. Seeing *benign* periostitis, however, can be helpful because malignant lesions will not cause benign periostitis. Some investigators with great experience in dealing with malignant bone tumors state that the only way benign periostitis can occur in a malignant lesion is if there is a concomitant fracture or infection. I have seen a few exceptions, but overall I think it is a valid statement.

Orientation or Axis of the Lesion

The orientation or axis of the lesion is a poor determinant of benign versus aggressive and seldom helps me to decide into which category the lesion should be placed. It has been said that if a lesion grows in the

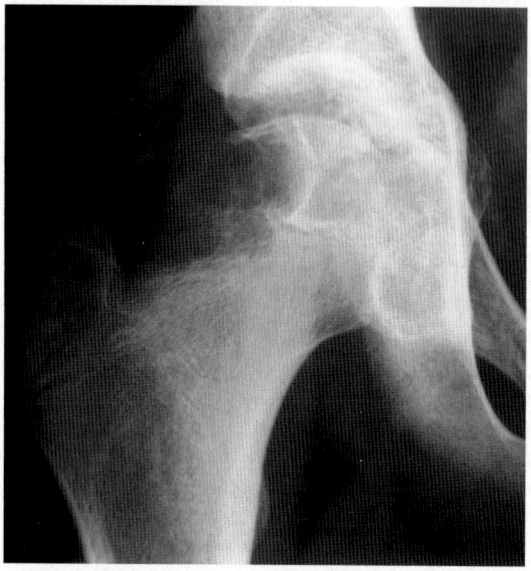

FIG. 3.1 **Apparent Cortical Destruction.** This benign chondroblastoma has noncalcified chondroid tissue replacing cortical bone in the proximal femur, which gives the lesion a destructive appearance. This is an example of cortical replacement rather than of cortical destruction, which can be very confusing if one uses cortical destruction as an aggressive or malignant key in differential diagnosis. Note that the zone of transition is narrow, as one would expect in a benign lesion such as this.

long axis of a long bone, rather than being circular, it is benign. Nonsense! Ewing sarcoma, an extremely malignant lesion, usually has its axis along the shaft of a long bone. Conversely, many fibrous cortical defects are circular yet totally benign. I see no reason to even consider the axis of a lesion as part of its radiologic evaluation.

Zone of Transition

Without question, the zone of transition is the most reliable indicator in determining benign versus malignant lesions. Unfortunately it also has some drawbacks, on which I will elaborate.

The zone of transition is the border between the lesion and the normal bone. It is said to be narrow if it is so well-defined that it can be drawn with a fine-point pen (Fig. 3.4). If it is imperceptible and cannot be clearly drawn, it is said to be wide (Fig. 3.5). Obviously all shades of gray lie in between, but most lesions can be characterized as having either a narrow or a wide zone of transition. If the lesion has a sclerotic border, it, by definition, has a narrow zone of transition.

If a lesion has a narrow zone of transition, it is a benign process. The exceptions to that are uncommon. If a lesion has a wide zone of transition, it is aggressive. Notice that I said aggressive and not malignant. As with aggressive periostitis, many benign lesions can have a wide zone of transition. A few of the same processes that can cause aggressive periostitis, and thereby mimic a malignant tumor, can have a wide zone of transition (i.e., infection and eosinophilic granuloma). They are aggressive in their radiographic appearance because they are fast-acting, aggressive lesions. The zone of transition is usually easier to characterize than the periostitis, plus it is always there to evaluate (or you wouldn't see a lesion), whereas many lesions, benign and malignant, have no periostitis. For these reasons, the zone of transition is the most useful indicator of whether a lesion is benign or malignant.

A lesion that consists of multiple small holes is said to be permeative. It has no perceptible border and therefore has a wide zone of transition. Round cell tumors such as multiple myeloma, primary lymphoma of bone (formerly called reticulum cell sarcoma), and Ewing sarcoma are typical of this type of lesion. However, infection and eosinophilic granuloma (Fig. 3.6) can have the same appearance.

The zone of transition only applies to lytic or predominantly lytic lesions. A blastic or sclerotic lesion will always appear to have a narrow zone of transition and may erroneously get into the benign differential even if it is malignant.

It is critical to be aware that the zone of transition is a plain film finding and cannot be used with magnetic resonance (MR) imaging. Many malignant tumors will appear to have narrow zones of transition on MR imaging exams and can mislead one into thinking a benign lesion is present (Fig. 3.7). The zone of transition can only be used with lytic lesions and on plain films.

DIFFERENTIATING TYPES OF TUMORS

Once it has been decided that a particular lesion is probably malignant, the differential is fairly straightforward. First of all, the list of malignant tumors is relatively short, and second, most tumors follow somewhat strict age groupings. Jack Edeiken, a famed skeletal radiologist, evaluated 4000 malignant bone tumors and found that they could be correctly diagnosed 80% of the time just by using the patient's age! He basically divides the tumors into decades of when they will affect a patient; for example, osteosarcoma and Ewing sarcoma are the only childhood primary malignant tumors of bone, and after the age of 40, only metastatic disease (mets), myeloma, and chondrosarcoma are common (Table 3.1). Although there are certainly outliers that are uncommon, these age guidelines are extremely useful. It is inappropriate to mention Ewing sarcoma in a 40-year-old or mets in a 15-year-old.

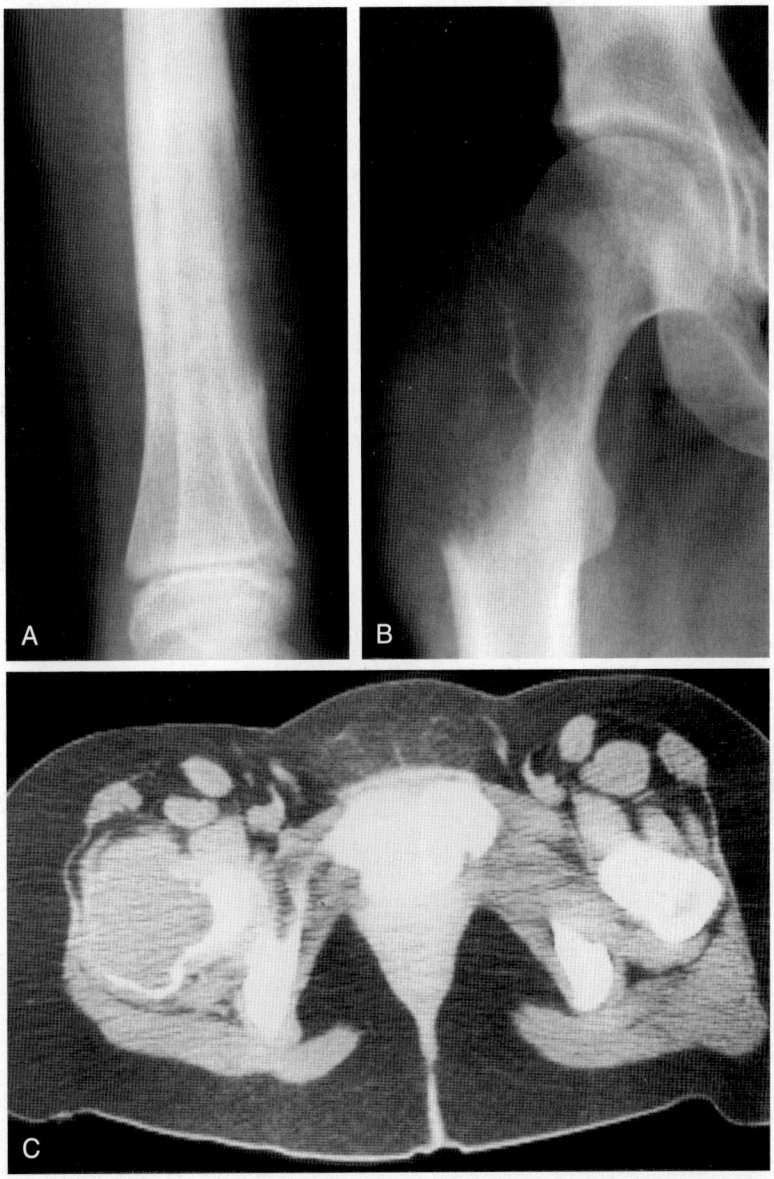

FIG. 3.2 (A) **Aneurysmal Bone Cyst.** This benign lesion has thinned the cortex to such a degree as to make it imperceptible on a plain radiograph. As in Fig. 3.1, this can be misconstrued as cortical destruction, giving the false impression of a malignant or very aggressive lesion. (B) **Giant Cell Tumor.** This lesion in the proximal femur has expanded and thinned the cortex to such a degree that it is imperceptible on the plain film. (C) On a CT scan through this region, a very thin cortex that was greatly expanded was identified. This giant cell tumor originated from the greater trochanter, which is an epiphyseal equivalent. Note that it has a well-defined but nonsclerotic zone of transition, as all giant cell tumors in long bones do.

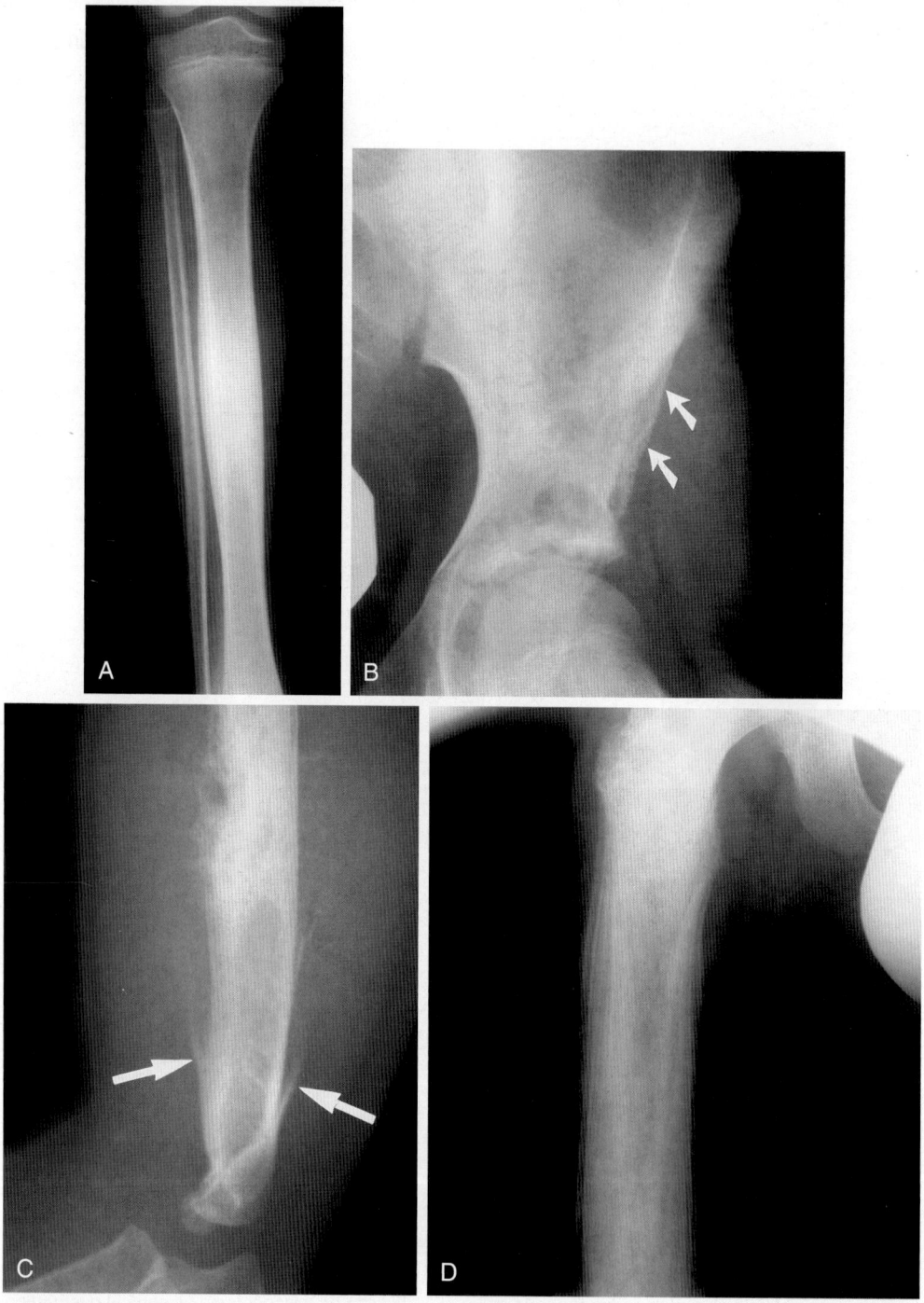

FIG. 3.3 **Benign Periostitis.** (A) An osteoid osteoma in the midshaft of the tibia has caused thick, wavy, dense periostitis, which is classic for benign type of periostitis. Malignant lesions are incapable of forming this type of periostitis and should not be considered in the differential. This type of periostitis is basically indistinguishable from callus formation in a fracture. (B) Thick, wavy periostitis *(arrows)* along the ilium in a child with a permeative lesion in the pelvis is characteristic for infection or eosinophilic granuloma. Ewing sarcoma was initially considered in the differential; however, the benign periostitis would make a malignant lesion very unlikely. Biopsy showed this lesion to be eosinophilic granuloma. (C) Aggressive periostitis. Amorphous, sunburst periostitis with a Codman's triangle *(arrows)* in a patient with a mixed lytic–sclerotic lesion of the humerus, which on biopsy was shown to be Ewing sarcoma. Although this type of periostitis is characteristic for a malignant lesion, it could also be seen with benign processes such as eosinophilic granuloma or infection. (D) Lamellated, or onion-skinned, periostitis is characteristic of an aggressive process, such as in this patient with Ewing sarcoma of the femur. Again, this aggressive type of periostitis could conceivably occur in a benign process such as infection or eosinophilic granuloma.

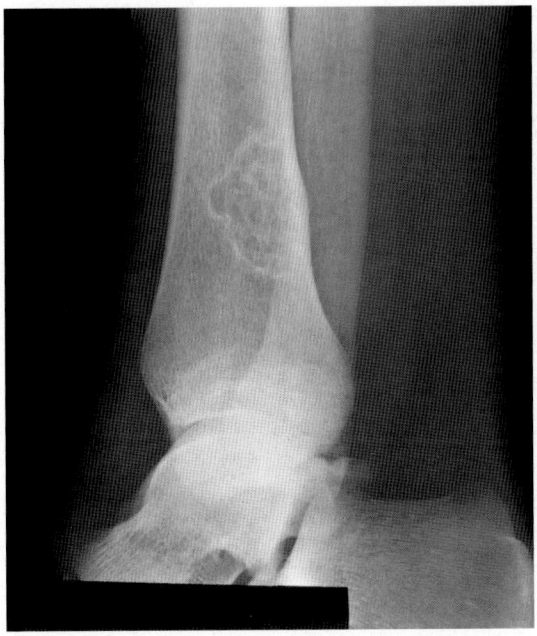

FIG. 3.4 **Narrow Zone of Transition.** The border of normal bone with a lesion is known as the zone of transition. When, as in this example of a nonossifying fibroma, the border can be drawn with a fine-point pen, it is said to be a narrow zone of transition, which is characteristic of a benign lesion. A narrow zone of transition may or may not have a sclerotic border.

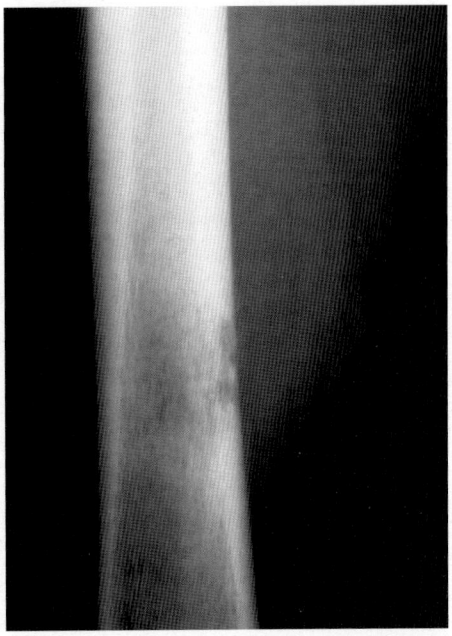

FIG. 3.5 **Wide Zone of Transition.** A lytic permeative process is seen in the midshaft of the femur in this patient. On biopsy, it was found to be a malignant fibrous histiocytoma. The zone of transition in this lesion is said to be wide, as it cannot be easily drawn with a fine-point pen. A permeative lesion such as this, by definition, has a wide zone of transition.

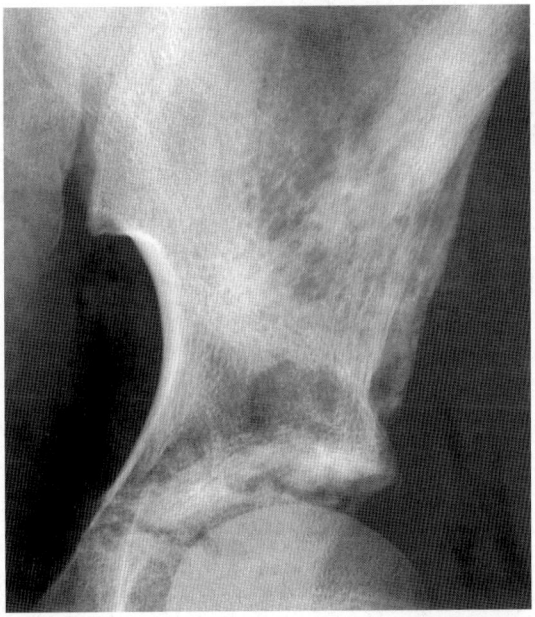

FIG. 3.6 **Permeative Pattern.** A permeative pattern is defined as multiple small irregular holes in bone, and indicates an aggressive process. Ewing sarcoma typically has a permeative pattern; however, infection and eosinophilic granuloma, as in this example, can also have a permeative pattern. This is a fine-detailed film of the same case shown in Fig. 3.3B.

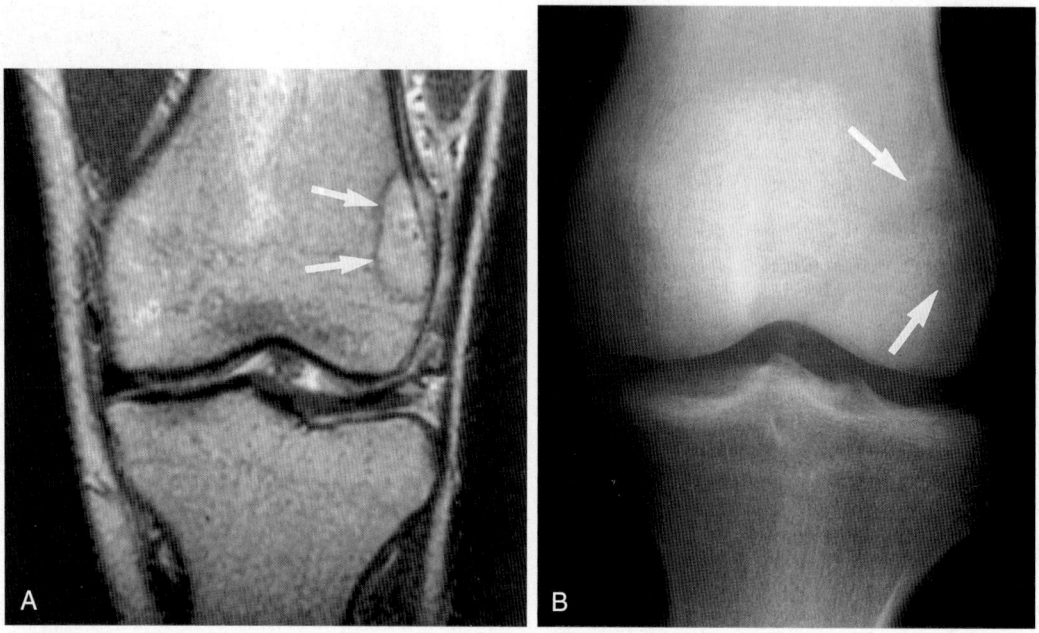

FIG. 3.7 **Zone of Transition on Magnetic Resonance (MR) Imaging.** (A) A T2-weighted MR image of the knee in this child with knee pain shows a well-defined lesion *(arrows)* with a low signal border suggesting a narrow zone of transition with a sclerotic border. Because the knee pain was described as probably related to the menisci, this lesion was felt to be an incidental, benign process, such as a nonossifying fibroma. However, the plain film (B), obtained later, shows a barely discernible lytic lesion with a wide zone of transition *(arrows)*. This lesion was, in fact, painful, and the differential diagnosis, based solely on the plain film, would include osteosarcoma—the eventual histologic diagnosis. The zone of transition can only be used on plain films—it is invalid on MR imaging.

TABLE 3.1
Malignant Tumors and Patient Age

Age	Tumor
1–30	Ewing
	Osteosarcoma
30–40	Fibrosarcoma and malignant fibrous histiocytoma
	Malignant giant cell tumor
	Primary lymphoma of bone
	Parosteal sarcoma
40+	Mets
	Myeloma
	Chondrosarcoma

Obviously, if a 15-year-old has a known primary tumor, then mets must be considered—in fact, *any* bone lesion, regardless of its appearance, could be a met and would be suspicious in a patient with a known primary tumor.

MR imaging should be routinely employed in the workup of malignant tumors. MR imaging will show the full bony and soft tissue extent and can identify the position of the larger adjacent vessels, making angiography unnecessary. Routine use of gadolinium (Gd-DTPA) with tumors does not appear to be justified, as it currently seems to give no additional information over noncontrast-enhanced studies.

Rather than give a description of characteristics of every malignant tumor, which is available in any of the leading skeletal radiology texts, let me make a few points on many of the primary malignant tumors of bone that I think may be helpful in their diagnosis.

Osteosarcoma

The most common malignant primary bone tumor is an osteosarcoma. Although it typically occurs toward the end of a long bone, it may occur anywhere in the skeleton with enough frequency so that location is not a helpful discriminator. Osteosarcomas are usually destructive, with obvious sclerosis

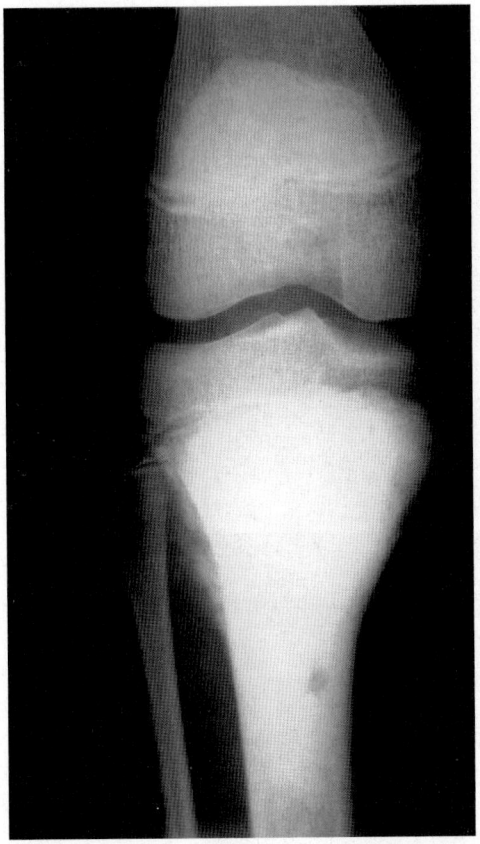

FIG. 3.8 **Osteosarcoma.** An extremely sclerotic lesion in the proximal tibia of a child is noted, which is characteristic for an osteogenic sarcoma.

present from either tumor new bone or reactive sclerosis (Figs. 3.8 and 3.9); however, on occasion they can be entirely lytic (Fig. 3.10). These are usually so-called telangiectatic osteosarcomas. There are many types and classifications of osteosarcomas, but it serves little purpose to the radiologist to try to distinguish between most of them.

These tumors occur almost exclusively in patients under the age of 30. Although some texts claim there is a second peak of osteosarcomas in patients around age 60, I, and others, do not believe this to be correct. Some osteosarcomas occur in older patients who have malignant degeneration of Paget's disease, and some occur secondary to prior irradiation; but de novo osteosarcomas in the older age group are uncommon.

Parosteal Osteosarcoma

A type of osteosarcoma that should be distinguished from the central osteosarcoma is the parosteal osteosarcoma. A parosteal osteosarcoma originates from the periosteum of the bone and grows outside the bone (Fig. 3.11). It often wraps around the diaphysis without breaking through the cortex. It occurs in an older age group than the central osteosarcomas and is not as aggressive. Treatment used to consist of merely shaving the tumor off the bone it originated from; however, recurrence rates were so high that now wide-bloc excisions are performed. Once a parosteal osteosarcoma violates the cortex of the adjacent bone, some consider it to be as aggressive as a central osteosarcoma and is treated in a similar fashion (i.e., amputation or radical excision). Therefore the radiologist needs to evaluate the lesion for invasion of the adjacent cortex to help determine treatment and prognosis. This is best done with CT or MR imaging (Figs. 3.11B and C).

A common location for parosteal osteosarcomas to arise is from the posterior femur, near the knee. A lesion that can mimic an early parosteal osteosarcoma in this location is a so-called cortical desmoid (Fig. 3.12). A cortical desmoid is an avulsion injury that is totally benign but can appear somewhat aggressive. Unfortunately it can appear malignant histologically, so biopsy can lead to disastrous consequences. Amputations for benign cortical desmoids being mistaken for malignancies have occurred. (See Chapter 4 for further points on cortical desmoids.) Another lesion that can be mistaken for a parosteal osteosarcoma is an area of myositis ossificans (Fig. 3.13). Like cortical desmoids, areas of myositis ossificans can be histologically mistaken for malignancies with disastrous consequences. Therefore differentiation is vital. Fortunately, differentiation between parosteal osteosarcoma and myositis ossificans is fairly easily done radiographically. (See Chapter 4 for differential points between parosteal osteosarcoma and myositis ossificans.)

Another type of osteosarcoma that often gets mentioned by residents in their differential of a parosteal osteosarcoma is a periosteal osteosarcoma. It should not get such attention. First, it's extremely rare, with fewer than 50 such lesions reported in the literature. Second, and most significantly, periosteal osteosarcomas do not resemble parosteal osteosarcomas (Fig. 3.14). Therefore mentioning both of these lesions in the same differential is inappropriate and simply means that the resident doesn't know what a periosteal osteosarcoma looks like. It's such a rare lesion that I teach residents not to worry about it—don't mention it. Radiology is hard enough without remembering all the rare lesions that might be seen once in a lifetime—if at all.

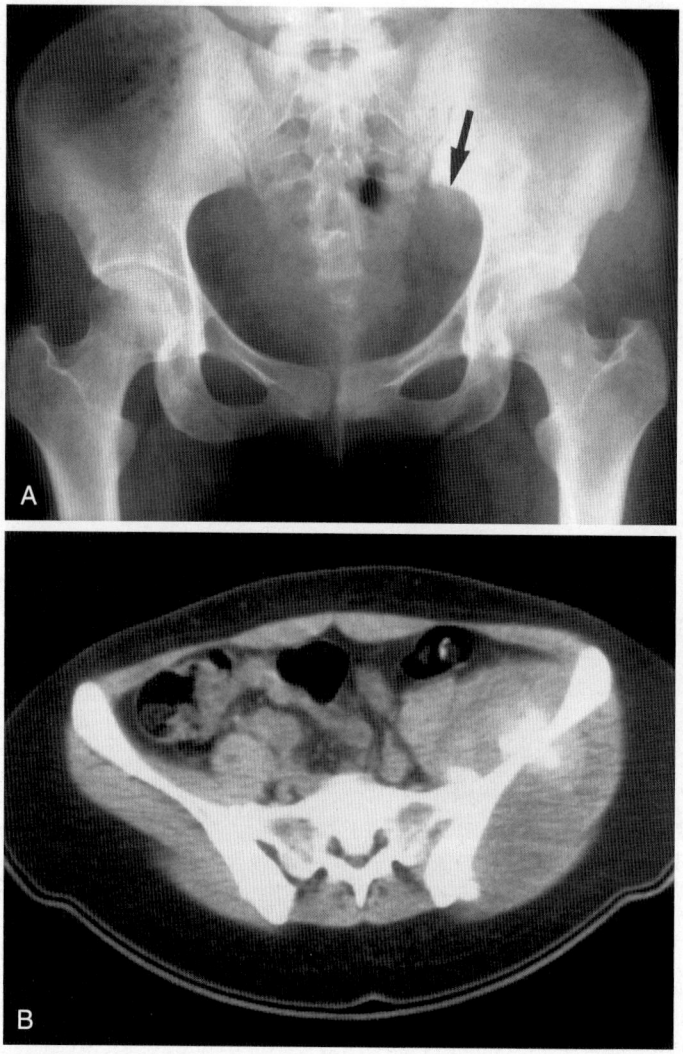

FIG. 3.9 **Osteosarcoma.** (A) A subtle sclerotic lesion is seen in the left ilium adjacent to the sacroiliac joint that was initially diagnosed as osteitis condensans ilii, a benign entity. Because of persistent pain the patient returned for a follow-up visit, and a small amount of cortical destruction on the pelvic brim was noted *(arrow)*. (B) A computed tomography (CT) scan was performed, which showed a large soft tissue mass and tumor new bone around the ilium, which is characteristic for an osteogenic sarcoma.

Ewing Sarcoma

The classic Ewing sarcoma is a permeative (multiple small holes) lesion in the diaphysis of a long bone in a child (Fig. 3.3D). However, only about 40% of these tumors occur in the diaphysis, with the remainder being metaphyseal or diametaphyseal or in flat bones. They do tend to be found primarily in children and adolescents, although a significant number occur in patients who are in their 20s, especially in flat bones. Although most often permeative in appearance, they can elicit reactive new bone, which can give the lesion a partially sclerotic or "patchy" appearance (Figs. 3.3C, 3.15, and 3.16). Ewing sarcomas often have an onion-skinned type of periostitis, but they can also have periostitis that is sunburst or amorphous in character (Fig. 3.16). Rarely, if ever, will a Ewing sarcoma have benign-appearing periostitis (thick, uniform, or wavy). If benign periostitis is present, other lesions should be considered instead, such as infection or eosinophilic granuloma.

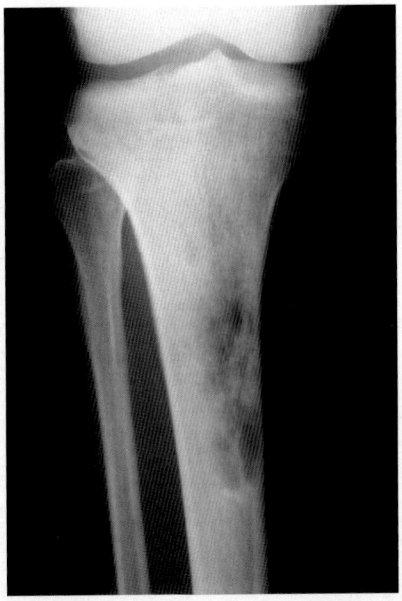

FIG. 3.10 **Lytic Osteosarcoma.** An ill-defined lytic lesion was noted in the proximal tibia of a 20-year-old with pain. This lesion has a differential diagnosis of eosinophilic granuloma (EG), infection, Ewing sarcoma, and osteogenic sarcoma. Biopsy showed it to be a lytic osteogenic sarcoma.

A knee jerk differential diagnosis for a permeative lesion in a child should be Ewing sarcoma, infection, and eosinophilic granuloma. These three entities can appear radiologically identical. I exclude Ewing sarcoma from the differential if I can see definite benign periostitis or if I can see a definite sequestrum of bone. In this differential list, only eosinophilic granuloma and infection can have benign periostitis or a sequestrum. Presence or absence of a soft tissue mass is not helpful in distinguishing between these three lesions. Presence of symptoms is not helpful, as all three entities can be symptomatic; however, it would be unusual to find an asymptomatic Ewing sarcoma.

Chondrosarcoma

Chondrosarcomas have a number of appearances that at times make them difficult to diagnose with any assurance. They most frequently occur in patients over age 40. An eminent bone radiologist once told me that if a pathologist makes the diagnosis of chondrosarcoma in a child, get another pathologist. Although it is very uncommon, chondrosarcomas occasionally occur in children; usually they are from malignant degeneration of an osteochondroma (Fig. 3.17) but do not have to be. I reserve the diagnosis of a chondrosarcoma for patients over the age of 40 unless they have an obvious enchondroma or osteochondroma that is painful or has a destructive appearance.

Probably the most difficult lesion for a bone pathologist to deal with is an enchondroma. It can be extremely difficult histologically to differentiate a low-grade chondrosarcoma from an enchondroma. Because low-grade chondrosarcomas do not metastasize, some pathologists call them "active" enchondromas. The diagnosis of chondrosarcoma usually initiates radical excision and therapy, although it is debatable (and somewhat controversial) as to whether a low-grade chondrosarcoma is even a malignant tumor. For these reasons, I usually reserve the diagnosis of "possible chondrosarcoma" for those lesions that are painful or show definite aggressive characteristics, such as periostitis and destruction. The truth of the matter is that neither radiologists nor pathologists can reliably distinguish between enchondromas and many chondrosarcomas (Fig. 3.18). MR imaging can be very helpful in distinguishing between a benign enchondroma and a chondrosarcoma. If a soft tissue mass or edema is present, it is unlikely to be an enchondroma.

Chondrosarcoma should be considered in the diagnosis anytime there is a lytic, destructive lesion with amorphous, snowflake calcification in an older patient (over 40) (Fig. 3.19). Without the presence of the calcified chondroid matrix, the lesion is indistinguishable from any other aggressive lytic lesion, such as mets, plasmacytoma, fibrosarcoma, malignant fibrous histiocytoma (MFH), or infection. Usually the radiologist can only give a long differential diagnosis such as this, which is entirely acceptable. A biopsy of the lesion will have to be performed at any rate, so it is not necessary for the radiologist to make the diagnosis. This is the case with most malignant tumors. The radiologist does play an important role, however, in suggesting additional lesions that might masquerade as malignancies and in imaging the lesion to show such features as the full extent, the presence of a soft tissue component, and metastases. As mentioned earlier, MR imaging plays an invaluable role in this regard and should be performed on every potential malignant bone lesion.

Malignant Giant Cell Tumor

Giant cell tumors are rarely malignant if mets is the marker for malignancy. It is said that approximately 15% of giant cell tumors are malignant; however, that is based on how often they recur, which is not a valid marker for

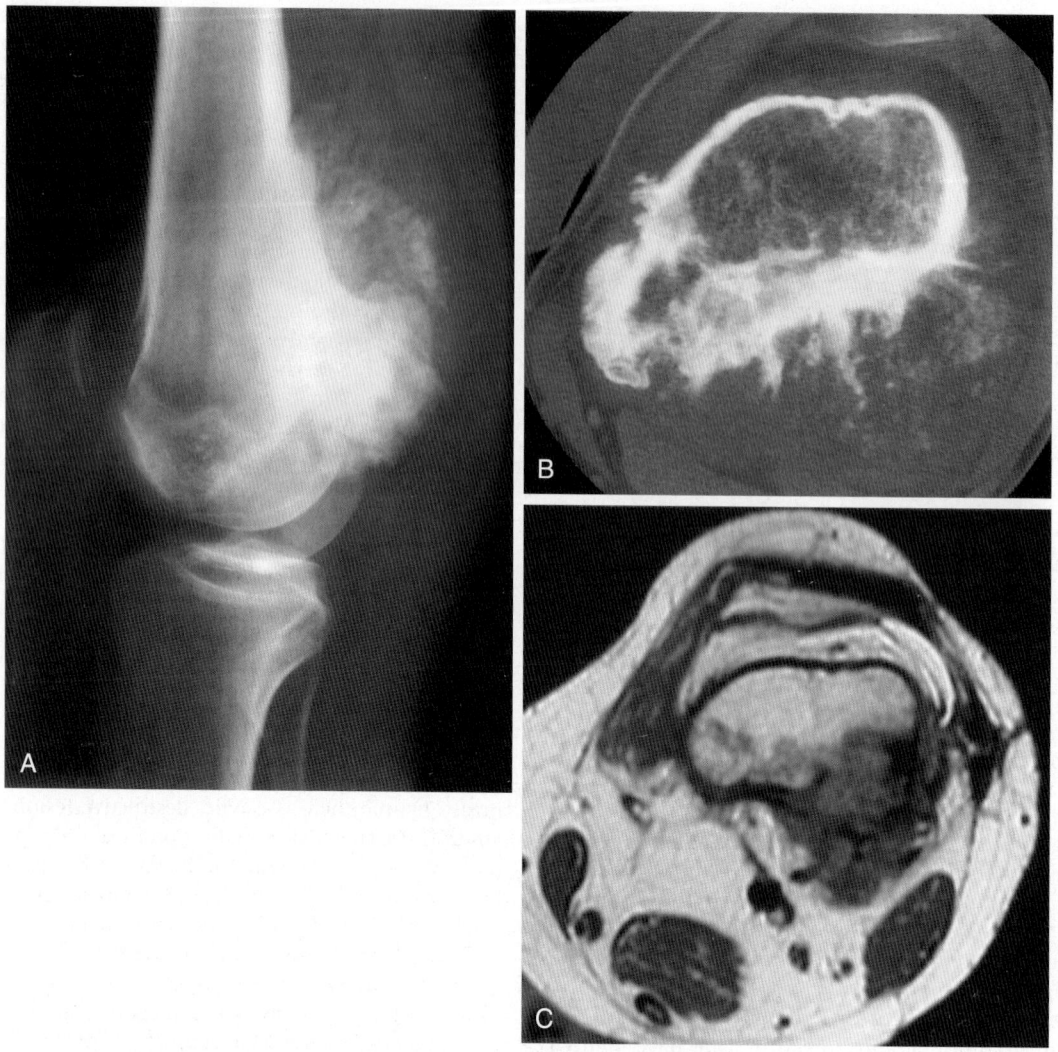

FIG. 3.11 **Parosteal Osteogenic Sarcoma.** (A) A lateral film of the distal femur shows a large calcific mass with an ill-defined, fluffy, calcific periphery growing off the posterior femur. The location and appearance are characteristic for a parosteal osteogenic sarcoma. (B) A computed tomography (CT) scan through this lesion shows cortical and medullary involvement, which indicates a more sinister lesion, with treatment and prognosis similar to that of a central osteogenic sarcoma. Without intramedullary involvement, a parosteal sarcoma has a favorable prognosis. (C) A proton density magnetic resonance (MR) image in another patient with a parosteal osteosarcoma shows involvement of the marrow.

malignant. Unfortunately there does not seem to be any way to foretell which giant cell tumor will become malignant. Benign and malignant giant cell tumors appear radiologically identical (see Chapter 2). They also are histologically similar. So how is the diagnosis made? If metastases (usually to the lung) occur, the tumor is considered malignant. Malignant giant cell tumors tend to occur primarily in the fourth decade of life.

Malignant Fibrous Histiocytoma

Malignant fibrous histiocytomas (MFHs) are the most common soft tissue sarcoma and do not commonly occur as primary bone tumors. Osseous MFHs are lytic malignant tumors that do not produce osteoid or chondroid matrix. They usually do not elicit reactive new bone and, therefore are almost always lytic in appearance. This lytic appearance may take any form,

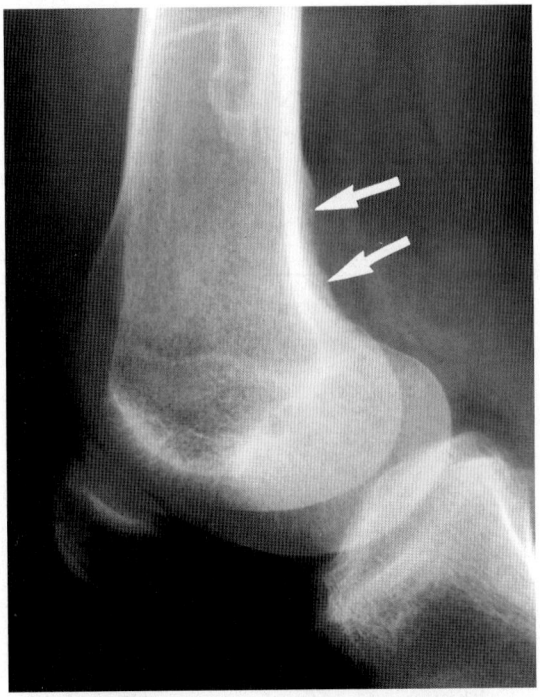

FIG. 3.12 **Cortical Desmoid.** Irregular periostitis *(arrows)* off the medial supracondylar ridge of the distal femur is pathognomonic for a small avulsion of the adductor muscles and is called a cortical desmoid. Biopsy of this lesion can easily result in a mistaken diagnosis of a sarcomatous lesion and should therefore be avoided. A cortical desmoid should not be confused with an early parosteal osteogenic sarcoma on radiographs, as it will then lead to an unnecessary biopsy, perhaps with dire consequences. An incidental finding is a nonossifying fibroma seen just proximal to the cortical desmoid.

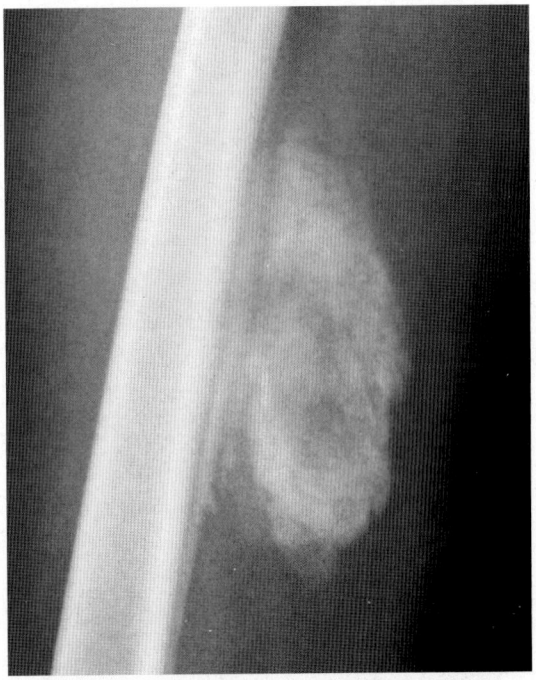

FIG. 3.13 **Myositis Ossificans.** This lesion is often confused with parosteal osteogenic sarcoma, since at first glance, it has a close resemblance. However, myositis ossificans, as in this example, will demonstrate calcification that is densest in the periphery and well-defined, whereas parosteal osteogenic sarcoma has calcification that is most concentrated centrally and ill-defined in the periphery. Myositis ossificans is another lesion that can be confused with a malignant lesion on biopsy and therefore should be radiographically rather than surgically diagnosed.

from permeative to moth-eaten (Figs. 3.20 and 3.21) to a fairly well-defined area of lysis (Fig. 3.22). This can make radiographic diagnosis very difficult.

The age range for MFH is quite broad, but they tend to predominate in the fourth decade. Also, desmoids and MFHs tend to be the only tumors that are not consistently high in signal on T2-weighted MR images (Fig. 3.23).

Desmoid

A desmoid tumor (not to be confused with a cortical desmoid—see Chapter 4) is a half-grade fibrosarcoma. It has also been called a desmoplastic fibroma or aggressive fibromatosis. These lesions, like MFHs, are lytic but are usually fairly well-defined because of their slow growth. They often have benign periostitis present that has thick spicules, or "spikes," and normally have a multilocular appearance (Figs. 3.24). They are slow growing and seldom metastasize, but they can exhibit inexorable tumor extension into surrounding soft tissues with disastrous results. Like fibrosarcoma and MFHs, these lesions can exhibit a bony sequestrum (Fig. 3.24).

Primary Lymphoma of Bone (Reticulum Cell Sarcoma)

Primary lymphoma of bone (formerly called reticulum cell sarcoma) has a radiologic appearance identical to that of Ewing sarcoma (i.e., a permeative or moth-eaten pattern) (Fig. 3.25). It tends to occur in an older age group than does Ewing sarcoma, and whereas the Ewing sarcoma patient is typically systemically symptomatic, the primary lymphoma of bone patient is often asymptomatic. In fact, primary lymphoma of bone is the only malignant tumor that can involve a large amount of bone while the patient is systemically asymptomatic.

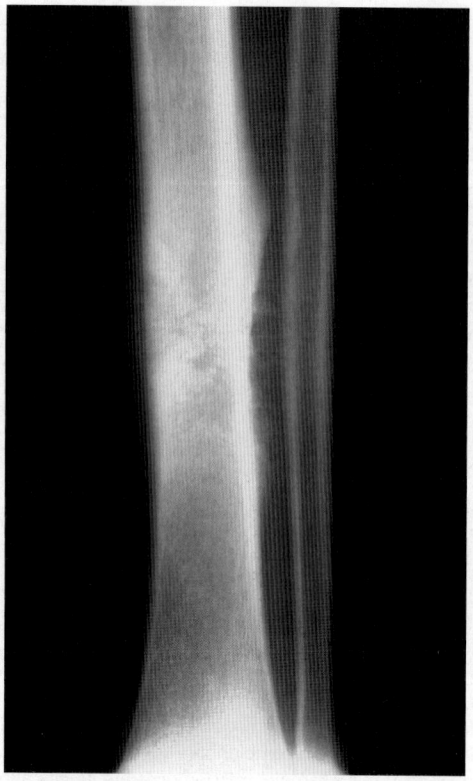

FIG. 3.14 **Periosteal Osteogenic Sarcoma.** Unlike the parosteal osteosarcoma, the periosteal osteogenic sarcoma does not have large amounts of calcification in soft tissues. It typically has a saucerized configuration with periostitis that resembles hair on end or is sunburst, as in this example. Although this lesion is very malignant, it inexplicably will not invade the medullary space. Although parosteal and periosteal sarcomas originate from the same point and have similar names, they do not have a similar radiographic appearance.

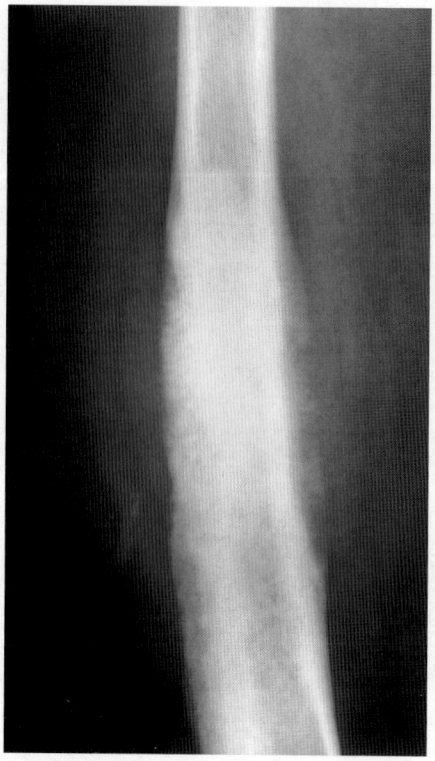

FIG. 3.15 **Ewing Sarcoma.** A mixed lytic–sclerotic lesion in the femur of a child with periostitis that is amorphous and sunburst, such as in this example, is characteristic of a Ewing sarcoma. An osteosarcoma could have a similar appearance.

Metastatic Disease

Metastatic lesions must be included in *any* differential diagnosis of a bone lesion in a patient over the age of 40. They can have virtually any appearance: they can mimic a benign lesion (see Chapter 2) or a primary bone tumor. Judging the origin of the tumor from the appearance of the metastatic focus can be difficult—if not impossible—although some appearances are fairly characteristic. For instance, multiple sclerotic foci in a male are probably prostatic metastases (Fig. 3.26), although lung, bowel, or almost any other organ tumor could present in the same way. In a female, the same picture would probably result from breast metastases. The only primary tumor that virtually never presents with blastic mets is renal cell carcinoma. Typically, an expansile lytic metastasis should be either renal or thyroid in origin (Fig. 3.27), although there are many exceptions to this rule.

Myeloma

Like metastases, myeloma should be considered only in a patient over the age of 40, although some radiologists use age 35 for the lower limits of myeloma. Myeloma typically has a diffuse permeative appearance that can mimic a Ewing sarcoma or a primary lymphoma of bone (Fig. 3.28). It frequently involves the calvarium (Fig. 3.29). Because of the age criteria, Ewing sarcoma and myeloma are not in the same differential, however. Rarely, myeloma can present with multiple sclerotic foci that resemble diffuse mets. Myeloma is one of the only lesions that is not characteristically "hot" on a radionuclide bone scan; therefore radiologic "bone surveys" are performed instead of radionuclide bone scans when evidence of myeloma is found clinically.

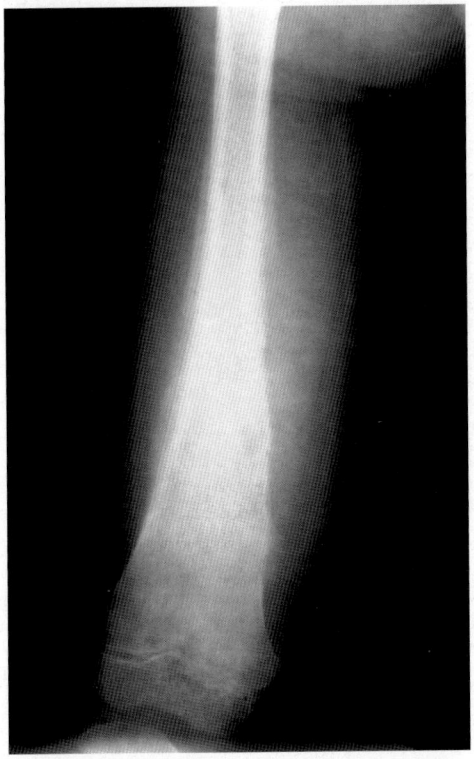

FIG. 3.16 **Ewing Sarcoma.** This is a predominantly sclerotic process with large amounts of sunburst periostitis in the diaphysis of a femur that, on biopsy, was found to be Ewing sarcoma.

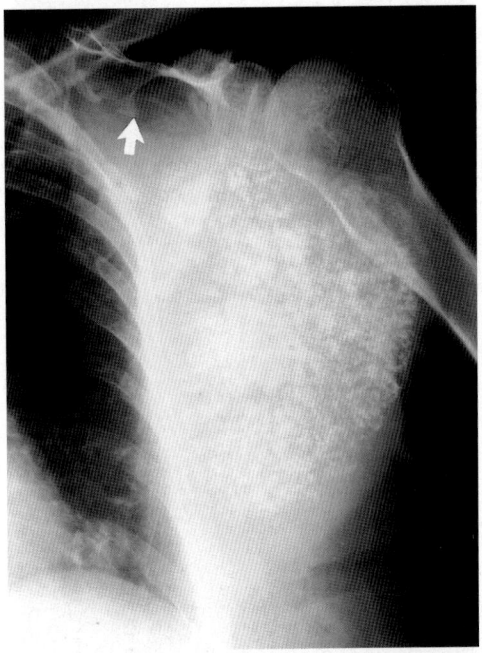

FIG. 3.17 **Chrondrosarcoma.** A large soft tissue mass with typical chondroid matrix is seen in this young adult with a history of multiple osteochondromatosis. A sessile osteochondroma is seen off the proximal humerus, and another osteochondroma is seen protruding off the scapula *(arrow)*. The chrondrosarcoma in the axilla presumably arose from a prior benign osteochondroma that has undergone malignant degeneration.

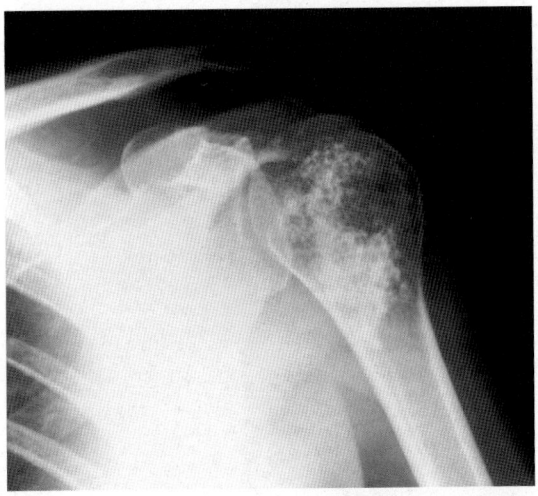

FIG. 3.18 **Chondrosarcoma.** Typical snowflake, punctate, amorphous calcification in the proximal humerus is seen, which is typical of an enchondroma. The patient, however, had pain associated with this lesion, and on biopsy it was found to be a chondrosarcoma.

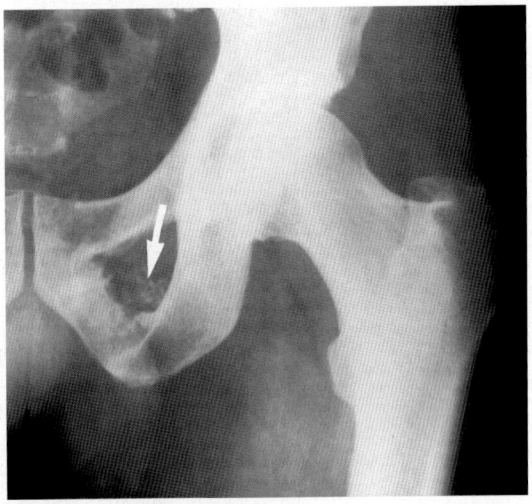

FIG. 3.19 **Chondrosarcoma.** An amorphous, irregular calcification is seen in a lesion arising in the ischium *(arrow)*. This is fairly typical for a chondrosarcoma.

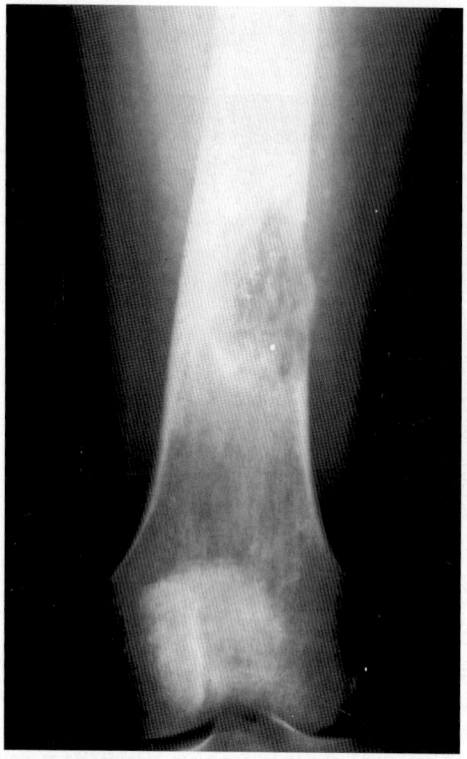

FIG. 3.20 **Malignant Fibrous Histiocytoma (MFH).** An ill-defined lytic lesion that is permeative or moth-eaten is seen in the diaphysis of the femur. On biopsy it was shown to be an MFH.

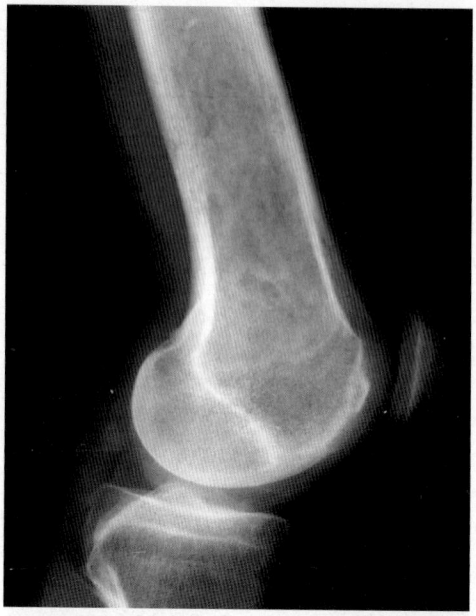

FIG. 3.21 **Malignant Fibrous Histiocytoma (MFH).** A moth-eaten or permeative process in the distal femur, with some involvement of the posterior cortex, is seen on this lateral radiograph. In a patient under the age of 30, a Ewing sarcoma, eosinophilic granuloma, or infection would be the differential diagnosis. In a patient over the age of 30, infection and MFH would be more common. A 1-degree lymphoma of bone could have a similar appearance.

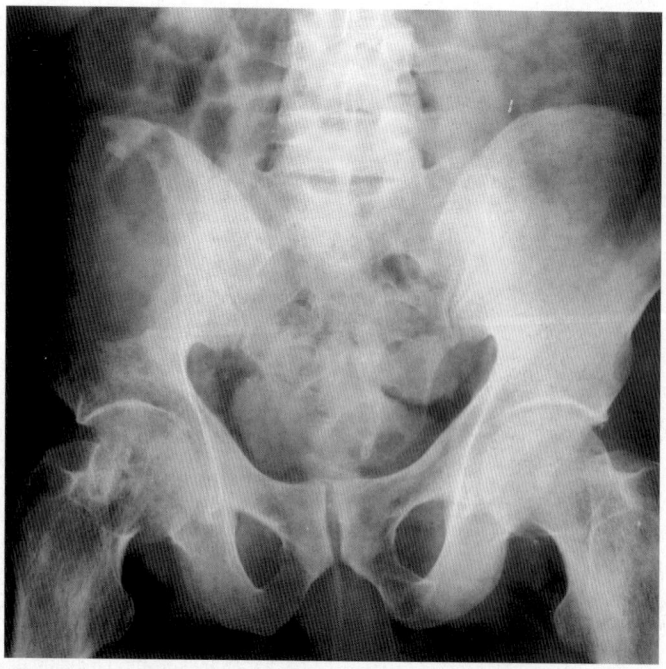

FIG. 3.22 **Malignant Fibrous Histiocytoma (MFH).** A large, fairly well-defined destructive process of the entire right iliac wing is noted. On biopsy this was shown to be an MFH. An MFH can be very slow growing and will occasionally have a narrow zone of transition, such as this.

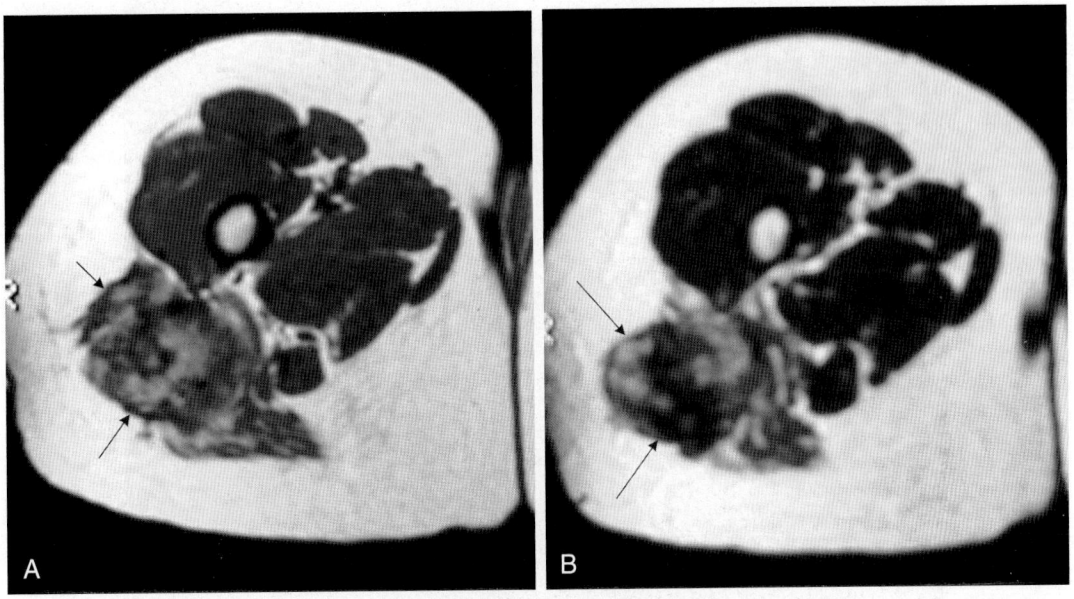

FIG. 3.23 **Desmoid.** A large soft tissue mass *(arrows)* is seen in the right buttock, which is low signal on both the T1-weighted (A) and the T2-weighted (B) images. This is typical for a soft tissue desmoid tumor.

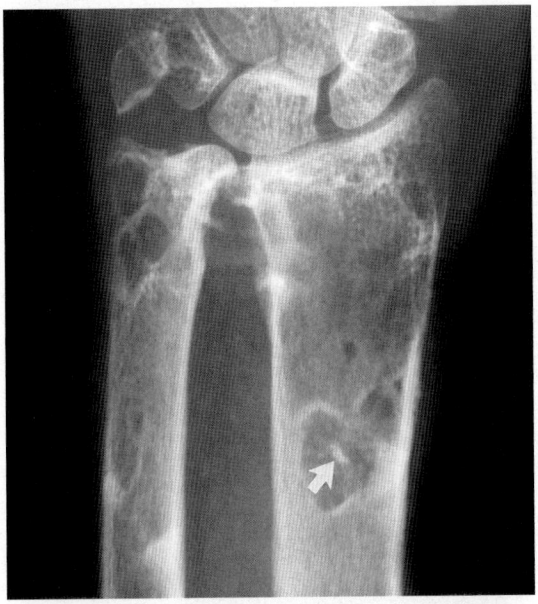

FIG. 3.24 **Desmoid Tumor.** A lytic destructive process involving both bones of the distal forearm is noted, with at least one portion demonstrating a sequestrum *(arrow)*. A desmoid tumor is a fibrosarcomalike lesion, and fibrosarcomas are known to occasionally demonstrate bony sequestra in the same manner as will osteomyelitis, lymphoma, and eosinophilic granuloma.

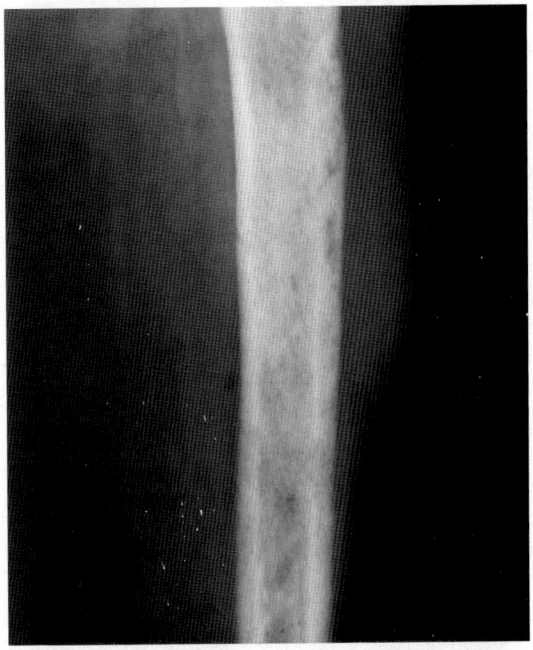

FIG. 3.25 **Primary Lymphoma of Bone.** A diffuse permeative pattern throughout the humerus in this 35-year-old patient is characteristic of primary lymphoma of bone.

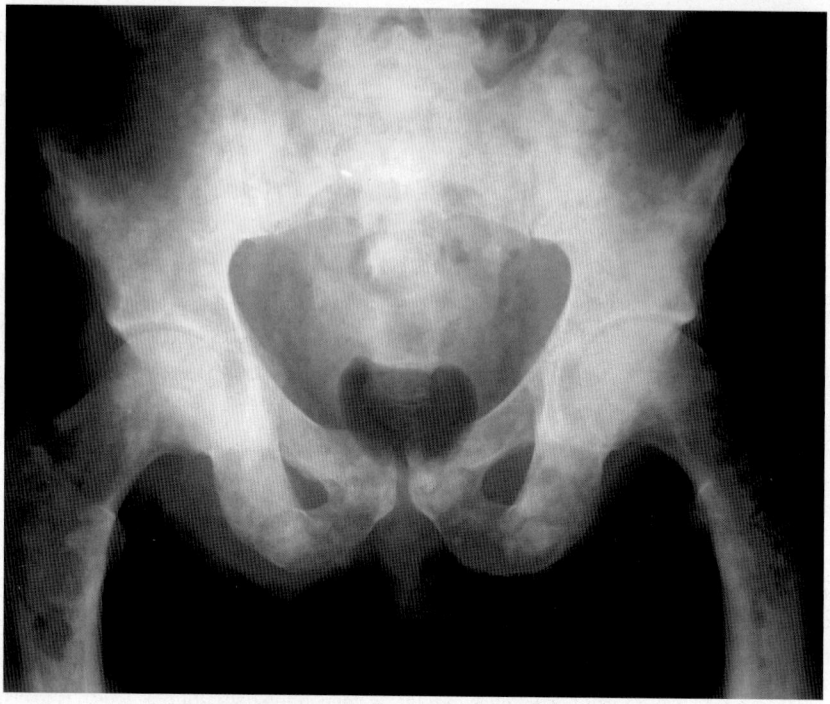

FIG. 3.26 **Metastatic Prostate Carcinoma.** Diffuse blastic metastases are seen throughout the pelvis and proximal femurs, with a lytic destructive lesion seen in the right proximal femur. Prostate metastases tend to be blastic, but as shown here they can occasionally be lytic.

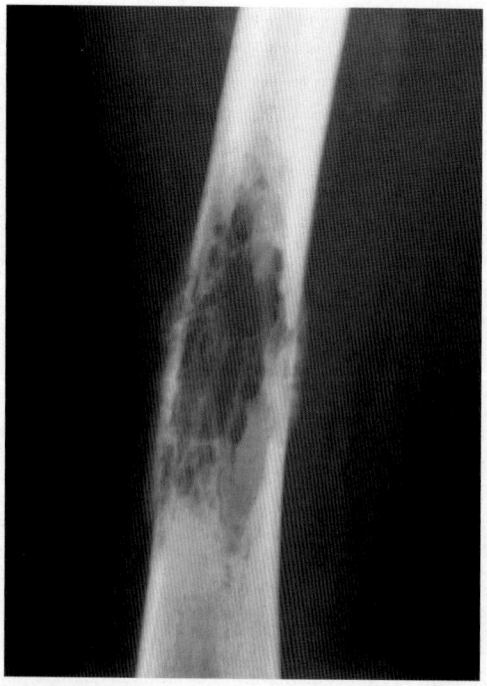

FIG. 3.27 **Metastatic Renal Cell Carcinoma.** A lytic lesion in the diaphysis of the femur is noted, which is characteristic for renal cell carcinoma. Up to one-third of renal cell carcinomas initially present with a bony metastasis. Renal cell carcinoma virtually never presents with a blastic metastatic focus.

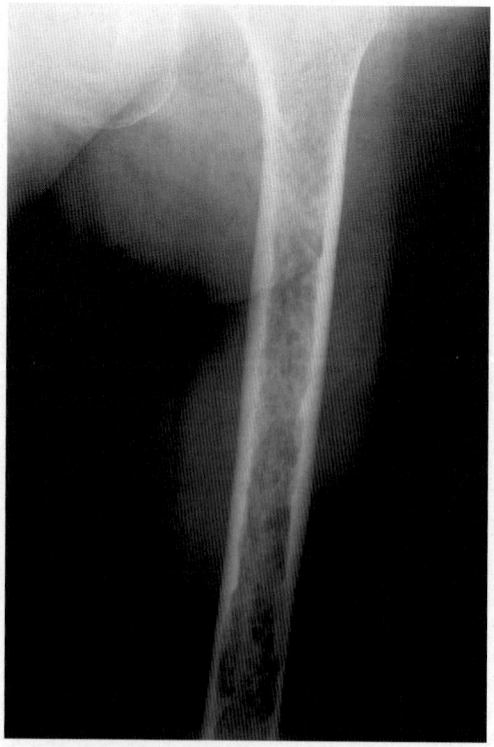

FIG. 3.28 **Multiple Myeloma.** A diffuse moth-eaten pattern is seen throughout the diaphysis of the femur in this 45-year-old patient, which is characteristic for myeloma. Primary lymphoma of bone could have a similar appearance.

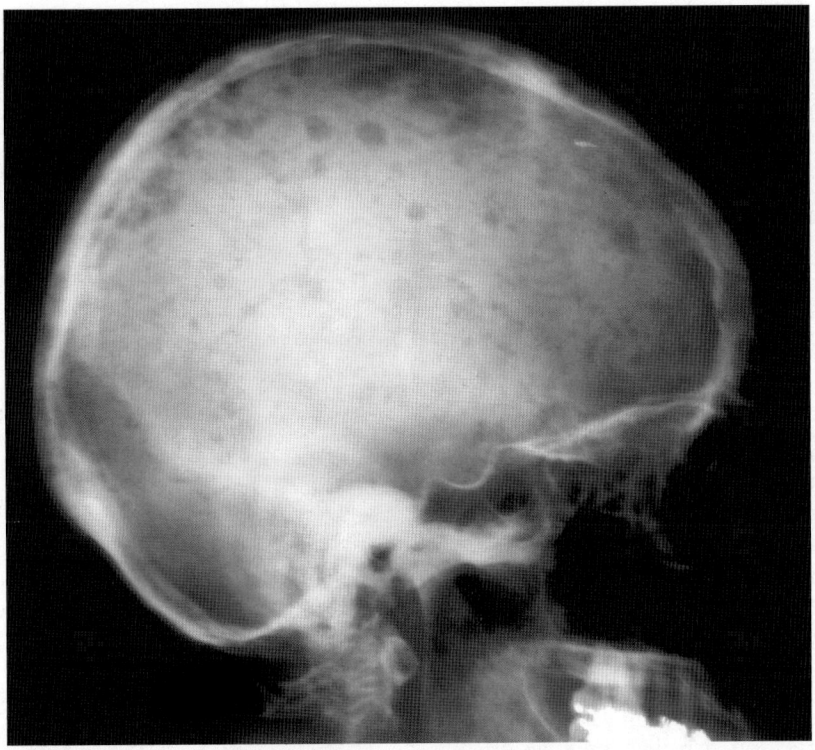

FIG. 3.29 **Multiple Myeloma.** A lateral view of the skull shows multiple lytic lesions in the calvarium, which is a characteristic appearance of multiple myeloma.

Occasionally, myeloma will present with a lytic bone lesion called a plasmacytoma. This lesion can mimic any lytic bone lesion, benign or aggressive in its appearance; it can precede other evidence of myeloma by up to 3 years. It can be solitary or multiple, although some insist it must be solitary to be considered a plasmacytoma, and when it is multifocal, it is myeloma. Whatever. It has an appearance on MR imaging in the vertebral body that is virtually pathognomonic. It resembles the cadaveric section of a brain with which every medical student is familiar, hence the name "minibrain" appearance (Fig. 3.30).

Soft Tissue Tumors

Most radiology residents feel uneasy when faced with the differential diagnosis of a soft tissue tumor. They will give elaborate description with plenty of pertinent and not-so-pertinent negatives, such as "no calcifications are seen," "no bony destruction is noted," and "no obliteration of fat planes is apparent." Then, when faced with finally giving a differential, few can give an authoritative list of the possibilities. The reason for this is quite simple: there is no authoritative, useful differential for soft tissue tumors, whether or not there is calcification, bony destruction, fat plane involvement, or whatever. You can play the odds and mention the two most common soft tissue tumors, MFH and liposarcoma, as the best candidates, but any cell type can produce a benign or malignant tumor and mimic any other soft tissue tumor. A lipoma can be separated out by the appearance of fat, but a liposarcoma may or may not have fat present. Therefore we are left to give descriptions of size and extent, and let the pathologist tell us the rest. Most of us are uncomfortable with this approach because our training has been to derive an answer—or at least a listing of probable lesions. This is just not possible for soft tissue tumors.

A few words about soft tissue tumors that may be helpful: as mentioned earlier, liposarcomas do not have to have fat visible in the tumor. There are at least three subtypes of liposarcomas, two of which have only small amounts of fat present. Synovial sarcomas, or synoviomas, only rarely, if ever, originate in a joint. They are often adjacent to joints. There are no malignant tumors that routinely need to be considered in

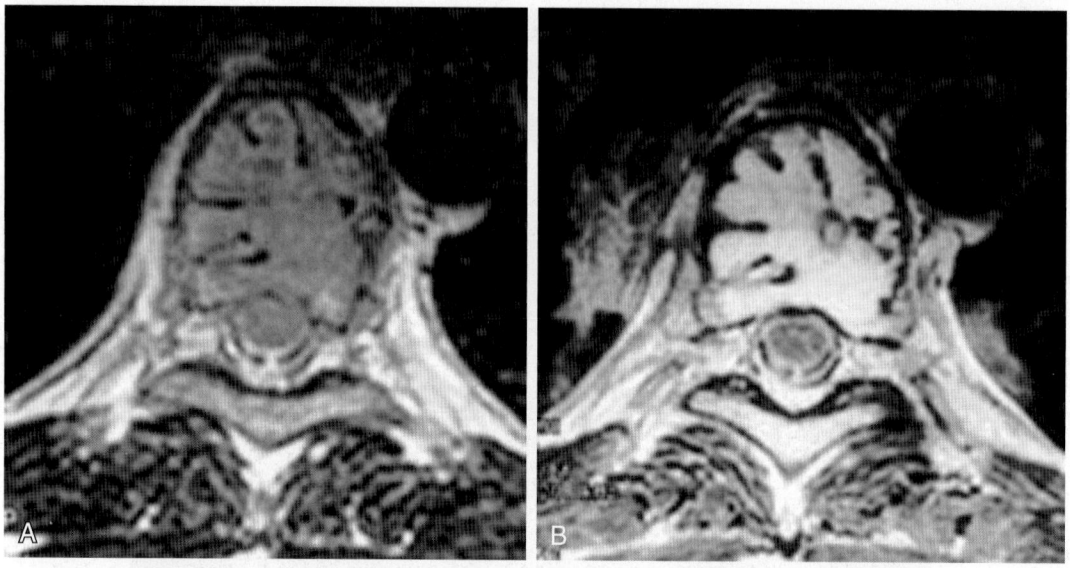

FIG. 3.30 **Magnetic Resonance (MR) Imaging Appearance of Plasmacytoma.** Axial proton density (A) and T2-weighted (B) images through a vertebral body with a plasmacytoma show a characteristic, if not pathognomonic, appearance of a "minibrain," which is seen only with plasmacytoma.

the differential diagnosis of joint lesions. Synovial osteochondromatosis is a benign joint lesion that occurs from metaplasia of the synovium and leads to multiple calcific loose bodies in a joint. This can histologically mimic a chondrosarcoma; therefore it is best diagnosed radiographically, since it has a pathognomonic radiographic appearance (Fig. 3.31). Up to 20% of the time, however, the loose bodies do not calcify, and the lesion then can mimic pigmented villonodular synovitis (PVNS) on plain films. With MR imaging, synovial osteochondromatosis can have a "tumefactive" appearance, with all the loose bodies packed together so tightly that it resembles a solid mass in the joint (Fig. 3.32). I have seen several cases where MR imaging suggested a tumor, and a subsequent biopsy was called chondrosarcoma and amputation was then performed. This assures a great 5-year survival, but the diagnosis should be made before a biopsy is performed so that a tumor is not in the differential.

PVNS is a benign synovial soft tissue process that causes joint swelling and pain and, occasionally, joint erosions (Fig. 3.33). Calcifications are virtually never associated with it.

Hemangiomas often have phleboliths associated with them and often cause "cortical holes" in adjacent bone that mimic a permeative pattern (Fig. 3.34). The permeative pattern of round cell lesions occurs in the intramedullary or endosteal part of the bone and can

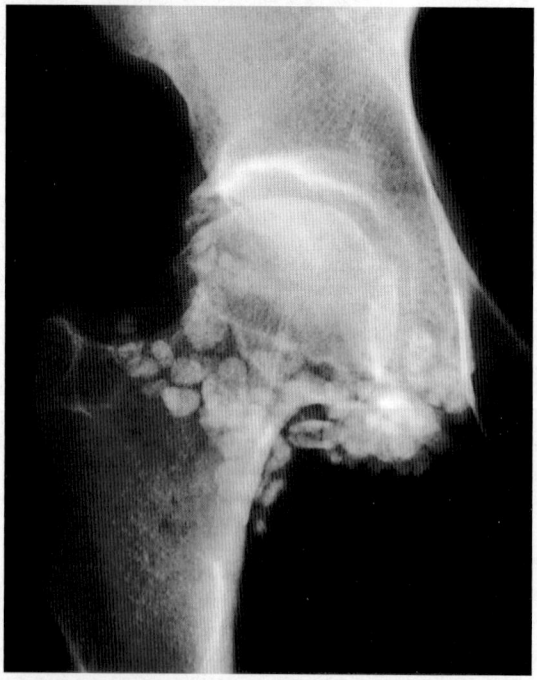

FIG. 3.31 **Synovial Osteochondromatosis.** Multiple calcific loose bodies in a hip joint such as this are virtually pathognomonic for synovial osteochondromatosis. Notice the erosions in the acetabulum. In up to 30% of cases, the loose bodies are nonossified. When nonossified, this process is indistinguishable from pigmented villonodular synovitis on plain films.

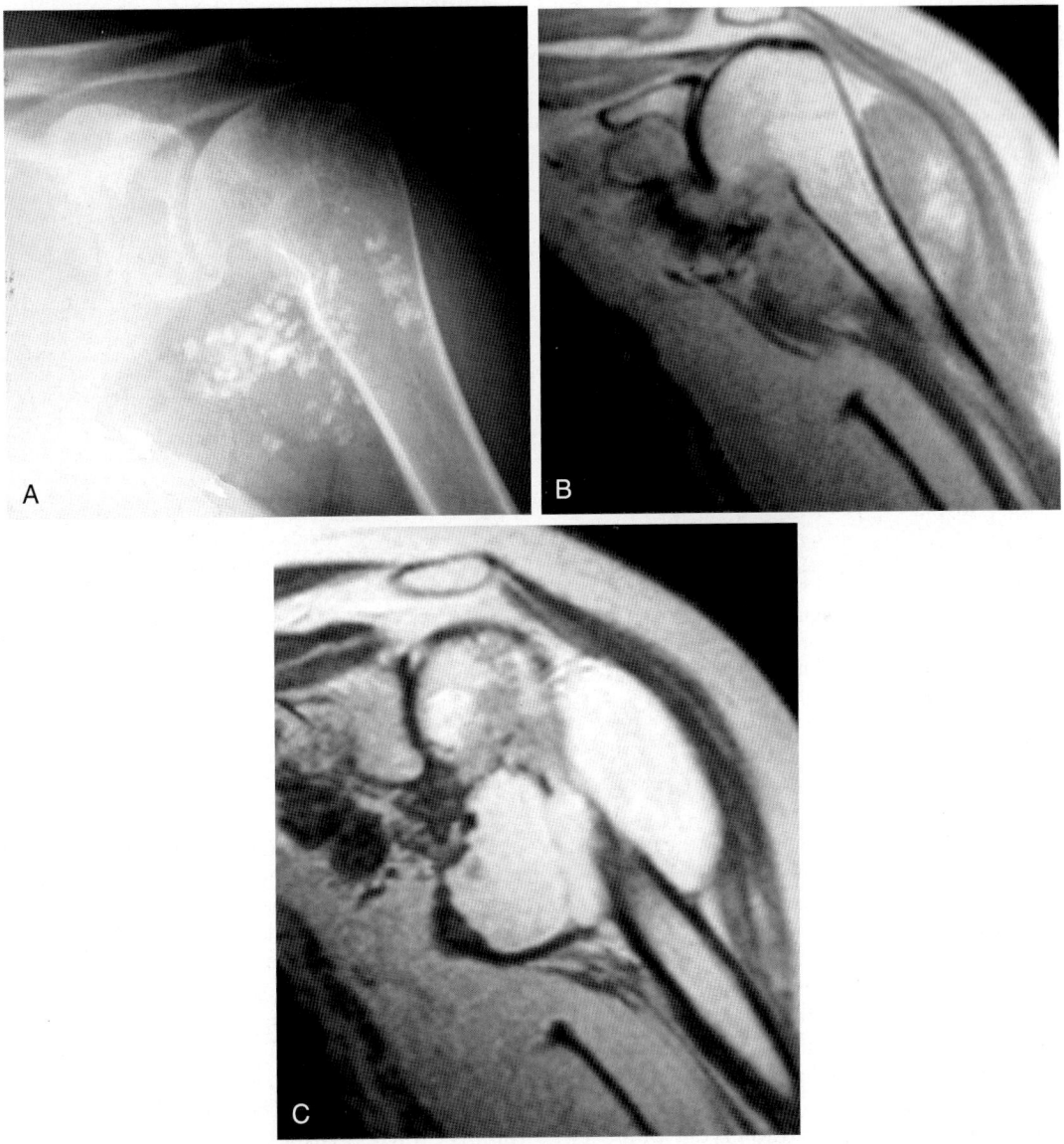

FIG. 3.32 **Tumefactive Synovial Osteochondromatosis.** (A) A plain film of the shoulder shows a partially calcified mass which is eroding the medial aspect of the humerus. Coronal proton-density (B) and T2-weighted (C) images of the shoulder reveal a large mass encircling the humeral head, which was interpreted as a sarcoma. A biopsy was performed and called "chondrosarcoma," which resulted in a forequarter amputation. The intra-articular nature of the mass was not appreciated until after the radical surgery, when it was correctly recognized as synovial chondromatosis.

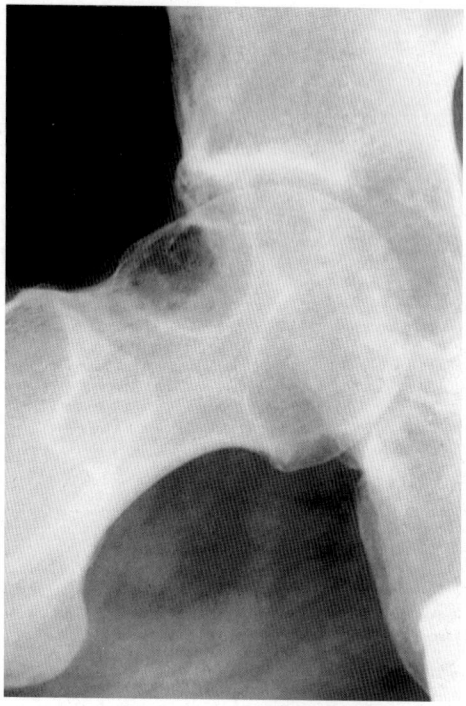

FIG. 3.33 **Pigmented Villonodular Synovitis (PVNS).** Large erosions in the femoral head and acetabulum are characteristic for pigmented villonodular synovitis; however, nonossified synovial osteochondromatosis could present like this.

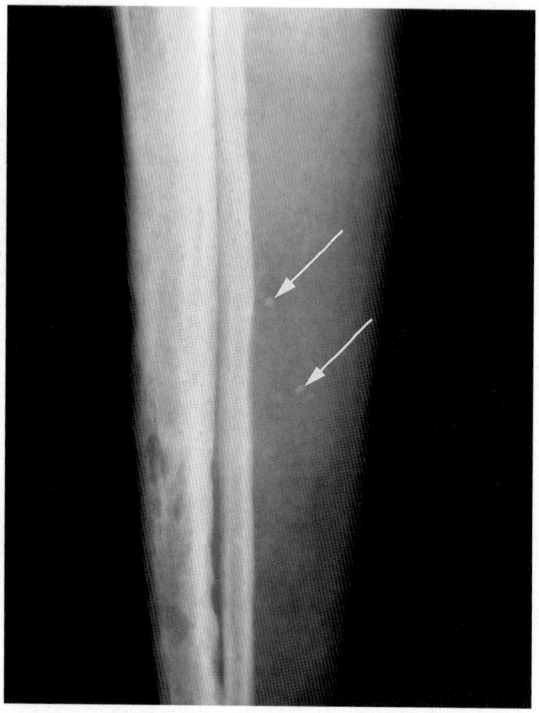

FIG. 3.34 **Hemangioma.** Multiple, irregular lytic lesions, predominantly cortical in nature, are seen in the tibia in this patient with a soft tissue mass. Cortical holes such as this occur almost exclusively in radiation and soft tissue hemangioma. Note the phleboliths in the posterior soft tissues *(arrows)*, which are often seen in hemangioma and make this an easy diagnosis.

be differentiated from "cortical holes" by the intact cortex (see Chapter 7, Metabolic Bone Disease).

Atypical synovial cysts, such as Baker's cysts around the knee, can present as a soft tissue mass and result in an unnecessary biopsy. On CT, these lesions may not be appreciated as fluid-filled lesions, and their association with a joint can be easily overlooked. MR imaging will demonstrate a very high signal intensity with T2 weighting and may show some fluid in the adjacent joint with an identical signal (Fig. 3.35). Differentiation of a solid mass from a ganglion is one of the few uses of Gd-DTPA in musculoskeletal MR imaging. A solid tumor will diffusely enhance with gadolinium, whereas a ganglion will have rim enhancement only. Intravenous contrast should be given whenever a mass that looks like a fluid collection or cyst is seen in a location atypical for a cyst or ganglion. Two tumors that typically mimic fluid on T2-weighted MR images are synovial sarcoma and neural tumors (neurofibromas and schwannomas) (Fig. 3.36).

A hematoma can present as a focal mass and be misdiagnosed on MR imaging as a tumor. If high signal is present on a T1WI, blood products should be considered, but keep in mind that tumors often have bleeding within, so that alone won't indicate a hematoma. Also, blood may or may not have high T1 signal. Gadolinium can be misleading in hematomas, as some enhancement can occur in long-standing hematomas, making one think it is a solid tumor. Heighthened suspicion for a hematoma should be present if a history of trauma or anticoagulation is elicited. A characteristic appearance for a hematoma is peripheral high T1 signal (Fig 3.37), but, while virtually pathognomonic, this is not always present.

A common mistake many make in giving IV contrast with MR imaging of tumors is to fat-suppress the postcontrast images and compare them with the non–fat-suppressed precontrast images. This can lead to an occasional misdiagnosis by assuming that all the high signal on the postcontrast image is from contrast enhancement, thereby making the call of a solid mass.

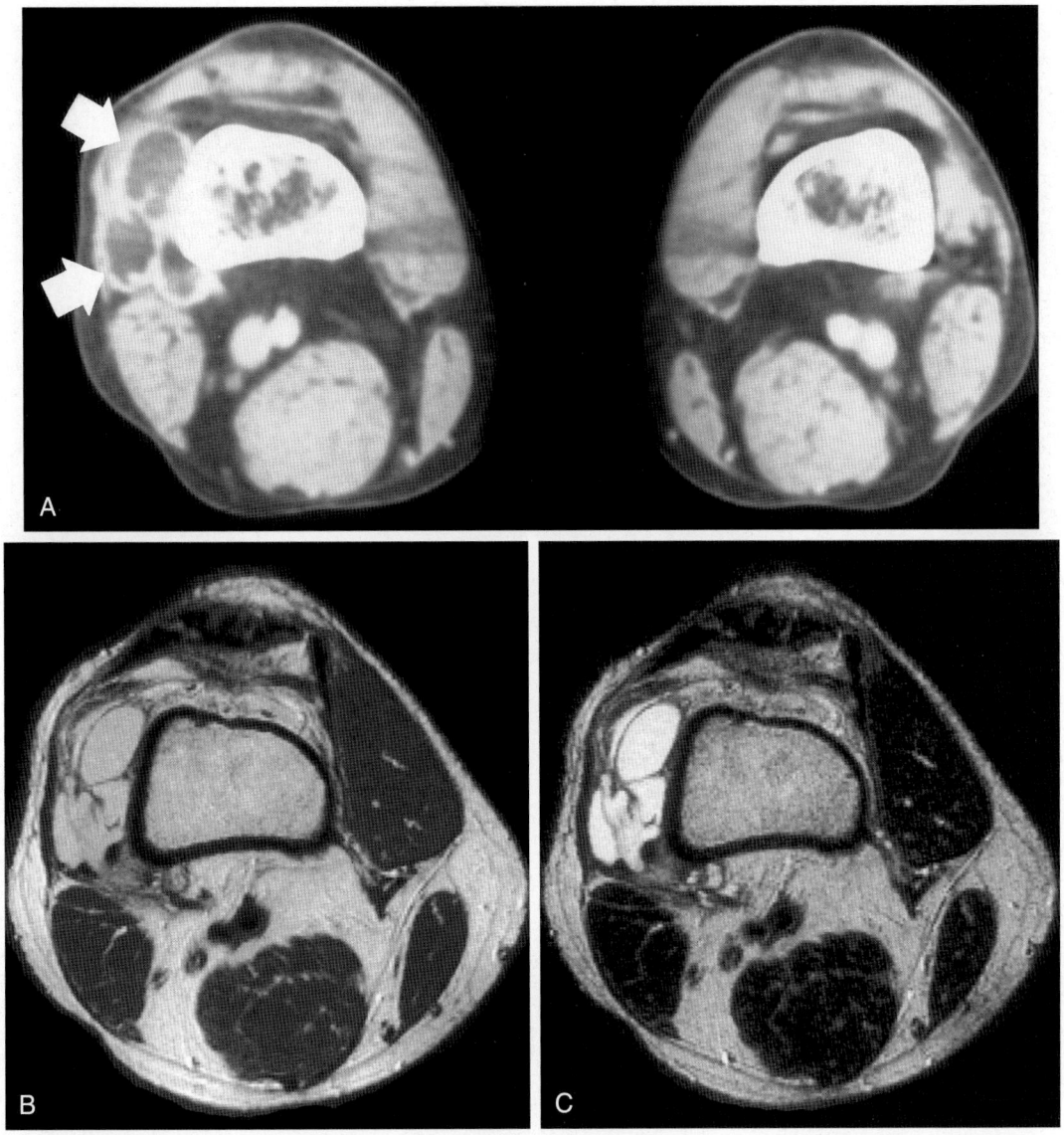

FIG. 3.35 **Atypical Synovial Cyst.** (A) Computed tomography (CT) scan through the distal femur in a patient with a soft tissue mass around the right knee shows a multilocular soft tissue mass adjacent to the distal right femur *(arrows)*. (B) A magnetic resonance (MR) imaging exam with T1 weighting through the same area as imaged in (A) shows intermediate-intensity signal in a multilocular soft tissue mass. (C) T2 weighting shows high-intensity signal in the lesion, which is characteristic for fluid. This was an atypical synovial cyst arising from the knee joint.

A fluid collection can sometimes appear to enhance on the postcontrast images simply as a result of the fat suppression (Fig. 3.38). When comparing pre- and postcontrast images, it is important to not change any imaging parameters except for giving gadolinium, or you won't know for sure what's causing the increased signal in the mass. There's no good reason to fat-suppress the postcontrast images—it simply makes for prettier pictures, but at the expense of an occasional misdiagnosis. If you must fat-suppress the postcontrast images, you must also fat-suppress the precontrast images so that you have only changed one variable.

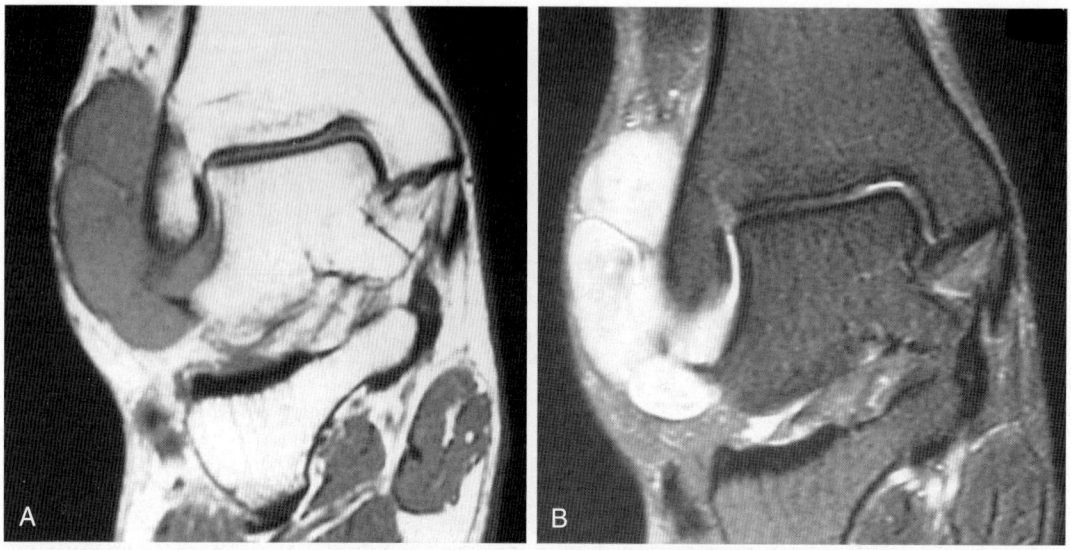

FIG. 3.36 **Schwannoma.** Coronal T1-weighted (A) and T2-weighted (B) images of an ankle in a young woman with a painful mass show a homogeneous mass that seems to emanate from the joint itself, suggesting an atypical ganglion. IV contrast should have been administered to determine if this were a solid or a cystic mass. At surgery, this was found to be a solid tumor, a benign schwannoma. It did not extend into the joint.

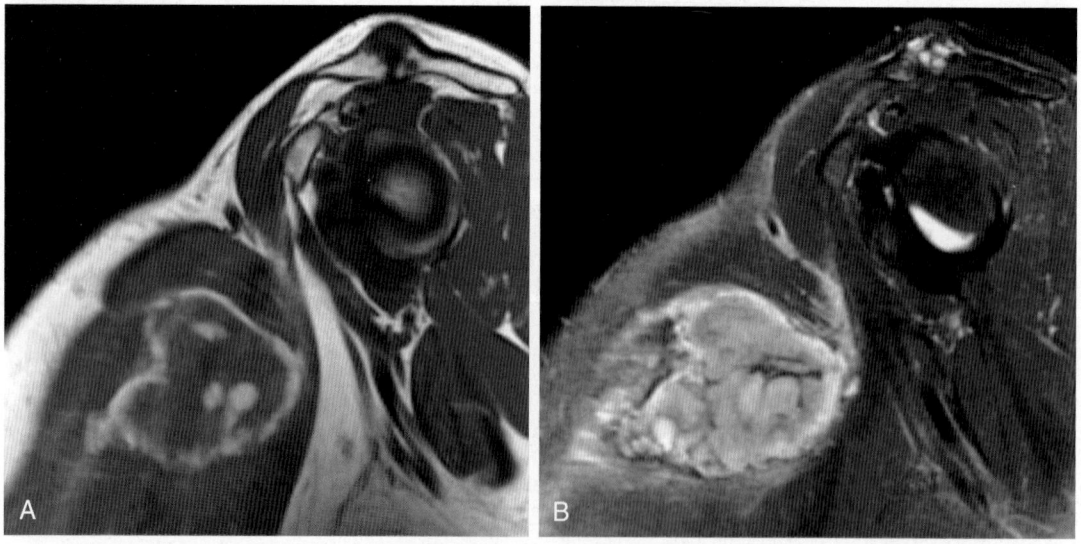

FIG. 3.37 **Hematoma.** (A) T1- and (B) T2-weighted sagittal images through the shoulder of an athlete with trauma to his pectoralis major shows a mass with surrounding high T1 signal that is pathognomonic for a hematoma. On the T2WI (B), it has the appearance of a sarcoma.

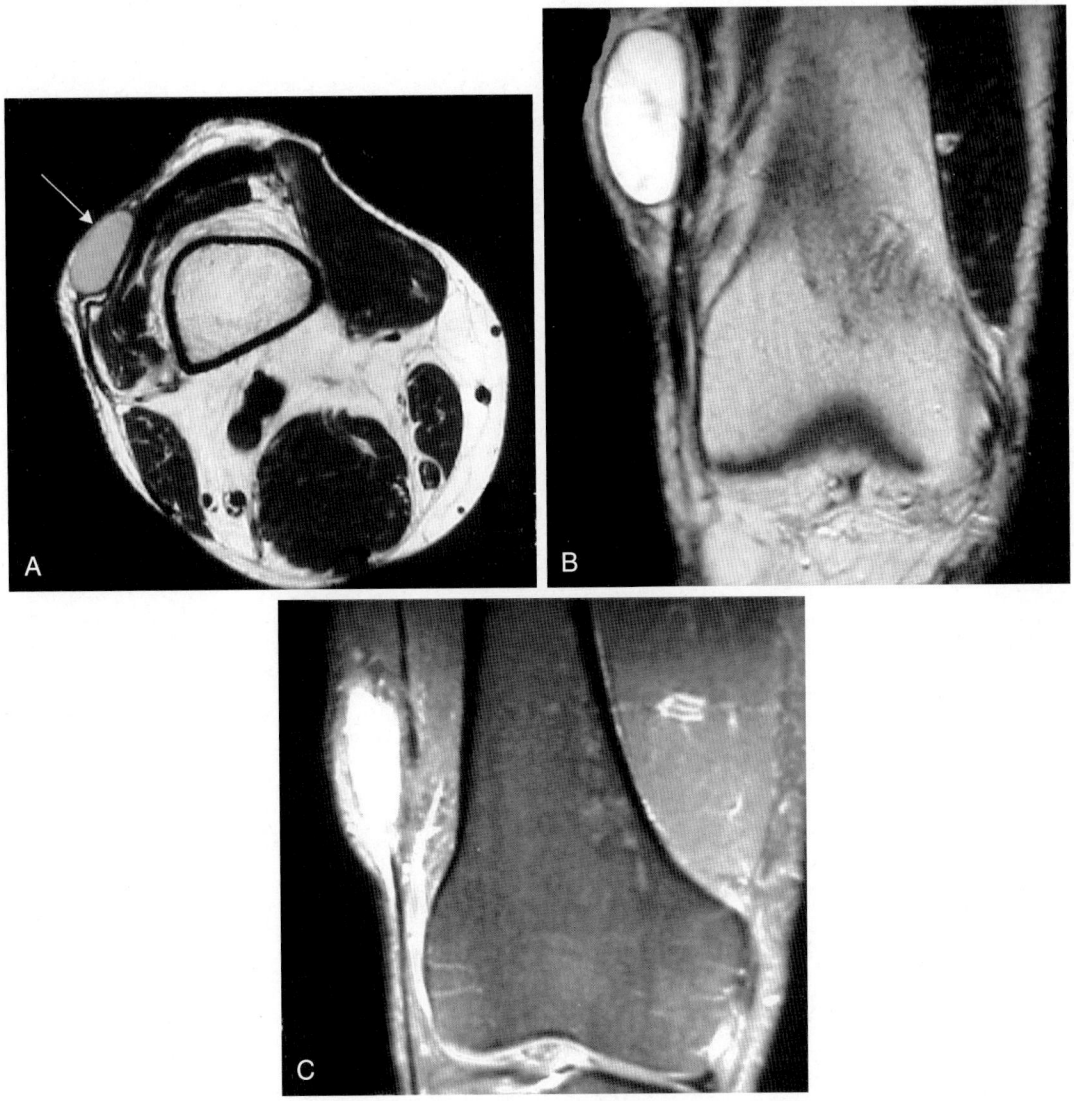

FIG. 3.38 **Hemorrhagic Cyst.** A 61-year-old man presented with a mass on his thigh, which was revealed to be of intermediate signal on an axial T1-weighted image (A) *(arrow)*. A coronal T2 weighted image shows marked high signal (B), which is homogeneous. Is this solid or cystic? A coronal T1-weighted image with fat suppression was performed after administration of gadolinium (C), which shows apparent diffuse enhancement indicating this is a solid mass. However, the increased signal cannot reliably be attributed to enhancement from the gadolinium because fat suppression was applied, which, in some instances, can make a mass appear brighter simply because of its relatively higher signal compared to the muscles. Notice on the T1 image in (A) that the mass is higher in signal than the muscles; therefore when fat suppression is applied, the next highest signal structure is the mass. Scaling the image then makes it appear bright, which can be misinterpreted as secondary to contrast enhancement. This was incorrectly called a solid tumor, and at surgery was found to be a hemorrhagic cyst.

CHAPTER 4

"Don't Touch" Lesions

Skeletal "don't touch" lesions are those processes that are so radiographically characteristic that a biopsy or additional diagnostic tests are unnecessary. Not only does the biopsy result in unnecessary morbidity and cost, but in some instances a biopsy also can be frankly misleading and lead to additional unnecessary surgery.

Most of our radiology training teaches us to give a differential diagnosis of a lesion, leaving it up to the clinician to decide between the various entities. For the "don't touch" lesions, however, a differential list is inappropriate, as that often makes the next step on the decision tree a biopsy. Because a biopsy of these lesions is not required for a final diagnosis, a radiologic diagnosis should be made without a list of differential possibilities. "Don't touch" lesions can be classified into three categories: (1) posttraumatic lesions, (2) normal variants, and (3) lesions that are real but obviously benign.

POSTTRAUMATIC LESIONS

Myositis ossificans is an example of a lesion on which a biopsy should not be performed because its aggressive histologic appearance can often mimic a sarcoma. Unfortunately, radical surgery has been performed based on the histologic appearance of myositis ossificans when the radiologic appearance was diagnostic. The typical radiologic appearance of myositis ossificans is circumferential calcification with a lucent center (Fig. 4.1). This is often best appreciated on computed tomography (CT) exam (Fig. 4.2). A malignant tumor that mimics myositis ossificans will have an ill-defined periphery and a calcified or ossific center (Fig. 4.3). Periosteal reaction can be seen with myositis ossificans or with a tumor. Occasionally the peripheral calcification of myositis ossificans can be difficult to appreciate; in such cases, a CT scan should help, or delayed films a week or two later are recommended. Biopsy should be avoided when myositis ossificans is a clinical consideration. Magnetic resonance imaging (MRI) in myositis ossificans can be misleading because the peripheral calcification may not be conspicuous and often has marked soft tissue edema surrounding it (Fig. 4.4).

Another posttraumatic entity in which a biopsy can be misleading is an avulsion injury. These injuries can have an aggressive radiographic appearance, but because of their characteristic location at insertion sites (e.g., antero–inferior iliac spine or ischial tuberosity), they should be recognized as benign (Figs. 4.5 and 4.6). Again, delayed films of several weeks will usually allow the problem case to become more radiographically and clinically clear. Biopsy can lead to the mistaken diagnosis of a sarcoma and should therefore be avoided. Any area that is undergoing healing can have a high nuclear–chromatin ratio and a high mitotic figure count, thereby occasionally simulating a malignancy.

A cortical desmoid is a process considered by many to be an avulsion off the medial supracondylar ridge of the distal femur. It occasionally simulates an aggressive lesion radiographically and on biopsy can look malignant.[1] In many instances, biopsy has led to amputation for this benign, radiographically characteristic lesion (Figs. 4.7 and 4.8). Cortical desmoids occur only on the posteromedial epicondyle of the femur. They may or may not be associated with pain and can have increased radionuclide uptake on bone scan. They may or may not exhibit periosteal new bone and usually occur in young people. Biopsy should be avoided in all cases. They are often seen as incidental findings on MRI and have a characteristic appearance (Fig. 4.9).

Trauma can lead to large, cystic geodes or subchondral cysts near joints that can be mistaken for other lytic lesions, and thus a biopsy is performed. Although the biopsy specimen is not likely to mimic a malignant process, it is nevertheless avoidable. Because geodes from degenerative disease almost always are associated with additional findings, such as joint space narrowing, sclerosis, and osteophytes, a diagnosis should be made radiographically (Figs. 4.10 and 4.11). However, on occasion, the additional findings are subtle and can be missed (Fig. 4.12). Geodes can also occur in the setting of calcium pyrophosphate dihydrate crystal disease (also known as CPPD or pseudogout), rheumatoid arthritis, and avascular necrosis.[2]

An entity that is often confused with metastatic disease to the spine is discogenic vertebral disease. It can mimic metastatic disease radiographically and

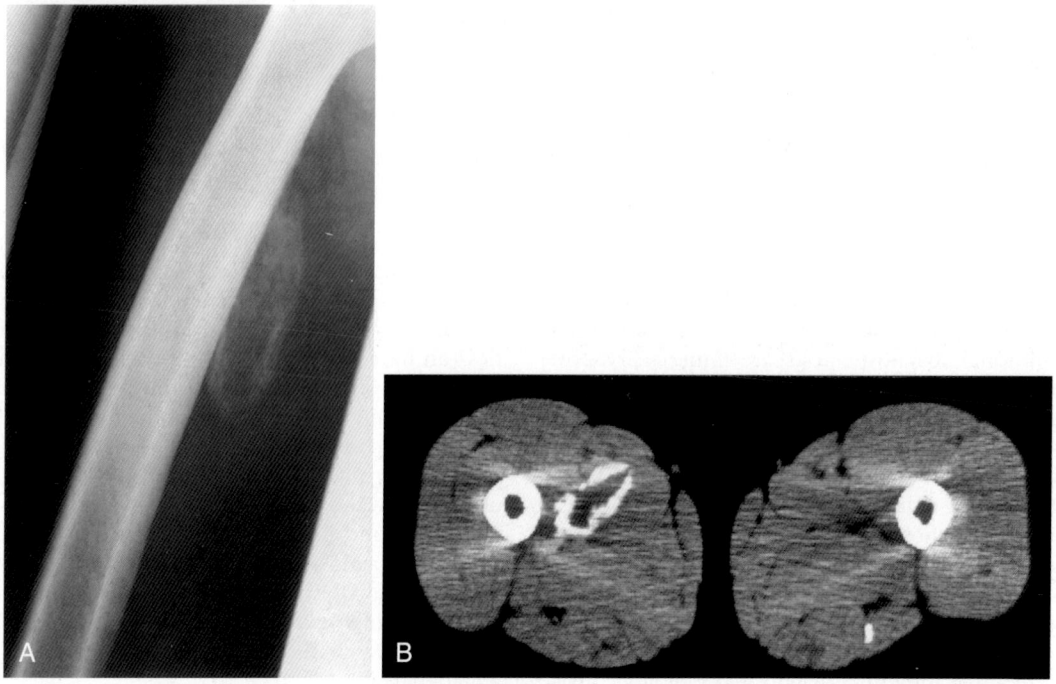

FIG. 4.1 **Myositis Ossificans.** (A) A plain film of the femur in this patient, who, presented with a soft tissue mass, shows a calcific density adjacent to the posterior cortex of the femur that is calcified primarily in its periphery. From seeing the plain film alone, it should not be difficult to say that this is peripheral, circumferential calcification; nevertheless, a computed tomography (CT) scan was obtained (B), and shows that the calcification is unequivocally peripheral. This is virtually diagnostic of myositis ossificans.

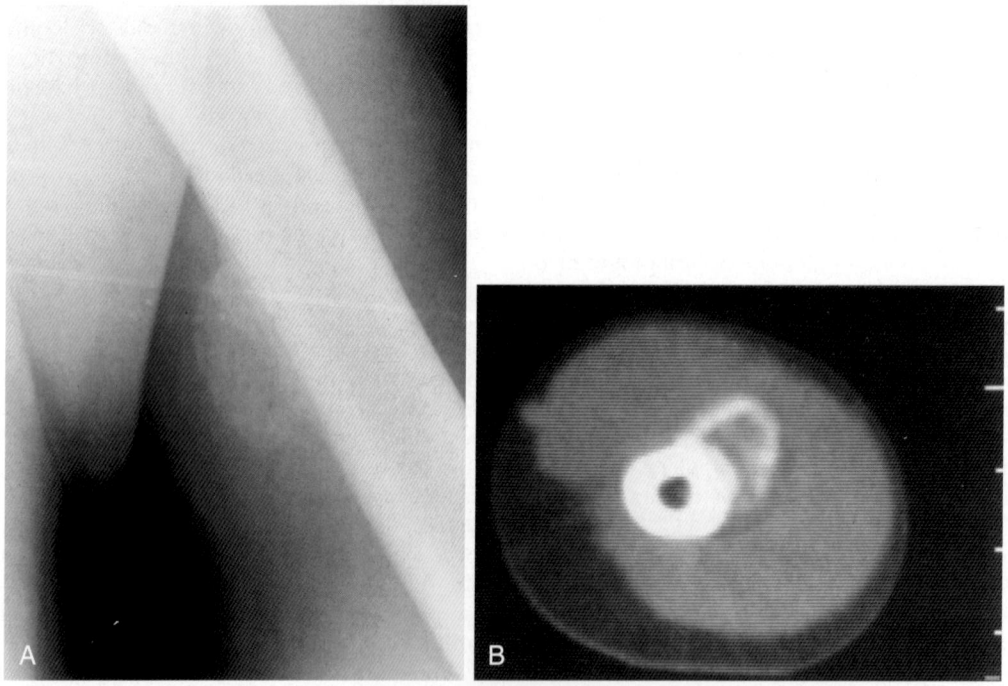

FIG. 4.2 **Myositis Ossificans.** (A) Hazy calcification is seen adjacent to the humeral shaft, with underlying periosteal reaction noted. It is difficult to ascertain whether or not the calcification is circumferential. (B) A computed tomography (CT) scan through this mass shows that the calcification is unequivocally circumferential, making the diagnosis of myositis ossificans a certainty.

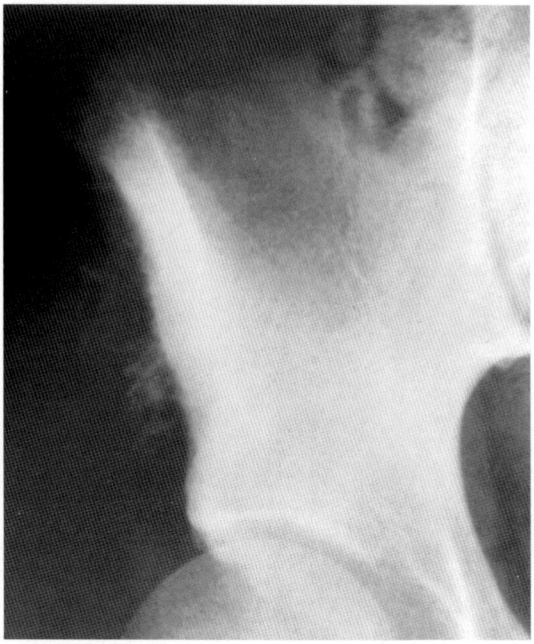

FIG. 4.3 **Osteogenic Sarcoma.** Hazy, ill-defined calcification is seen adjacent to the iliac wing in this patient that can be ascertained from the plain film to definitely not be circumferential. Even though a prior history of trauma was obtained in this case, myositis ossificans is not a consideration with this appearance of calcification. Biopsy showed this to be an osteogenic sarcoma.

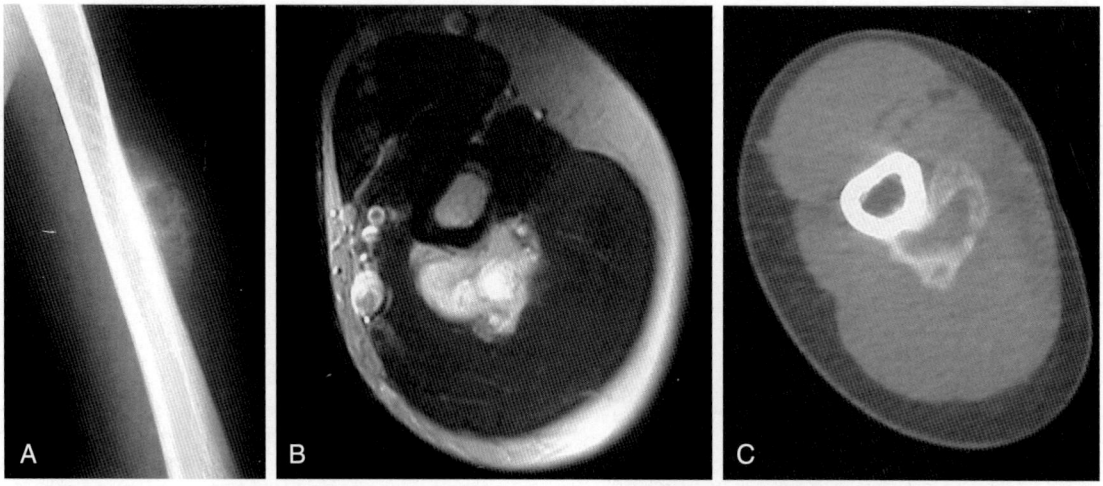

FIG. 4.4 **Myositis Ossificans.** (A) A plain film of the humerus in this 30-year-old man shows a calcific mass adjacent to the diaphysis of the humerus. The calcification is not clearly peripheral in nature, although the central portion is less well mineralized. (B) An axial T2-weighted image through the mass shows only a high signal mass without evidence of calcification. (C) A computed tomography (CT) scan through the mass demonstrates the typical peripheral calcification, which is virtually pathognomonic for myositis ossificans.

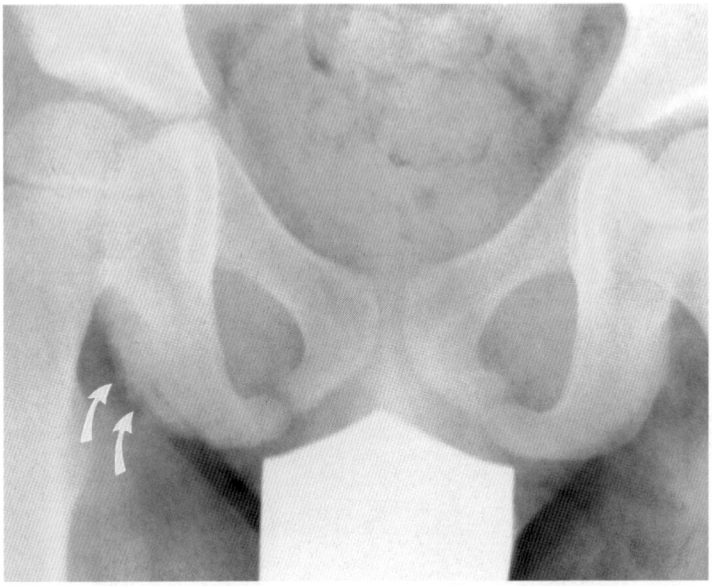

FIG. 4.5 **Avulsion Injury.** Cortical irregularity *(arrows)* at the ischial tuberosity in this patient with pain over this region raises the question of possible tumor. This is a classic appearance, however, for an avulsion injury from this region, and a biopsy should be avoided.

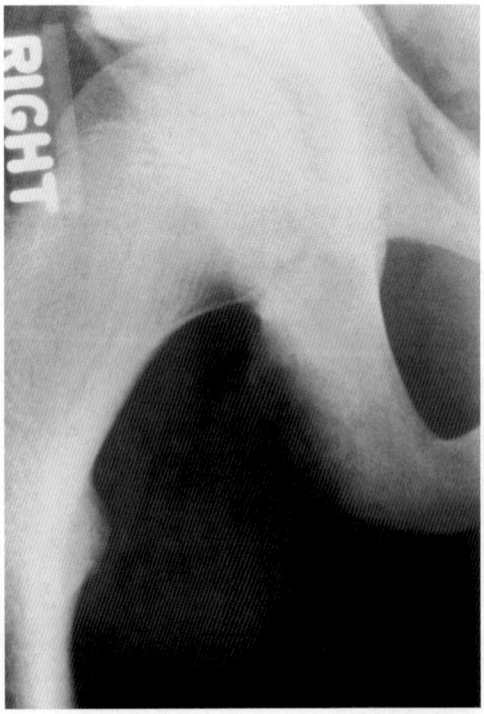

FIG. 4.6 **Avulsion Injury.** Cortical irregularity with a Codman triangle of periostitis is seen along the ischial tuberosity. This was at first thought to represent a malignancy. Because of the characteristic location, an avulsion injury was considered, and the lesion was observed. It healed without sequelae.

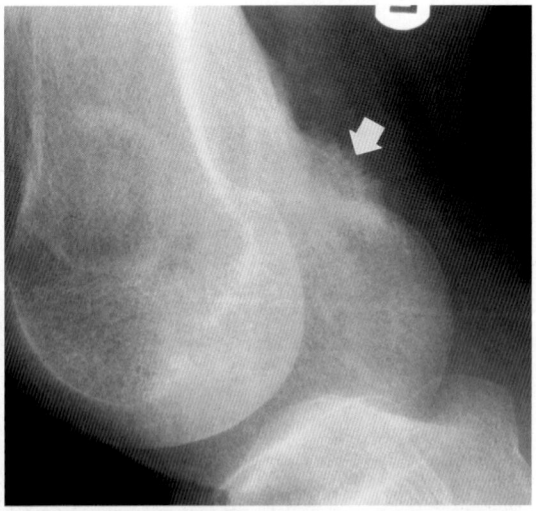

FIG. 4.7 **Cortical Desmoid.** A focal cortical irregularity is seen in the posterior aspect of the femur *(arrow)* with adjacent periostitis noted. Although a tumor such as an early parosteal osteosarcoma could perhaps have this appearance, the location and appearance are characteristic of a cortical desmoid, and a biopsy should not be performed.

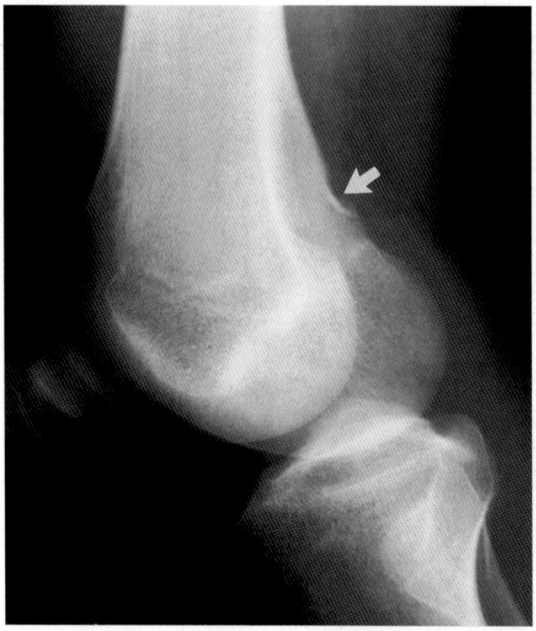

FIG. 4.8 **Cortical Desmoid.** A well-defined cortical defect is seen in the posterior distal femur *(arrow)*, which is a common appearance for a fairly well-healed cortical desmoid.

clinically, and unless the radiologist is familiar with this process, it can lead to an unnecessary biopsy.[3,4] Discogenic vertebral disease most often is sclerotic and focal (Fig. 4.13). It is adjacent to an end plate, and the associated disc space should be narrow. Osteophytosis is invariably present. It represents a variant of a Schmorl's node and should not be confused with a metastatic focus. On occasion it can be lytic or even mixed lytic–sclerotic. The typical clinical setting is a middle-aged woman with chronic low back pain. Old films often confirm the benign nature of this process. In the setting of disc space narrowing and osteophytosis, a biopsy of focal sclerosis adjacent to an end plate should not be performed.

Occasionally a fracture will be the cause of extensive osteosclerosis and periostitis, which can mimic a primary bone tumor (Fig. 4.14). Lack of immobilization can result in exuberant callus, which can be misinterpreted as aggressive periostitis or even tumor new bone. A biopsy in such a case might resemble a malignant lesion. Therefore any case associated with trauma should be carefully reviewed for a fracture.

Another traumatic process that can be misdiagnosed radiologically, leading to inappropriate treatment and morbidity, is a pseudodislocation of the humerus (Figs. 4.15 and 4.16). This results from a fracture with hemarthrosis, which causes distention of the joint and migration of the humeral head inferiorly. An axial or transscapular view shows that it is not anteriorly or posteriorly dislocated (the usual forms of shoulder dislocation), but merely inferiorly displaced. On an anteroposterior view, it can mimic a posterior dislocation. Often attempts are made to "relocate" the humeral head, which are both fruitless (because it is not dislocated) and painful. A fracture is invariably present, and if not seen on the initial films, it should be sought after with additional views. A transscapular or an axillary view is the key to making the diagnosis of a pseudodislocation. With either of these views, the humeral head can be seen to be normally positioned in relation to the glenoid, although it may appear somewhat inferiorly displaced. If necessary, the joint can be aspirated to confirm the presence of a bloody effusion and to show the normal position of the humeral head with no fluid in the joint.[5]

Costochondritis, or Tietze syndrome, can cause a bulbous swelling of a rib (Fig. 4.17) owing to periostitis, which can mimic a rib lesion. This condition is very painful and usually easily diagnosed clinically; however, with a bony lesion seen on radiographs, many clinicians may want a biopsy to rule out a malignant process. This would be a mistake, as with any posttraumatic or rapidly healing lesion, it can be difficult to categorize histologically. Because Tietze syndrome is a short-lived process, watchful waiting with repeat film in 2 to 3 weeks if the patient is not improved is probably indicated.

Sacral insufficiency fractures (see Chapter 5) are occasionally mistaken for an aggressive process such as metastatic disease, and should be easily recognized and not biopsied or irradiated (Fig. 4.18). Another fracture that can be mistaken for metastatic disease is a supra-acetabular insufficiency fracture. These can resemble a blastic metastatic process on plain films, but an MRI will show a fracture line that typically is curvilinear and parallel to the acetabulum (Fig. 4.19).

NORMAL VARIANTS

Numerous normal variants exist that are often confused with a pathologic process. This is best evidenced by the fact that several of the most popular radiology texts are atlases of normal variants.

A normal variant that has been described in the patella is a lytic defect in the upper outer quadrant called dorsal

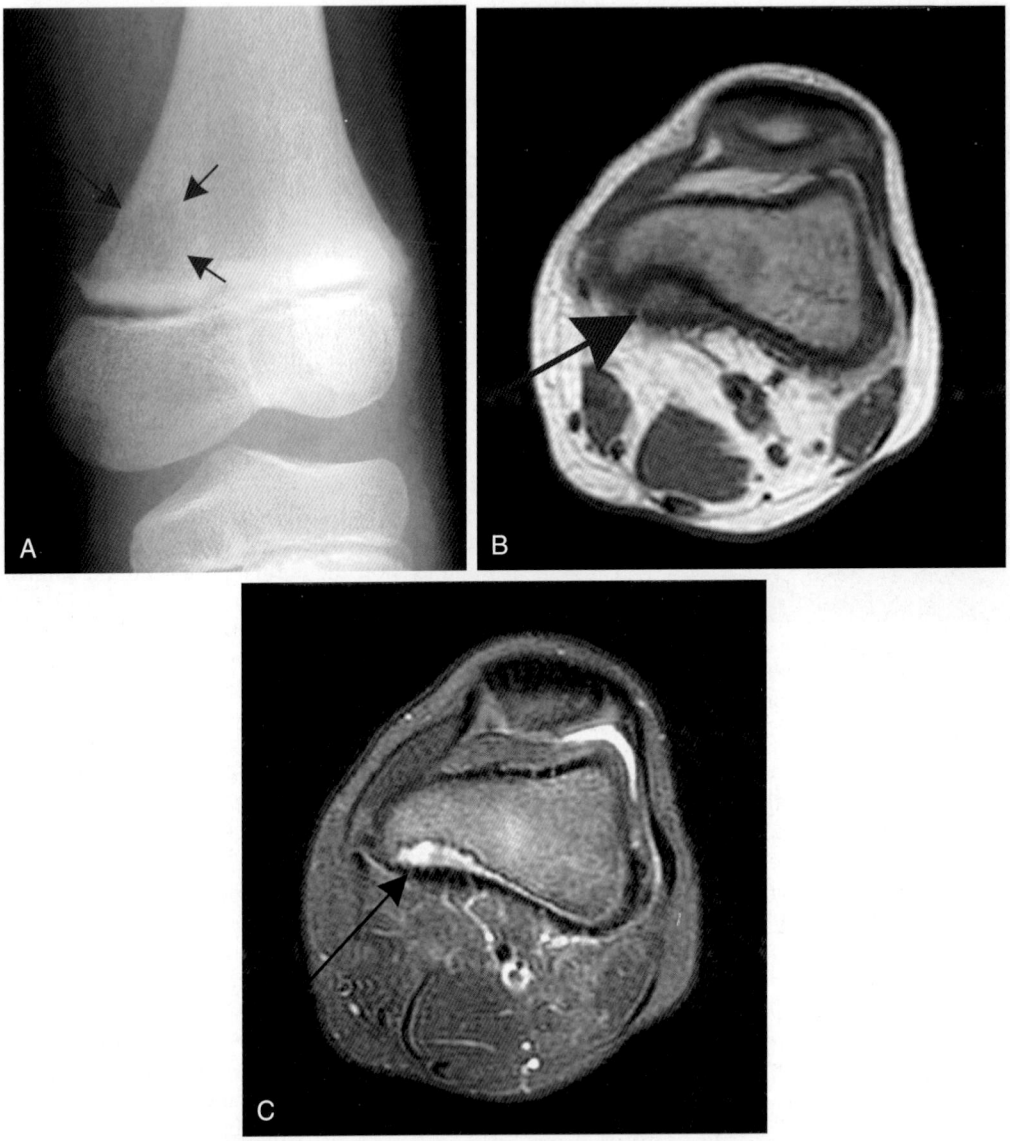

FIG. 4.9 **Cortical Desmoid.** (A) An anteroposterior (AP) film of the knee in a child shows a faint lytic lesion *(arrows)* in the medial aspect of the distal femur. Axial T1- (B) and T2-weighted (C) images through the lesion show a cortically based process *(arrows)* in the medial supracondylar ridge, which is characteristic for a cortical desmoid.

defect of the patella (Fig. 4.20).[6] It can mimic a focus of infection, osteochondritis dissecans, or a lytic lesion. It is a normal developmental anomaly, however, and because of its characteristic location, a biopsy of it should not be performed. When seen on an MR exam, it is diagnosed based on its characteristic location, as the signal characteristics are similar to tumor or infection (Fig. 4.21).

Another entity often confused with a lytic pathologic process is a pseudocyst of the humerus (Fig. 4.22). This is merely an anatomic variant caused by the increased cancellous bone in the region of the greater tuberosity of the humerus, which gives this region a more lucent appearance on radiographs. With hyperemia and disuse caused by rotator cuff problems or any other shoulder disorder, this area of lucency may appear strikingly more

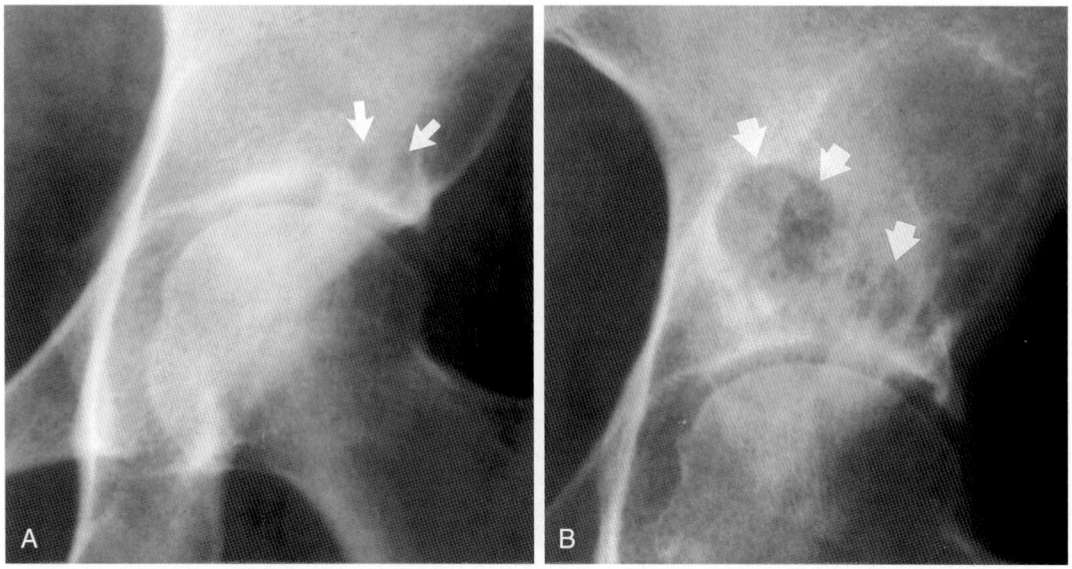

FIG. 4.10 **Geode.** (A) A plain film of the hip in this older patient with hip pain shows a lytic lesion in the supra-acetabular region *(arrow)*, which has a benign appearance. Mild osteoarthritis was felt to be present (when compared to the opposite hip, joint space narrowing and mimimal sclerosis were seen); hence this was felt to be a subchondral cyst or geode. (B) Several years later, the same hip shows a large lytic lesion *(arrows)* that still appears benign. The osteoarthritis has increased in severity. However, because of the growth of the lesion, it was biopsied and found to be a geode. A biopsy should have been avoided.

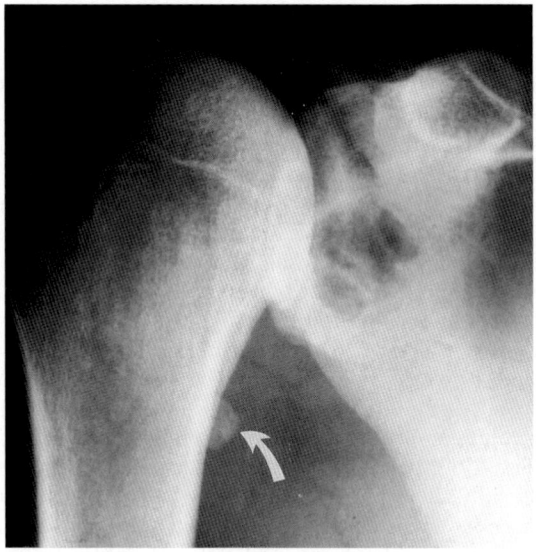

FIG. 4.11 **Geode.** A large cystic lesion was found in the shoulder in this middle-aged weight lifter, and the possibility of a metastatic process was considered. Because the humeral head has sclerosis and osteophytosis as well as a loose body in the joint *(arrow)*, degenerative disease of the shoulder was diagnosed; this makes the cystic lesion almost certainly a geode or subchondral cyst, which made a biopsy unnecessary.

lucent and mimic a lytic lesion. Biopsies of many of these lesions have been done mistakenly, and in several cases have been repeated (Fig. 4.22C) after the initial pathology report stated "normal bone—no lesion in specimen." Because of the associated hyperemia from the shoulder disorder (be it rotator cuff or whatever), a bone scan can show increased radionuclide uptake and thus sway the surgeon to do a biopsy of this normal variant. It is radiographically characteristic in its location and appearance, and a biopsy of it should not be done.[7] Although other lesions, such as a chondroblastoma (Fig. 4.23), infection, or even a metastatic focus, could occur in a similar location, they do not have quite the same appearance as a pseudocyst of the humerus.

A normal variant of the cervical spine that may, in fact, be posttraumatic is an os odontoideum.[8] It is an unfused dens that may move anterior to the C-2 body with flexion and can mimic a fractured dens (Figs. 4.24 and 4.25). Many of these lesions require surgical fixation; some surgeons fuse every case, believing that they are all unstable. Radiologists should recognize that this process is not acute so as to save the patient from having Crutchfield tongs or a halo applied and from possible immediate surgical intervention. Most cases are seen after trauma, and if no neurologic deficits are present, these patients can be seen electively and spared

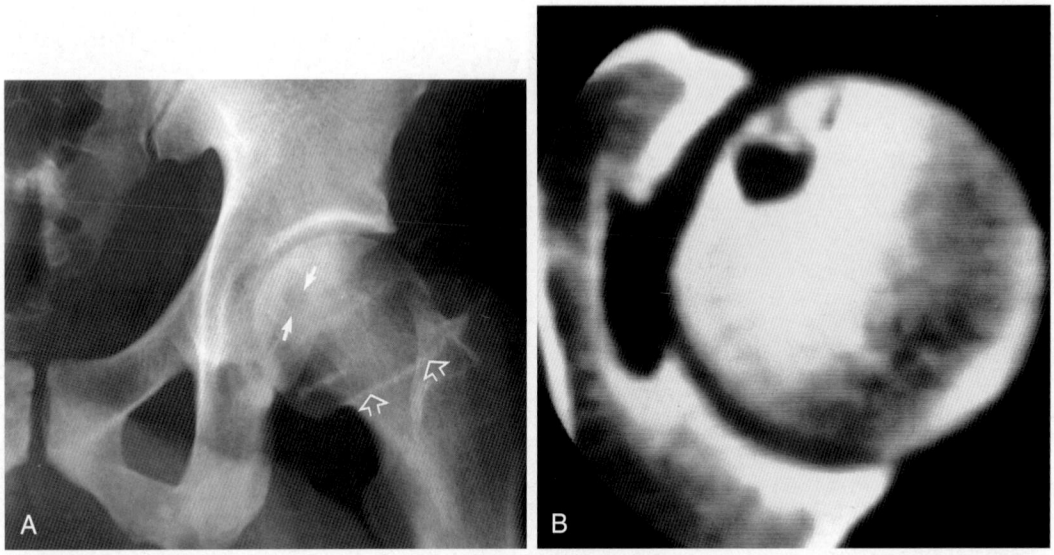

FIG. 4.12 **Geode.** (A) A cystic lesion was noted in the femoral head *(arrows)* of a young male with a painful hip. (B) A computed tomography (CT) scan through this area shows the subarticular nature and adjacent sclerosis. The differential diagnosis of infection, eosinophilic granuloma, and chondroblastoma was given. A ring of osteophytes *(open arrow heads)* was noted in retrospect on the plain film (A) in the subcapital region, which indicates degenerative disease of the hip. This is an extremely unusual presentation in a healthy 20-year-old male; however, it makes the lytic lesion in the femoral head almost certainly a subchondral cyst or geode. This was an active soccer player who had been playing with pain in his hip for several years after an injury that had caused the degenerative disease. Unfortunately, a biopsy was performed anyway, and a subchondral cyst or geode was confirmed.

the horrors and morbidity associated with treatment of the acutely fractured cervical spine. The radiologic signs for recognizing an os odontoideum are the smooth, often well-corticated inferior border of the dens and the hypertrophied, densely corticated anterior arch of C-1. This latter finding presumably represents compensatory hypertrophy and indicates a long-standing condition.[9]

Although unusual, osteopoikilosis, a benign familial process of multiple bone islands or small areas of osteosclerosis, has caused confusion by its similarity to metastatic disease (Fig. 4.26). Ordinarily osteopoikilosis has such a characteristic appearance that it will not be mistaken for another entity, and the predominance of sclerotic foci near the epiphyses should help to differentiate it from metastatic disease (Fig. 4.27).

OBVIOUSLY BENIGN LESIONS

Biopsies are frequently performed on some lesions that should be recognized radiographically as benign and left alone. These are lesions that should be diagnosed by the radiologist, not the pathologist. Listing a differential in such cases often spurs the surgeon to a biopsy, when in fact no biopsy should be necessary.

Perhaps the most commonly encountered lesion in this category is the nonossifying fibroma (NOF). It is identical to a fibrous cortical defect, but the term is usually reserved for defects larger than 2 cm. NOFs are, classically, lytic lesions that are located in the cortex of the metaphysis of a long bone that have a well-defined, often sclerotic, scalloped border with slight cortical expansion (Fig. 4.28) (also, see Chapter 2). They are almost exclusively found in patients under the age of 30, suggesting that the natural history of the lesion is involution. As they involute, they fill in with new bone (Fig. 4.29); hence they can have some increased radionuclide activity on bone scans. They are most often mistaken for an area of infection, eosinophilic granuloma, or aneurysmal bone cyst. NOFs are asymptomatic and have never been reported to be associated with malignant degeneration. On occasion, a pathologic fracture can occur through these lesions, but most surgeons do not advocate prophylactic curettage to prevent fracture, as with unicameral bone cysts. NOFs can be quite large but invariably have a benign appearance (Fig. 4.30), and

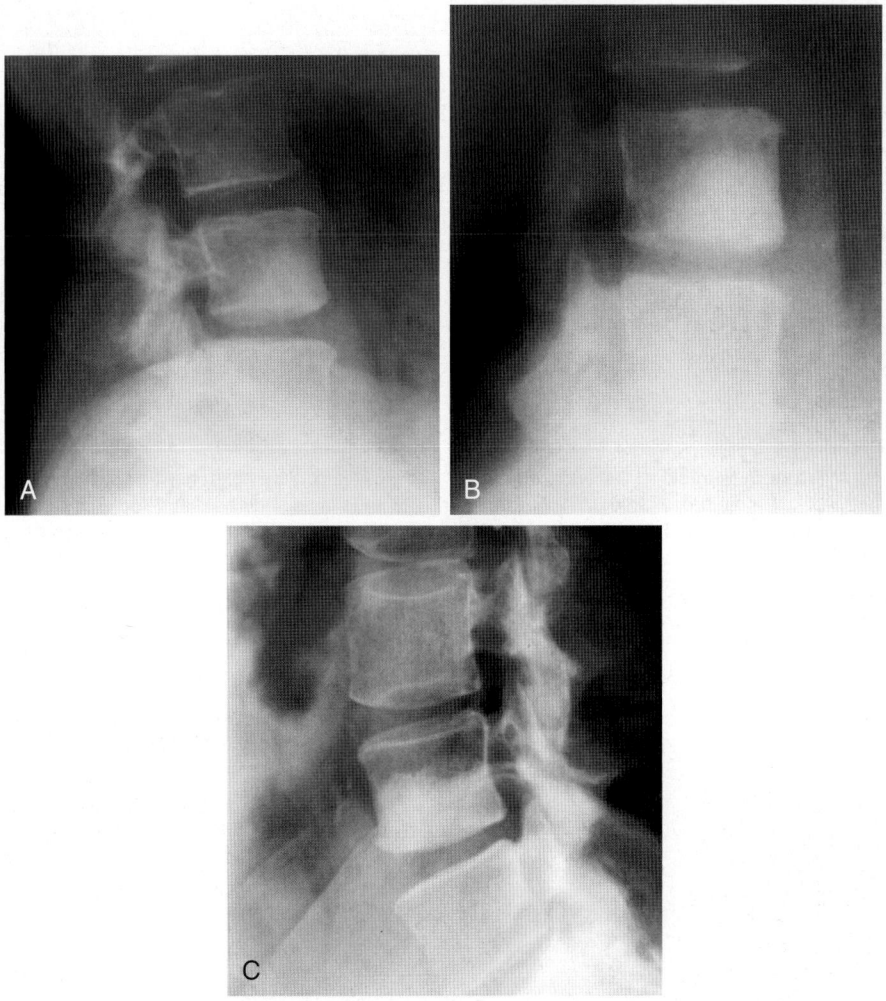

FIG. 4.13 **Discogenic Vertebral Sclerosis.** (A, B, C) These films all show patients with sclerosis on the inferior portion of the L-4 vertebral body associated with minimal osteophytosis and joint space narrowing at the adjacent disc space. This is the classic appearance for discogenic vertebral sclerosis, and a biopsy to rule out metastatic disease should not be performed.

biopsy should be avoided. The asymptomatic nature is imperative to help distinguish them from most of the other lesions in the differential and thereby preclude even giving a differential diagnosis. On occasion they are found to be multiple (Fig. 4.31), yet each lesion is so characteristic that they should be easily diagnosed.

Bone islands are not a radiographic dilemma when they are 1 cm or less. Occasionally, however, they grow to golf ball size and mimic sclerotic metastases (Fig. 4.32). They are always asymptomatic. Radiographically, two signs can be found to help distinguish giant bone islands from metastases: first, bone islands usually are oblong, with their long axis in the axis of stress on the bone (e.g., in a long bone, they align themselves along the axis of the diaphysis); second, the margins of a bone island, if examined closely, will show bony trabeculae extending from the lesion into the normal bone in a spiculated fashion.[10] (See Chapter 2.) This is characteristic of a bone island and helpful in differentiating it from more aggressive processes.

Unicameral bone cysts are often prophylactically packed so as to prevent fracture with subsequent deformity. When these cysts occur in the calcaneus, however, they should be left alone. They always occur in the anteroinferior portion of the calcaneus (Fig. 4.33), an area that does not receive undue stress. In fact, a pseudotumor of

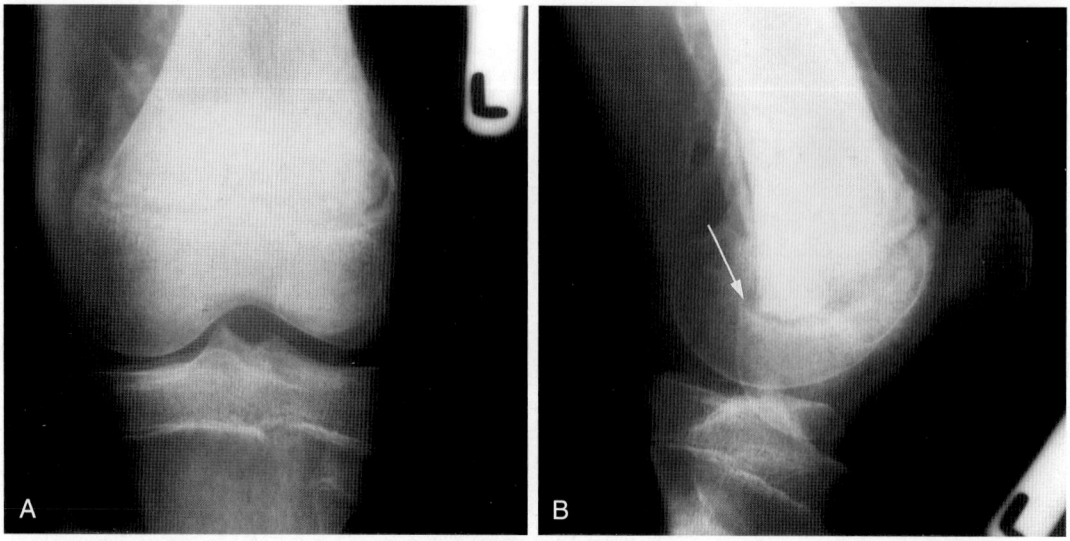

FIG. 4.14 **Fracture Mimicking Osteosarcoma.** (A) This 16-year-old had experienced pain around the knee for 2 weeks before these radiographs were taken. The knee films showed diffuse sclerosis and extensive periostitis about the distal femur, which was felt to be characteristic for an osteogenic sarcoma. The periosteal reaction, however, was felt to be much too thick, dense, and wavy to represent malignant type of periostitis. (B) A small offset of the epiphysis can be seen *(arrow)*, which indicates an epiphyseal slippage consistent with a Salter epiphyseal fracture. The patient had fallen off his bicycle and fractured his femur, yet continued to be active. The lack of immobility caused exuberant periostitis or callus with a large amount of reactive sclerosis, all of which mimicked an osteogenic sarcoma.

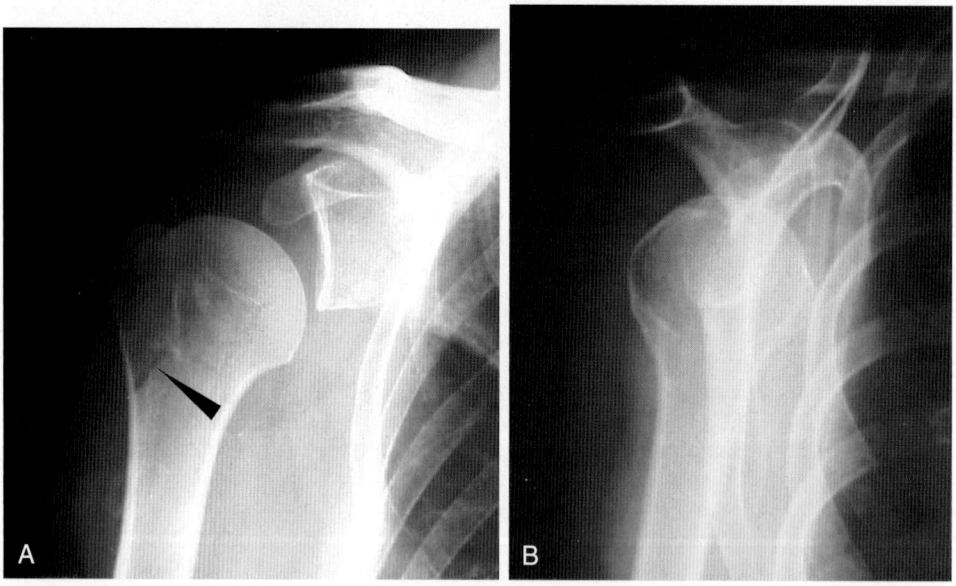

FIG. 4.15 **Pseudodislocation of the Shoulder.** (A) This patient experienced trauma to the shoulder, with resultant pain and immobility, and was thought to have a dislocation of the shoulder after the anteroposterior film was seen. The humeral head is inferiorly placed in relation to the glenoid; however, this is not the characteristic location of an anterior or posterior dislocation. (B) The transscapular view shows the humeral head to be situated normally over the glenoid without anterior or posterior dislocation. These findings are characteristic for a pseudodislocation caused by hemarthrosis, or blood in the joint, which allows the shoulder to be subluxed rather than dislocated. Aspiration of the blood will result in the humeral head returning to its normal position in relation to the glenoid; however, this is not usually necessary. When a pseudodislocation is seen, as in this example, search for an occult fracture should ensue. In this case, as seen on (A), a fracture *(arrow)* was initially missed.

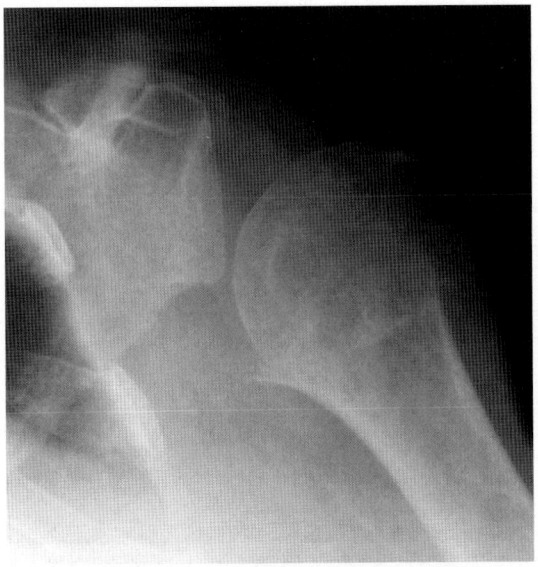

FIG. 4.16 **Pseudodislocation of the Shoulder.** The humeral head is inferiorly placed in relation to the glenoid. This is the characteristic location when a hemarthrosis is present. A minimally displaced fracture of the neck of the humerus with avulsion of the greater tuberosity has occurred, causing the hemarthrosis.

the calcaneus in the identical position is seen because of the absence of stress and resulting atrophy of bony trabeculae (Fig. 4.34). Calcaneal unicameral bone cysts are asymptomatic, only rarely fracture, and should not suffer the same fate as their counterparts in long bones. Calcaneal unicameral bone cysts seem to involute at a slower rate than those in long bones; hence they can be seen in patients older than 30. Also, as they involute, they occasionally undergo "lipidization," which is fatty infiltration. If imaged or biopsied during this stage, they get mistakenly diagnosed as an intraosseous lipoma. That is why many authors have called calcaneal unicameral bone cysts lipomas. Annually, around radiology oral boards time, residents ask me to explain why some texts refer to these lesions as unicameral bone cysts and others call them lipomas. In fact, they are all unicameral bone cysts. Many benign fibro-osseous lesions throughout the skeleton involute with fatty infiltration and get mistakenly called intraosseous lipomas.

Early in the course of its development, a bone infarct can have a patchy or a mixed lytic–sclerotic pattern or even resemble a permeative process as opposed to the classic appearance of a sclerotic, serpigenous peripheral border (Figs. 4.35 and 4.36). In a patient with bone pain and a permeative bone lesion, many aggressive

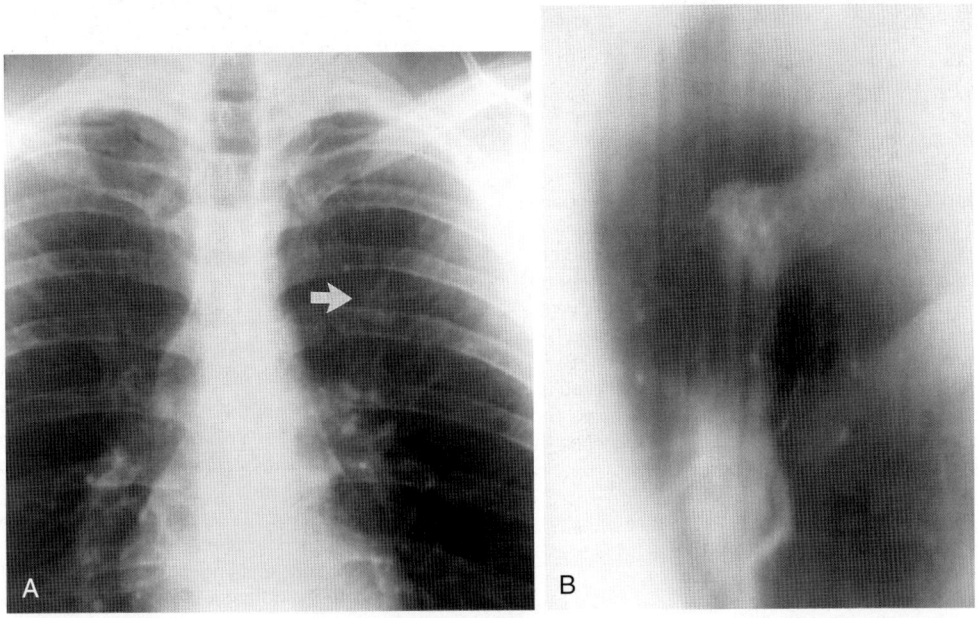

FIG. 4.17 **Costochondritis.** (A) A young male with point tenderness over the anterior chest wall had a chest radiograph that revealed a nodular density *(arrow)* that appeared attached to the second rib. (B) Tomograms of this area show a nodular density with speckled calcification at the distal end of the rib *(arrows)*, which was thought to possibly represent an osteochondroma. Any chondroid lesion that is painful should be suspicious for malignant degeneration, and a biopsy was planned for this patient. The clinical findings, however, were classic for costochondritis or Tietze syndrome, which rapidly cleared; therefore biopsy was cancelled. Costochondritis can cause periostitis and bulbous swelling of the ribs, as in this example, and a biopsy should not be performed.

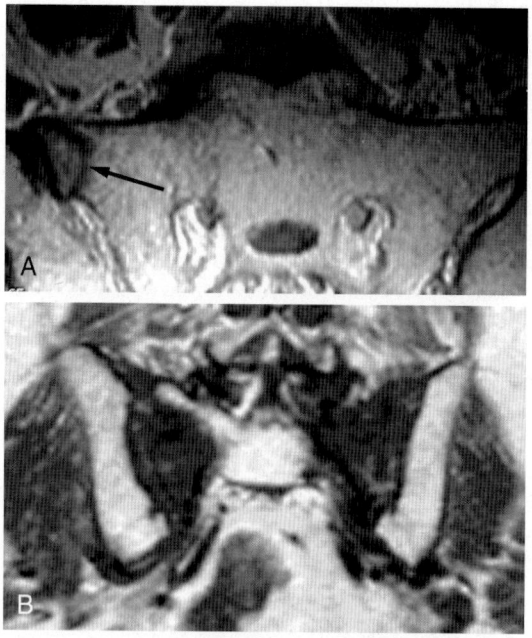

FIG. 4.18 **Sacral Insufficiency Fracture.** (A) A woman with a history of breast cancer presented with sacral pain and linear low signal adjacent to the sacroiliac (SI) joint was seen *(arrow)*. This was called an insufficiency fracture by the radiologist; however, a bone scan was interpreted as possible metastatic disease. Therefore she underwent radiation therapy. She had worsening sacral pain, and a magnetic resonance imaging (MRI) 6 months later (B) shows bilateral sacral insufficiency fractures. Radiation is one of the causative factors for insufficiency fractures and, in this case, caused additional pain and suffering when the initial imaging exam was diagnostic.

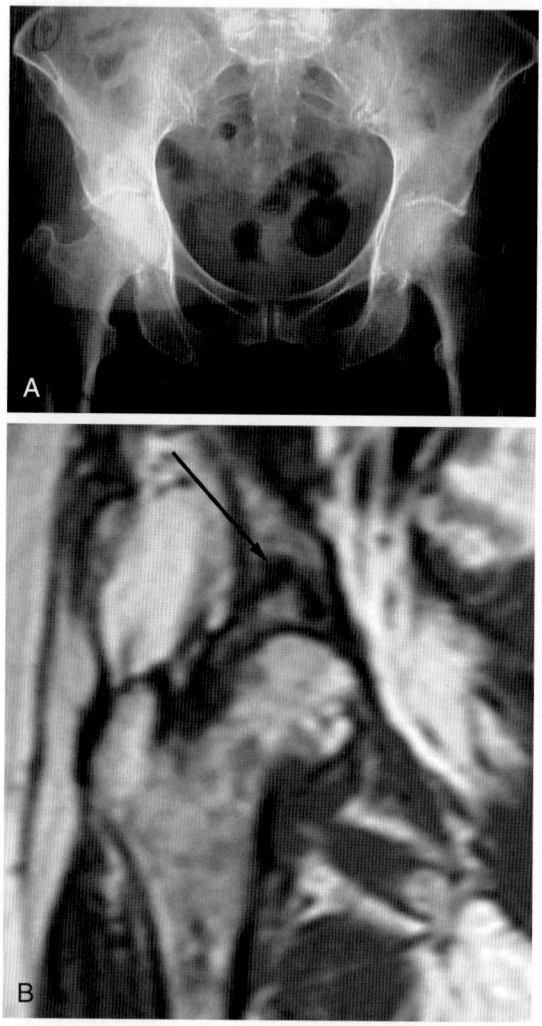

FIG. 4.19 **Supra-Acetabular Insufficiency Fracture.** (A) An elderly woman with a history of breast cancer presented with right hip pain and had an ill-defined area of sclerosis in the right supra-acetabular region (compare with the opposite side). A biopsy was requested, but the radiologist thought this might represent an insufficiency fracture. Magnetic resonance imaging (MRI) was obtained (B) that revealed a curvilinear fracture line *(arrow)*, which is characteristic for a supra-acetabular insufficiency fracture.

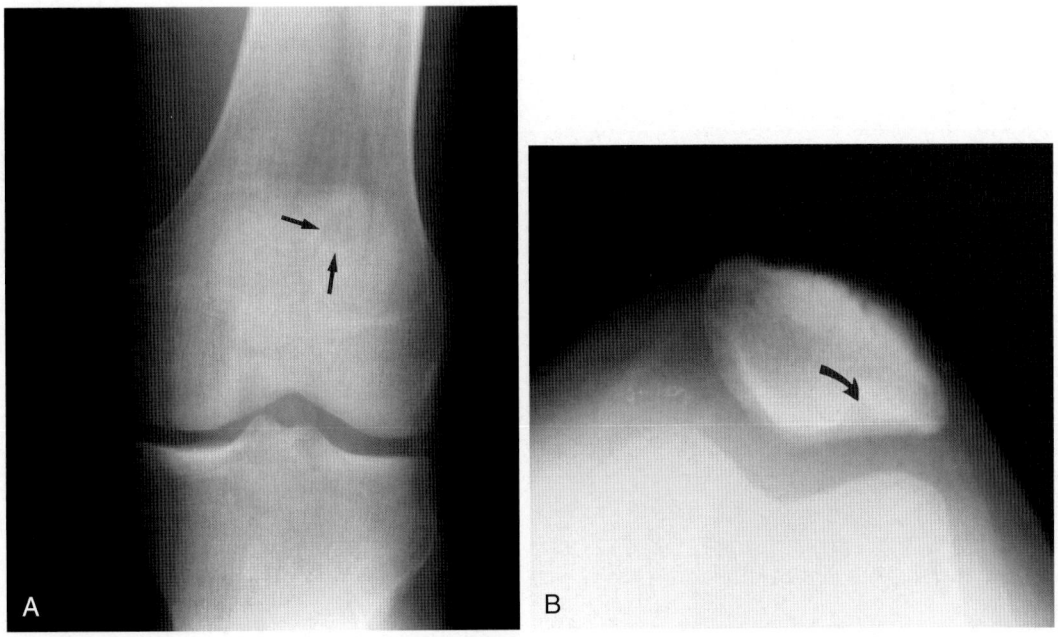

FIG. 4.20 **Dorsal Defect of the Patella.** A lytic defect in the upper outer quadrant of the patella (A) was seen in this patient *(arrows)*, which is characteristic for a normal variant called dorsal defect of the patella. It occurs only in the upper outer quadrant and should be asymptomatic. It lies adjacent to the articular surface as shown on the sunrise view (B).

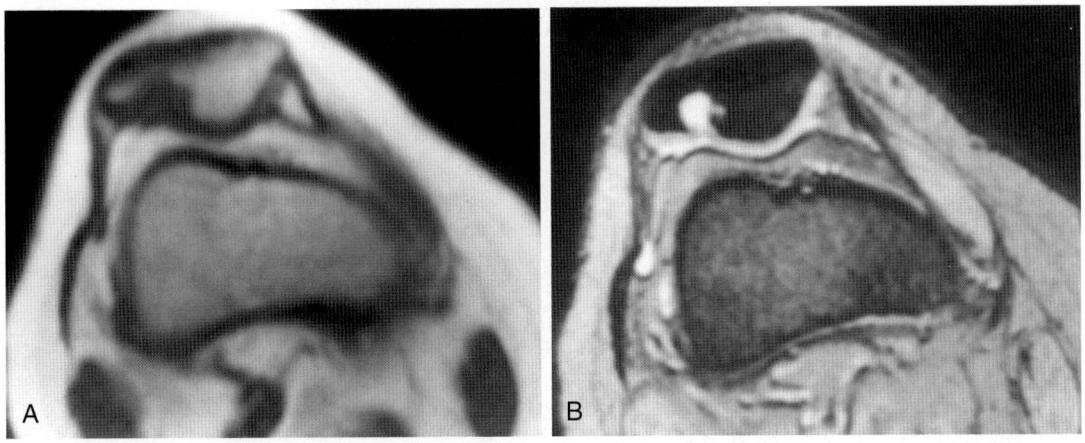

FIG. 4.21 **Magnetic Resonance (MR) Images of Dorsal Defect of the Patella.** (A) T1-weighted and (B) T2-weighted axial MR images through the patella in a patient with a lytic lesion in the upper outer quadrant of the patella shows low signal on the T1 image, which is high signal on T2. This is a characteristic appearance for a dorsal defect of the patella because of its location.

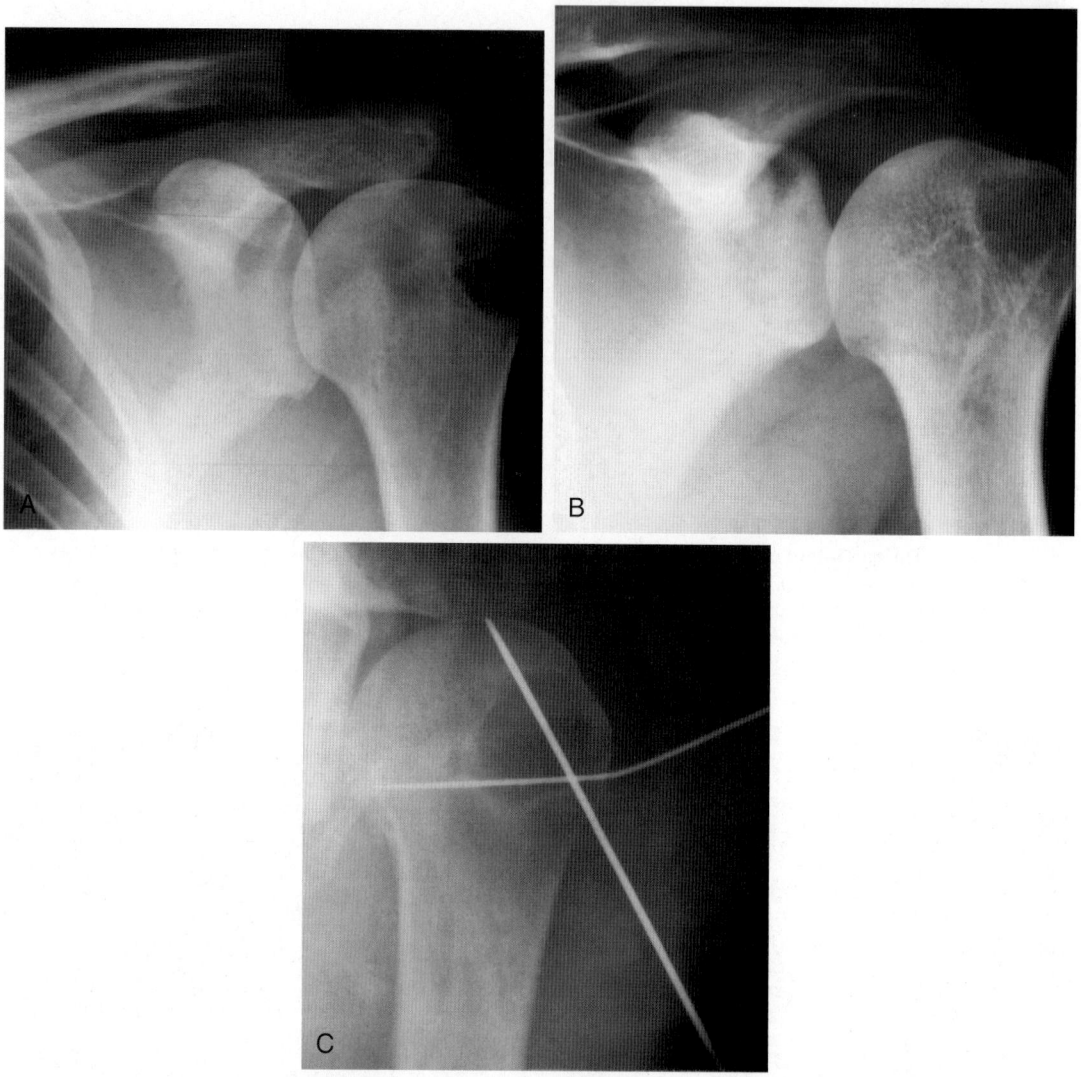

FIG. 4.22 **Pseudocyst of the Humerus.** (A, B, C) A well-defined lytic process is seen in the greater tuberosity in each of these examples. In each case it was believed to represent a lytic lesion. These patients were all symptomatic, and several had increased radionuclide uptake on isotope bone scan. The location and appearance, however, are characteristic for a pseudocyst of the humerus, which merely represents decreased cortical bone in this region. This becomes more pronounced when pain in the shoulder is present and hyperemia or disuse osteoporosis occurs. Biopsies of several of these examples were performed, and a biopsy was repeated in the example in (C) when the first biopsy was reported as "normal bone," and the surgeons assumed that they had missed the lesion. It was localized with K-wires at the second surgery to make certain it was not missed. This is an intra-operative film.

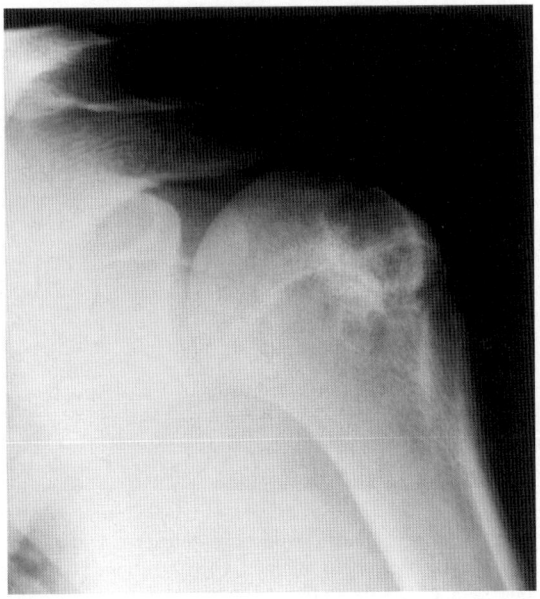

FIG. 4.23 **Chondroblastoma.** A well-defined lesion in the greater tuberosity of the humerus that has a sclerotic margin is easily distinguished from the prior examples of pseudocyst of the humerus. This was found to be a chondroblastoma.

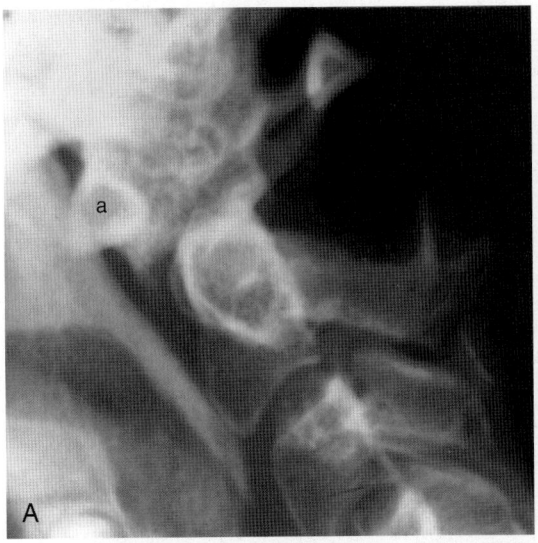

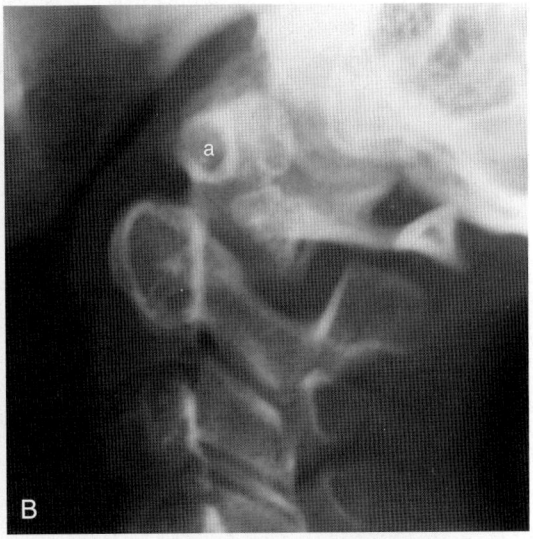

FIG. 4.24 **Os Odontoideum.** Flexion (A) and extension (B) views show that the anterior arch (*a*) of the C-1 vertebrae has moved markedly posterior in relation to the body of C-2 in extension. The odontoid or dens is difficult to see but appears to be separated from the body of C-2. Because of the smooth borders of the separated dens and because of the cortical hypertrophy of the anterior arch of C-1, this can safely be called an os odontoideum, which is a congenital or long-standing posttraumatic abnormality rather than an acute fracture. Obviously these patients should have no neurologic problems, yet in many instances the lesions are still felt to be unstable and are surgically fused. Surgery, if indicated, can be done on an elective basis.

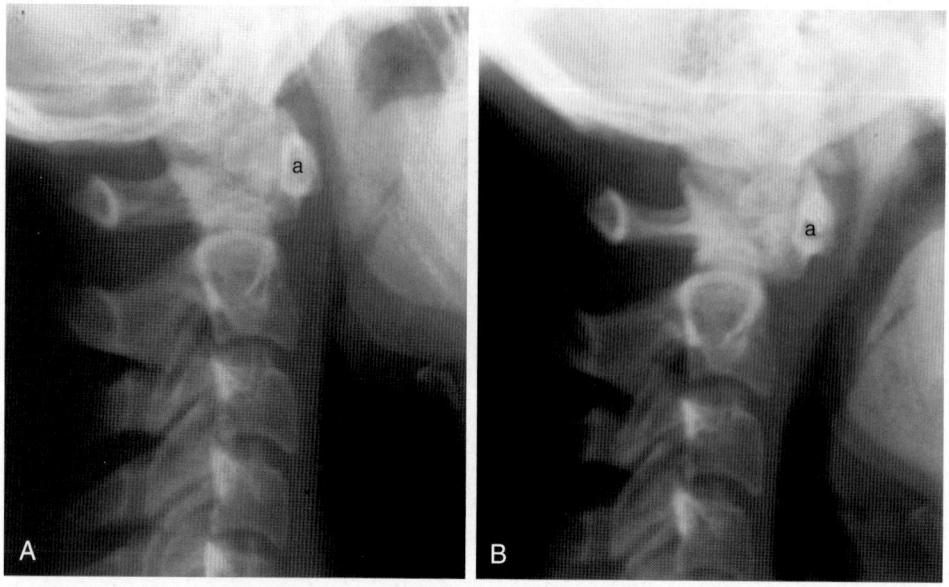

FIG. 4.25 **Os Odontoideum.** Extension (A) and flexion (B) show extreme motion of the anterior arch (a) of C-1 as compared with the C-2 vertebral body. The dens is difficult to find in this example but is certainly not attached to the C-2 body. Again, the smooth margins where the dens should be attached and the cortical hypertrophy of the anterior arch of C-1 make this a congenital or long-standing process consistent with an os odontoideum rather than an acute fracture.

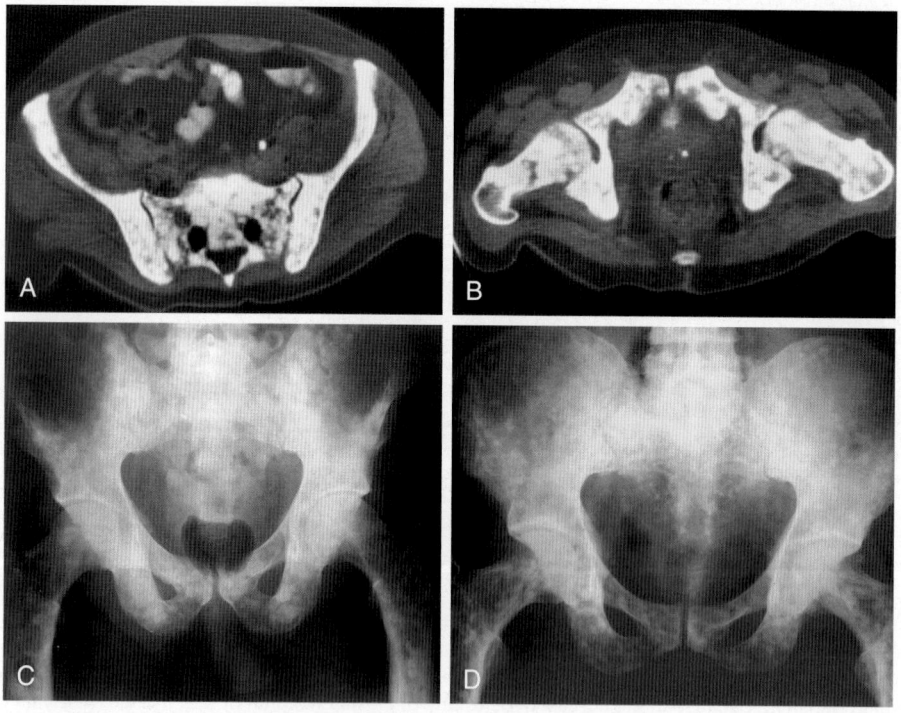

FIG. 4.26 **Diffuse Metastatic Disease Mimicking Osteopoikilosis.** (A, B) A computed tomography (CT) scan through the pelvis and hips shows diffuse sclerotic foci consistent with metastatic disease. One examiner felt that this might represent the sclerotic foci of osteopoikilosis, however, which is a benign familial process. (C) An anteroposterior view of the pelvis shows a similar appearance; however, a destructive lytic lesion is seen in the right proximal femur, which makes metastatic disease more likely. This patient had metastatic prostate carcinoma. Compare this with (D) in a patient with known osteopoikilosis, and it is easy to see how the two entities can be confused. Clinical history is vital in the distinction.

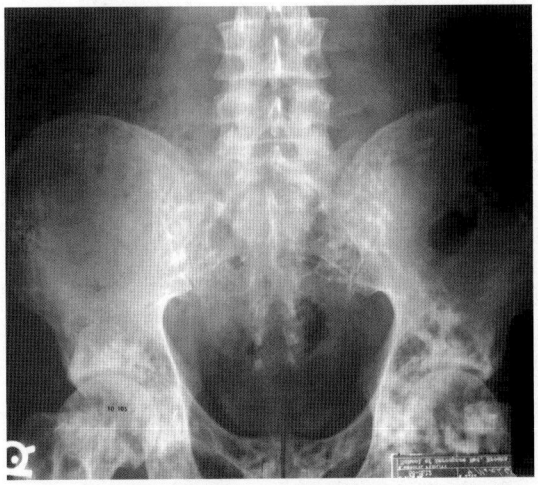

FIG. 4.27 **Osteopoikilosis.** A more typical example of osteopoikilosis is shown in this example, in which the sclerotic foci are predominantly around the joints rather than diffusely spread throughout the bones.

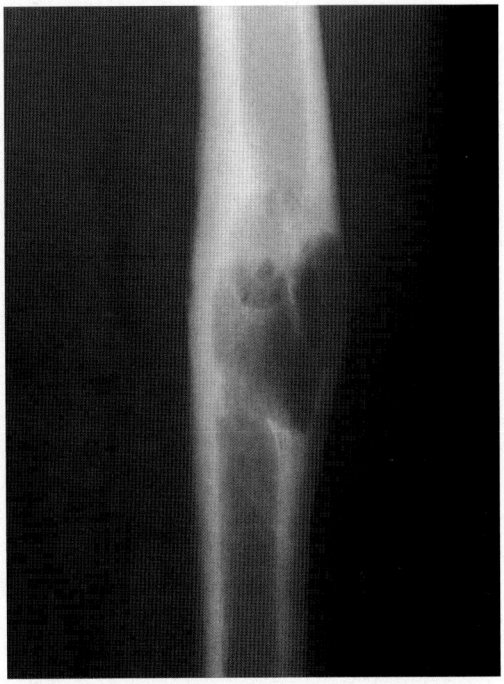

FIG. 4.28 **Nonossifying Fibroma.** A well-defined, slightly expansile lytic lesion is seen in a long bone, which is characteristic for a nonossifying fibroma. Unfortunately a biopsy of the lesion was performed, and the diagnosis was surgically confirmed.

disorders head the differential list and a biopsy soon ensues. If this process can be noted to be multiple and in the diametaphyseal region of a long bone, especially if the patient has an underlying disorder such as sickle cell anemia or systemic lupus erythematosus, areas of early bone infarction should be considered. In several instances, the MRI appearance of an infarct has saved patients from biopsy when the plain films were equivocal (Fig. 4.37).[11]

A commonly encountered lytic lesion on the lateral aspect of the femoral neck was first described by Michael Pitt as a synovial herniation pit.[12] It has taken on the appropriate eponym of a "Pitt's pit." It is felt to be caused by surface erosion of the synovium and soft tissues around the hip, but its exact etiology is unknown. It has a characteristic plain film and MR appearance primarily because of its location and benign appearance (Fig. 4.38). They are found much more frequently in patients with fermo-acetabular impingement, a process in which the femoral neck abuts the rim of the acetabulum when the hip is abducted (see Chapter 13). It is thought this likely results in cystic changes in the underlying femoral neck—a Pitt's pit.

CONCLUSION

These are but a few of the many examples in skeletal radiology in which the well-trained radiologist can be of invaluable assistance to the clinician and the patient by helping to avert a needless biopsy. Dozens of other examples are nicely shown in normal variant textbooks, which are widely available. Because of the potential harm in performing a needless biopsy, these examples are stressed. When these lesions are encountered by the radiologist, a differential diagnosis should not be

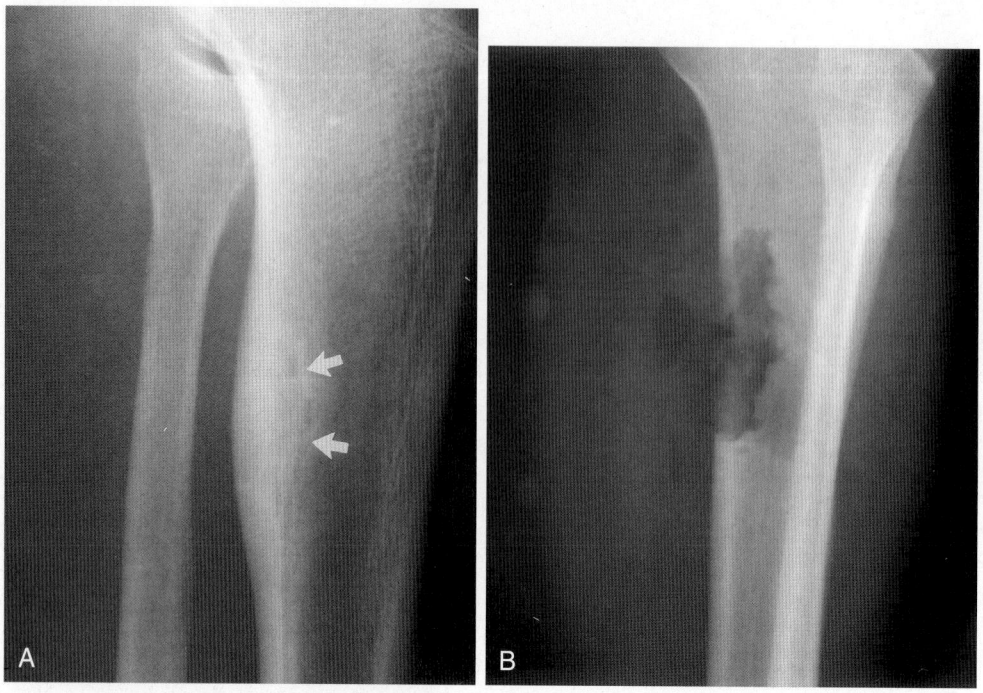

FIG. 4.29 **Resolving Nonossifying Fibroma.** (A) A minimally sclerotic, slightly expansile process is seen in the posterior proximal tibia *(arrows)*. This was felt by the surgeons to represent a focus of infection or an osteoid osteoma, even though the patient was asymptomatic. This is a characteristic appearance for a disappearing or resolving nonossifying fibroma. The postsurgical appearance, which went on to a pathologic fracture, is shown in (B). Surgery confirmed a nonossifying fibroma.

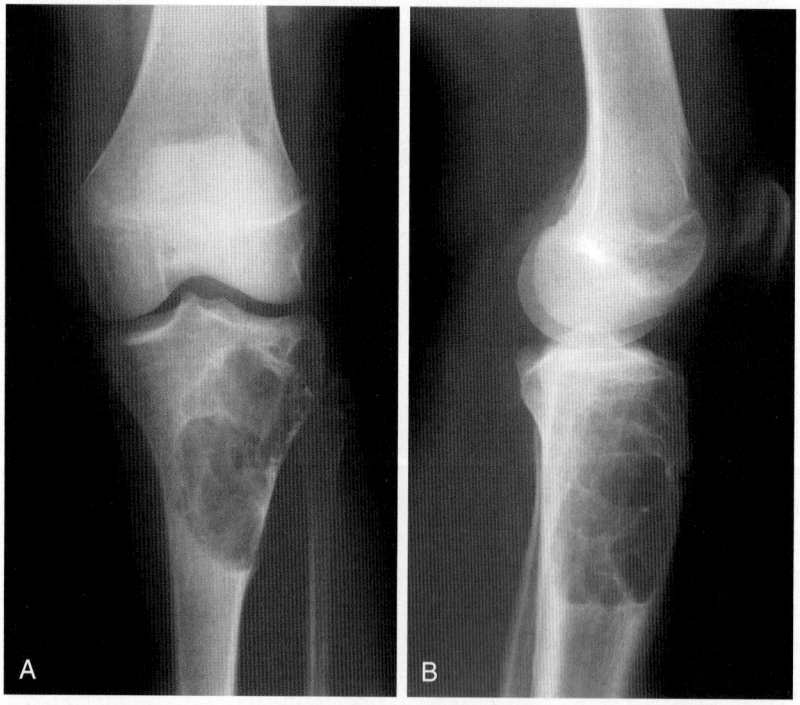

FIG. 4.30 **Nonossifying Fibroma.** (A and B) This well-defined, minimally expansile lytic lesion of the proximal tibia is characteristic for a nonossifying fibroma. It was felt by several radiologists to be a giant cell tumor; however, it has a sclerotic border and does not abut the tibial articular surface. Even though the patient was asymptomatic, a biopsy was performed and the diagnosis of a nonossifying fibroma was confirmed.

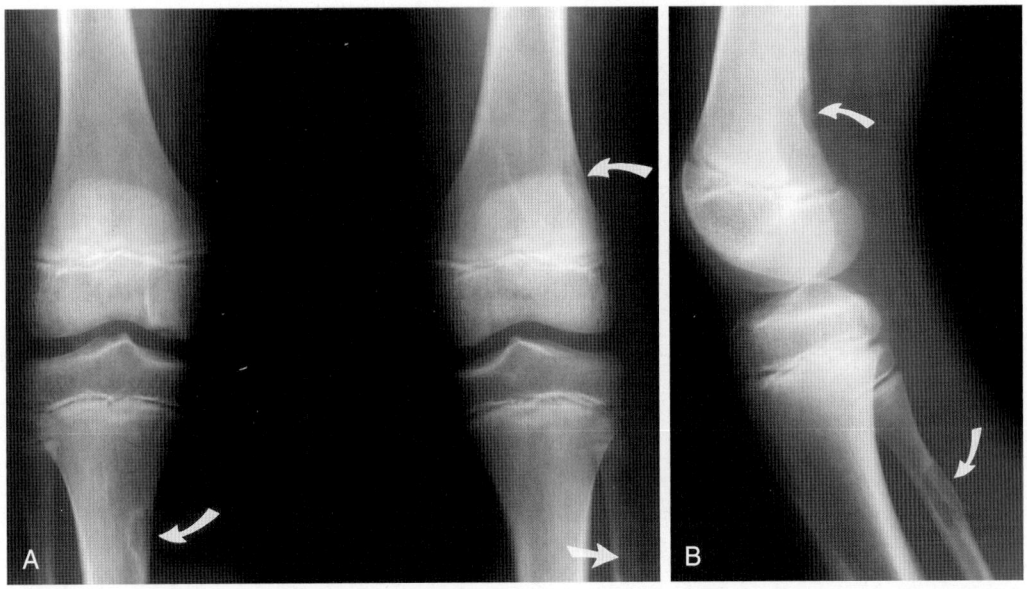

FIG. 4.31 **Multiple Nonossifying Fibromas.** Multiple well-defined lytic lesions *(arrows)* are seen around the knees in this patient on the anteroposterior (A) and lateral (B) views, each of which is characteristic for a nonossifying fibroma.

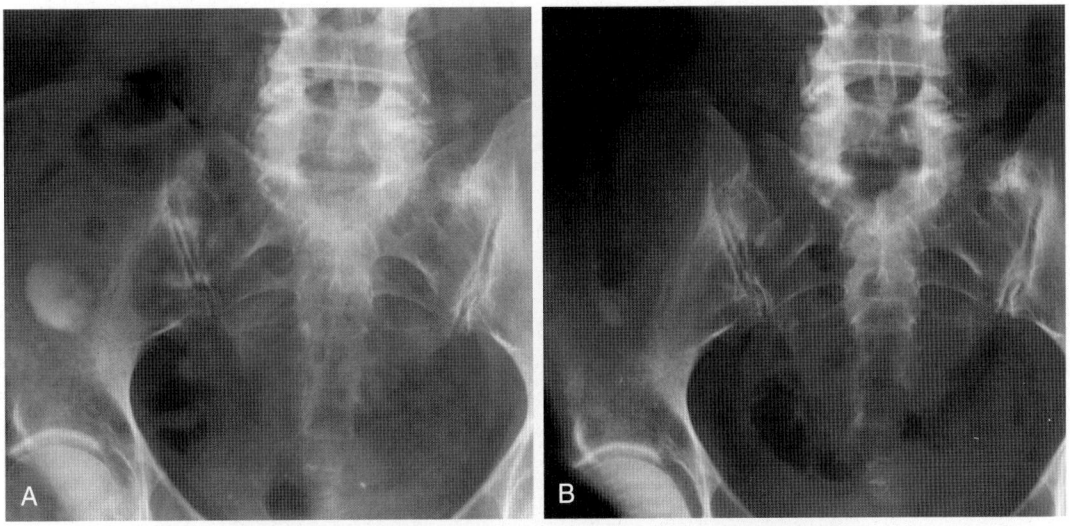

FIG. 4.32 **Giant Bone Island.** (A) A large sclerotic focus is seen in the right iliac wing *(arrow)*, which was thought to possibly represent an area of metastasis. (B) Old films from 5 years earlier were obtained, which showed a similar but much smaller process (arrow). This is characteristic for a growing bone island. Note in (A) how the lesion is somewhat spherical or oblong in the lines of trabecular stress, which is characteristic of a bone island.

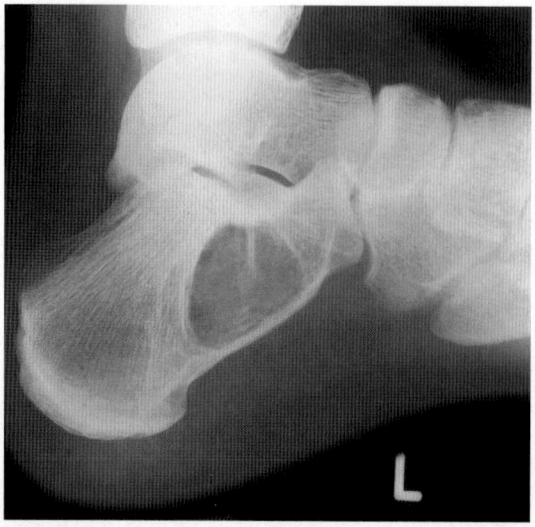

FIG. 4.33 **Unicameral Bone Cyst.** A well-defined lytic lesion on the anteroinferior portion of the calcaneus, as in this example, is virtually pathognomonic for a unicameral bone cyst or simple bone cyst. Because this is an area of diminished stress, it is thought not to be necessary to prophylactically curettage and pack this lesion in an effort to avoid a pathologic bone fracture, which is occasionally done in the femur and humerus with unicameral bone cysts.

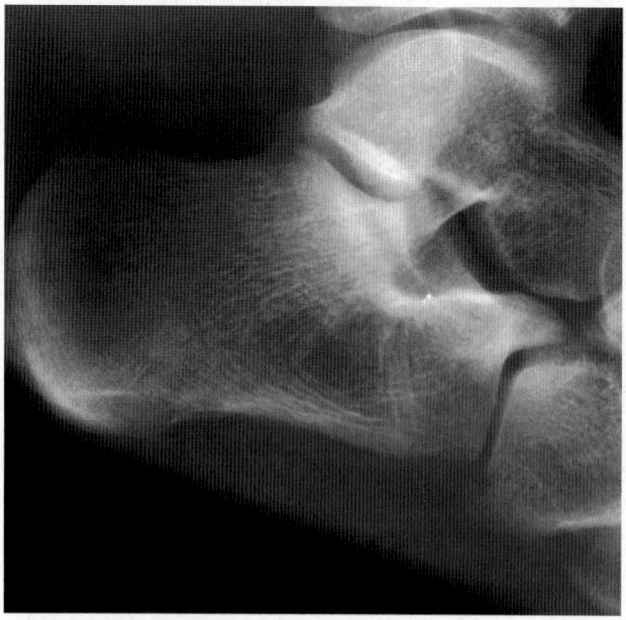

FIG. 4.34 **Pseudocyst of the Calcaneus.** An area of radiolucency is seen in the anteroinferior portion of the calcaneus that is similar to the example in Fig. 4.33 but is not as well defined. This is a pseudocyst similar to the pseudocyst of the humerus that results from diminished stress through this region.

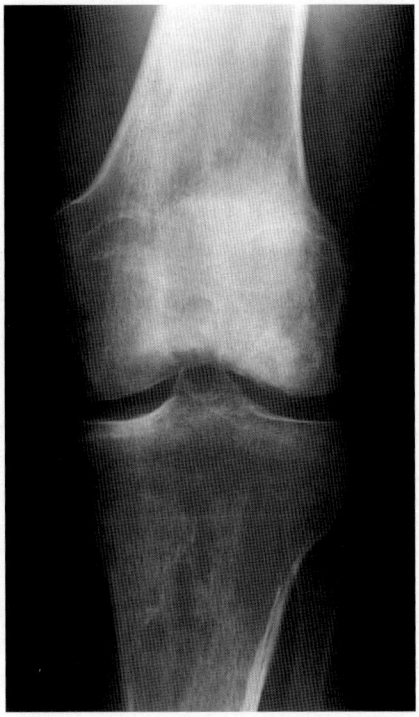

FIG. 4.35 **Early Bone Infarct.** Patchy demineralization is seen in the distal femur and proximal tibia in this patient with systemic lupus erythematosus. The opposite leg was similarly involved. This is characteristic for early bone infarcts and should not be confused with infection or metastatic disease.

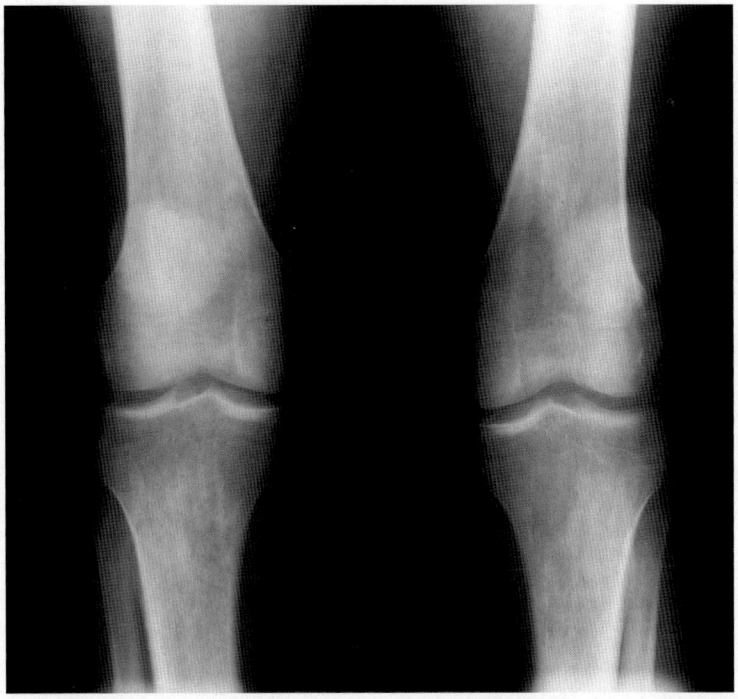

FIG. 4.36 **Bone Infarct.** A mixed lytic–sclerotic process is seen in the distal femurs and proximal tibias bilaterally in this patient with systemic lupus erythematosus. Because of pain in these regions, a biopsy was performed, and bone infarct was confirmed. With this characteristic location and this appearance, even though suggestive of a more aggressive process, a biopsy of these lesions should not be performed.

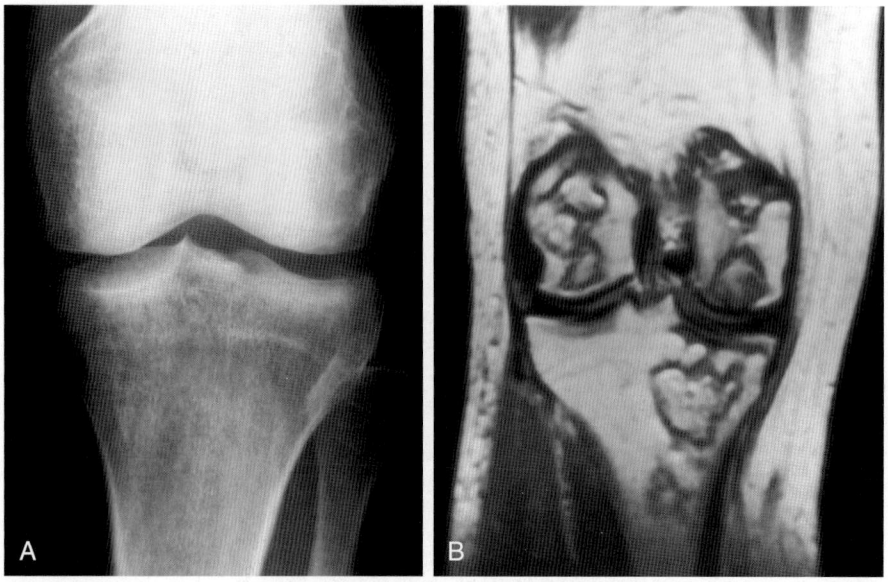

FIG. 4.37 **Bone Infarct.** (A) A plain film of the knee shows faint patchy sclerosis in the proximal tibia that was at first thought to be infection or malignancy. (B) Magnetic resonance imaging (MRI) shows the characteristic serpiginous border seen with bone infarct. MRI can on occasion better characterize the ill-defined early bone infarct, as in this example.

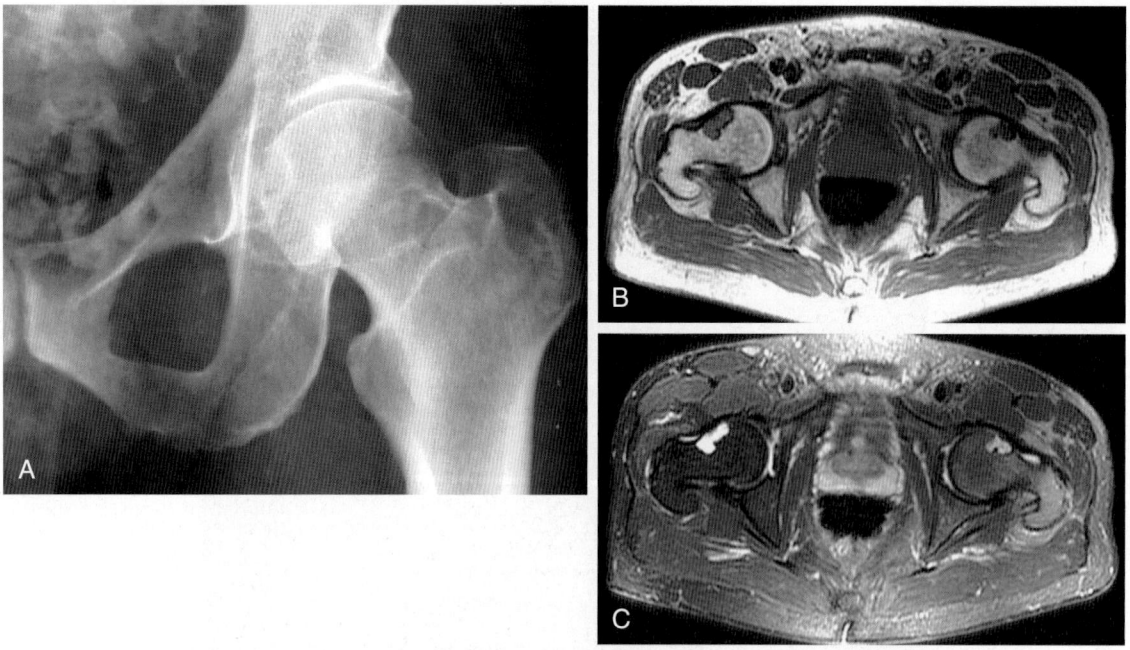

FIG. 4.38 **Pitt's Pit.** (A) A plain film of the left hip shows a well-defined lytic lesion in the lateral aspect of the femoral neck. It has a sclerotic border. This is a characteristic appearance of a synovial herniation pit, also called a Pitt's pit. (B) T1-weighted and (C) T2-weighted magnetic resonance (MR) axial images through the hips show bilateral lesions with low-signal T1 and high-signal T2, which is typical for Pitt's pits.

offered, as it will merely lead the surgeon to a biopsy in an attempt to reach a diagnosis. A biopsy in many of these entities not only is unnecessary, but also can be misleading.

REFERENCES

1. Barnes G, Gwinn J. Distal irregularities of the femur simulating malignancy. *AJR*. 1974;122:180.
2. Resnick D, Niwayama G, Coutts RD. Subchondral cysts (geodes) in arthritic disorders: pathologic and radiographic appearance of the hip joint. *AJR*. 1977;128:799.
3. Martel W, Seeger FJ, Wicks JD, et al. Traumatic lesions of the discovertebral junction in the lumbar spine. *AJR*. 1976;127:457.
4. Lipson S. Discogenic vertebral sclerosis with calcified disc. *New Engl J Med*. 1991;325:794–799.
5. Helms C, Richmond B, Sims R. Pseudodislocation of the shoulder: a sign of an occult fracture. *Emer Med*. 1986;18:237–241.
6. Goergen TG, Resnick D, Greenway G, et al. Dorsal defect of the patella (DDP): a characteristic radiographic lesion. *Radiology*. 1979;130:333.
7. Helms C. Pseudocyst of the humerus. *AJR*. 1979;131:287–292.
8. Minderhoud JM, Braakman R, Penning L. Os odontoideum: clinical, radiological and therapeutic aspects. *J Neurol Sci*. 1969;8:521.
9. Holt RG, Helms CA, Munk PL, Gillespy III T. Hypertrophy of C-1 anterior arch: useful sign to distinguish os odontoideum from acute dens fracture. *Radiology*. 1989;173:207–209.
10. Onitsuka H. Roentgenologic aspects of bone islands. *Radiology*. 1977;124:607.
11. Munk PL, Helms CA, Holt RG. Immature bone infarcts: findings on plain radiographs and MR scans. *AJR*. 1989;152(3):547–549.
12. Pitt M, Graham A, Shipman J, Birkby W. Herniation pit of the femoral neck. *AJR*. 1982;138:1115–1121.

CHAPTER 5

Trauma

Radiology of trauma to the skeletal system is such a large topic that entire volumes have been devoted to it. Lee Rogers has written the definitive work in his excellent book entitled *Radiology of Skeletal Trauma*,[1] and Jack and William Harris' outstanding book on *Radiology of Emergency Medicine*[2] is a must read for anyone dealing with a large emergency department population. The leading orthopedic treatise on fractures is Rockwood and Green's multivolume text.[3] The following is merely an overview of selected cases that residents and medical students should be exposed to that can be studied in greater detail by referring to the texts mentioned above.

Before starting with specific examples, the uninitiated or neophyte radiologist should keep a few key points in mind concerning radiology of trauma. First, have a high index of suspicion. Every radiologist in the world has missed fractures on radiographs because they were not sufficiently attuned to the fact that a fracture might be present. Oftentimes the history is either nonexistent or misleading, and the anatomical area of concern is therefore overlooked. When in doubt, examine the patient! Orthopedic surgeons seldom miss seeing fractures on radiographs because they have examined the patient, they know where the patient hurts, and they have a high index of suspicion. Second, always get two radiographs at 90 degrees to each other in every trauma case. A high percentage of fractures are seen only on one view [the anteroposterior (AP) or the lateral] and will therefore be missed unless two views are routinely obtained. Third, once a fracture is identified, don't forget to look at the rest of the film. About 10% of all cases have a second finding that often is as significant as, or even more significant than, the initial finding. Many fractures have associated dislocation, foreign bodies, or additional fractures, so be sure to examine the entire film.

SPINE

Examination of the Cervical Spine

The cervical spine (C-spine) is one of the most commonly radiographed parts of the body in a busy emergency department, and can present the most difficulty in interpretation. Usually a cross-table lateral of the C-spine is obtained first, so as not to unduly move the patient who might have a cervical fracture. If the lateral C- spine appears normal, the remainder of the C-spine series, which may include flexion and extension views (if the patient can cooperate), is obtained.

What do you look for on the lateral C-spine? First, make certain that all seven cervical vertebral bodies can be visualized. A number of fractures are missed because the shoulders obscure the lower C-spine levels (Fig. 5.1). If the entire C-spine is not visualized, repeat the film with the shoulders lowered.

What constitutes complete visualization of the C-spine? Many radiologists insist on seeing the top of the T1 vertebral body on the lateral view, while others will pass a C-spine lateral film if it includes any of the C-2 body. Most texts say the lateral view should show "C-1 through C-7." What does "through C-7" mean? I have no idea, but I was trained to accept a lateral C-spine film that included *any* of the C-7 body. It can be difficult to image the T-1 vertebral body in the majority of cases; therefore I feel it is acceptable to accept a lateral C-spine film with *any* of the C-7 vertebral body visible if the report includes the disclaimer that the C-7 to T-1 disc space is not seen and clinical correlation must be obtained to warrant additional films or a computed tomography (CT) of that area. In fact, this is a moot point in many practices who routinely acquire CT throughout the C-spine instead of plain films. Complete CT evaluation of the C-spine will probably evolve to be the standard of care, but is not yet widely accepted as the normal routine.

Next, evaluate five parallel (more or less) lines for step-offs or discontinuity as follows (Fig. 5.2A and B):

Line number 1 is in the prevertebral soft tissue. It extends down the posterior aspect of the airway; it should be several millimeters from the first three or four vertebral bodies and then move farther away at the laryngeal cartilage; it should be less than one vertebral body width from the anterior vertebral bodies from C-3 or C-4 to C-7; and it should be smooth in its contour.

Line 2 follows the anterior vertebral bodies and should be smooth and uninterrupted. Anterior osteophytes can encroach on this line and extend beyond it, and should therefore be ignored in drawing this line.

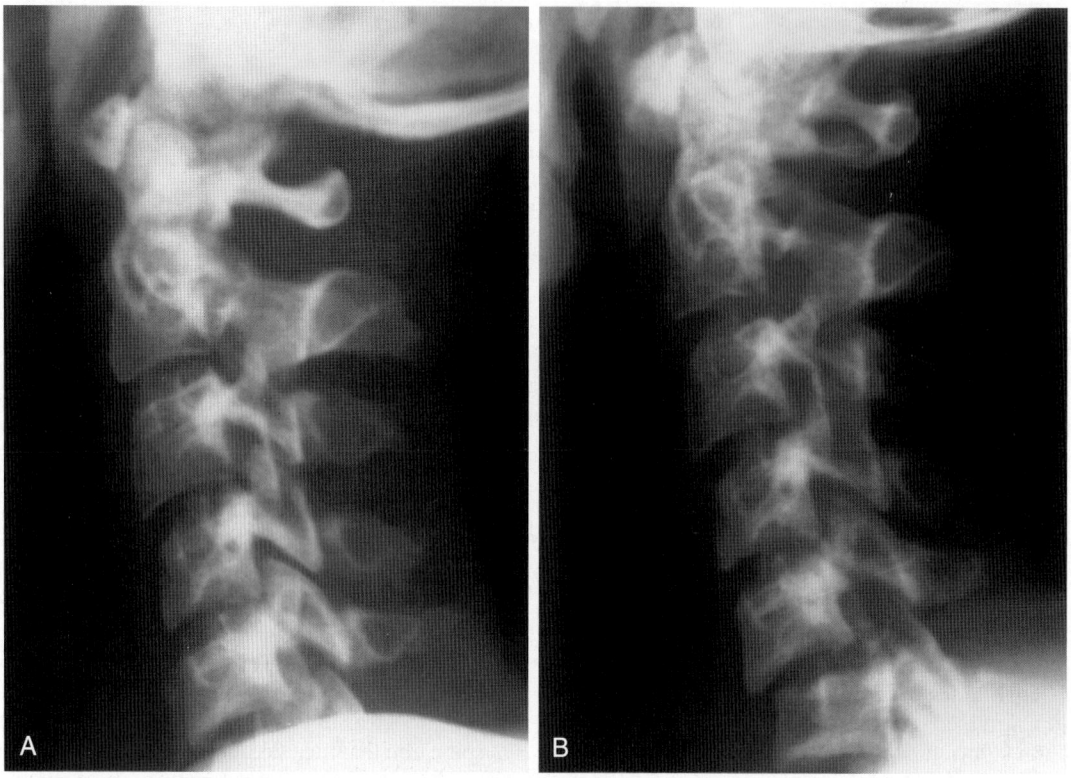

FIG. 5.1 **Shoulders Obscuring C-7.** This patient came to the emergency department after being injured as a result of diving into a shallow swimming pool. He had neck pain but no neurologic deficits. The initial radiograph obtained of the cervical spine (C-spine) (A) was interpreted as being within normal limits. However, because of high-riding shoulders, only five cervical vertebrae are visible. A repeat examination (B) with the shoulders lowered reveals a dislocation of C-5 on C-6. To visualize C-7, the shoulders were lowered even farther. The C-7 vertebral body must be visualized on every lateral C-spine examination in a trauma setting.

Interruption of the anterior vertebral body line is a sign of a serious injury (Fig. 5.1B).

Line 3 is similar to the anterior vertebral body line (line 2) except that it connects the posterior vertebral bodies. Like line 2, it should be smooth and uninterrupted; any disruption signifies a serious injury.

Line 4, called the spinolaminal line, connects the posterior junction of the lamina with the spinous processes. The spinal cord lies between lines 3 and 4; therefore any offset of either of these lines could mean that a bony structure is impinging on the cord. Severe neurologic deficits can result from very little force against the cord, and any bony structure lying on the cord must be recognized as soon as possible.

Line 5 is not really a line so much as a collection of points—the tips of the spinous processes. The spinous processes are quite variable in size and appearance, although C-7 usually has the largest. A fracture of one of the spinous processes, by itself, is not a serious injury, but it occasionally heralds other, more serious injuries. Also, who wants to miss a fractured spinous process, however innocuous, and then have the patient (after visiting another doctor) proclaim that you didn't see her "broken neck" on the radiograph?

After visually inspecting these five lines on the lateral C-spine, then inspect the C1–2 area a little more closely. Make certain that the anterior arch of C-1 is no greater than 2.5 mm from the dens (Figs. 5.3A and B). Any greater separation than this (except in children, in whom up to 5.0 mm is normal) is suspicious for disruption of the transverse ligament between C-1 and C-2 (Figs. 5.4A and B).

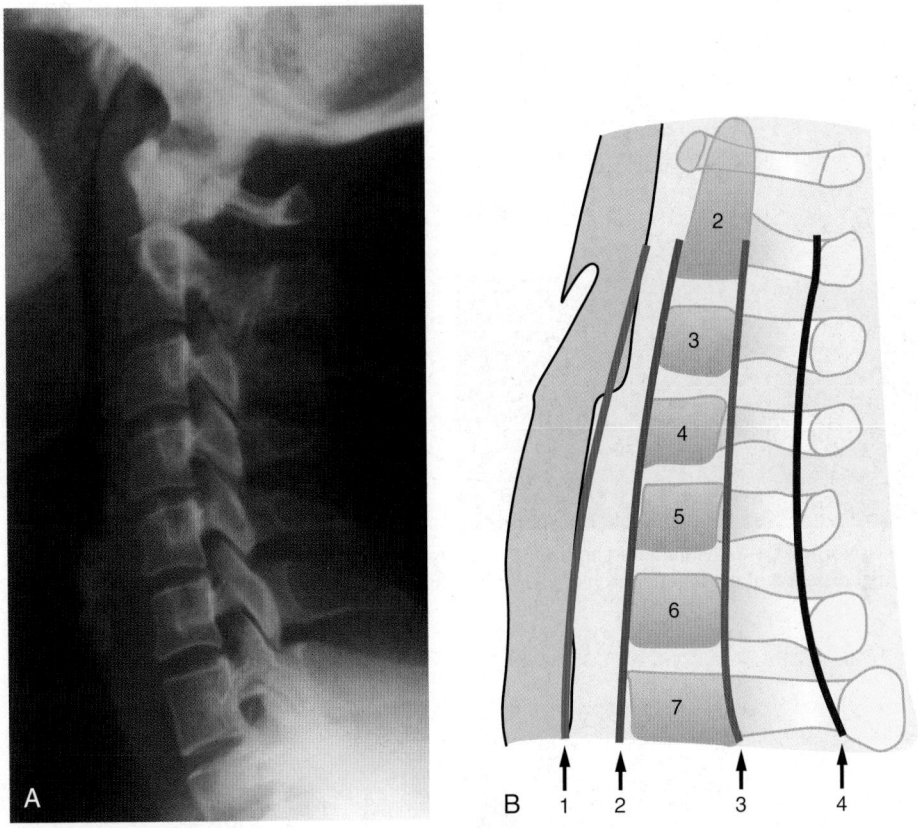

FIG. 5.2 **Normal Lateral Cervical Spine.** (A) Lateral radiograph of a normal cervical spine. (B) Diagrammatic representation of a lateral cervical spine (C-spine) showing four parallel lines that should be observed in every lateral C-spine examination. Line 1 is the soft tissue line that is closely applied to the posterior border of the airway through the first four or five vertebral body segments and then widens around the laryngeal cartilage and runs parallel to the remainder of the cervical vertebrae. Line 2 demarcates the anterior border of the cervical vertebral bodies. Line 3 is the posterior border of the cervical vertebral bodies. Line 4, called the spinolaminal line, is drawn by connecting the junction of the lamina at the spinous process. It represents the posterior extent of the central canal, which contains the spinal cord itself. These lines should generally be smooth and parallel, with no abrupt step-offs.

The disc spaces are examined next to see that there is no inordinate widening or narrowing, either of which could indicate an acute traumatic injury. If a disc space is narrowed, it will usually be secondary to degenerative disease. Make certain that associated osteophytosis and sclerosis are present, however, before assuming the narrowing is due to degenerative disease.

An examination of the lateral C-spine, as described above, can be done in less than 1 minute. If this view is normal, then the remainder of the examination can be completed, including flexion and extension views. It is imperative that the patient initiate the flexion and extension without help from the technician or anyone else. A patient, if conscious and semialert, will not injure himself with voluntary flexion and extension, and will have muscle guarding, preventing motion, if an injury is present. Even gentle pressure to aid in flexion or extension can cause severe injury if a fracture or dislocation is present.

I would like to stress the importance of learning to look at lateral spine films with anterior facing either right or left. Many radiologists can only interpret images facing one way, and become almost unable to function if the films are not placed on the viewbox in their preferred orientation. This is fine if they can control the film; however, in meetings where slides are shown, in books and journals, and on oral board exams, they cannot turn the film to

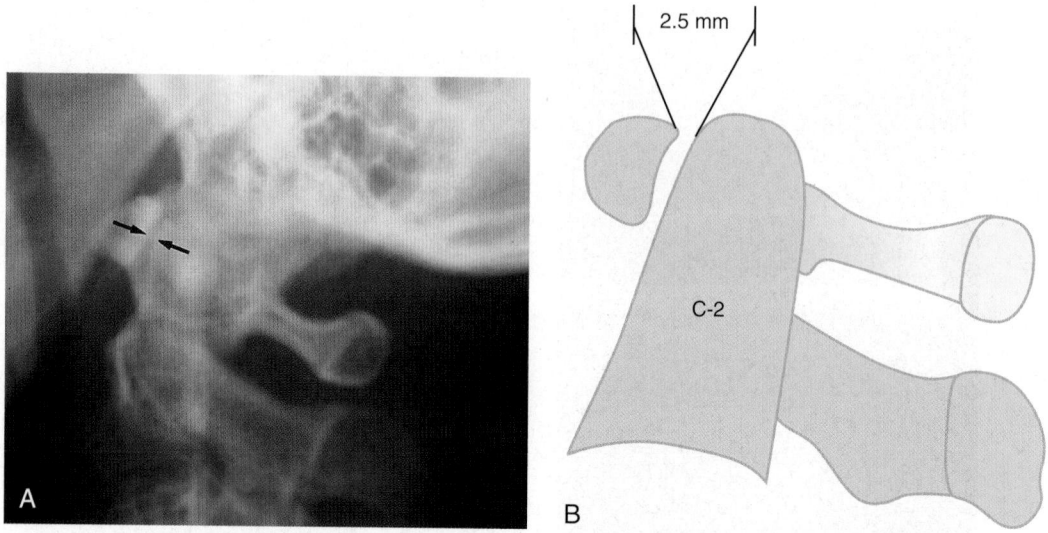

FIG. 5.3 **Normal C1-2.** A lateral radiograph (A) and drawing (B) of the upper cervical spine, showing the normal distance of the anterior arch of C-1 to be less than 2.5 mm from the odontoid process of C-2 *(arrows)*.

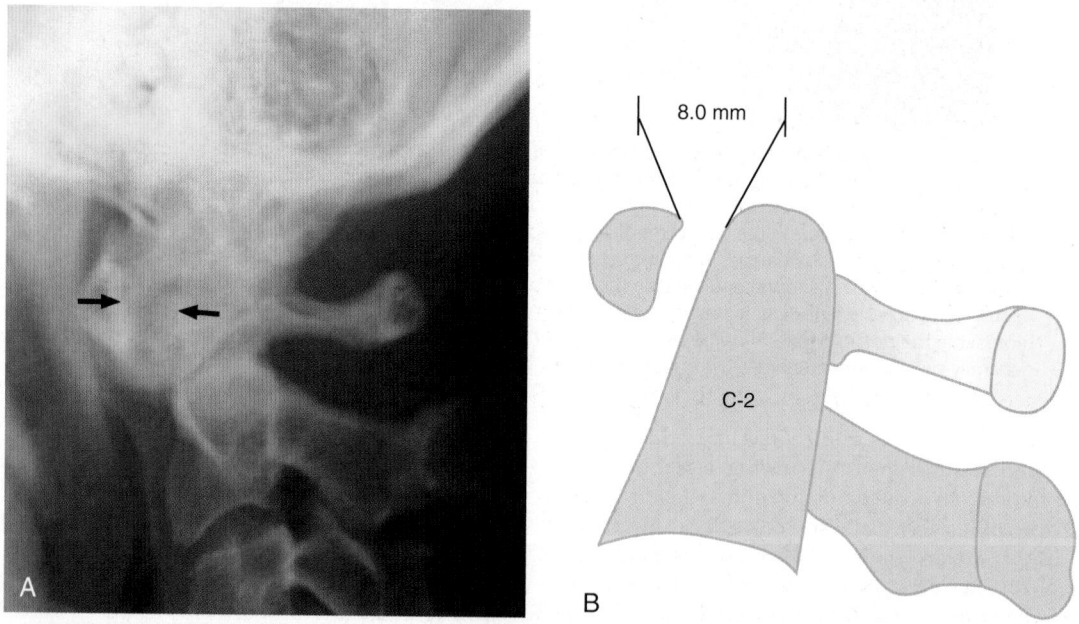

FIG. 5.4 **C1-2 Dislocation.** A lateral radiograph (A) and drawing (B) of the upper cervical spine in a patient with trauma to the neck, which shows that the anterior arch of C-1 is 9 mm anterior to the odontoid process of C-2 *(arrows)*. This is diagnostic of a dislocation of C-1 on C-2, and indicates rupture of the transverse ligaments, which normally hold these vertebral segments together.

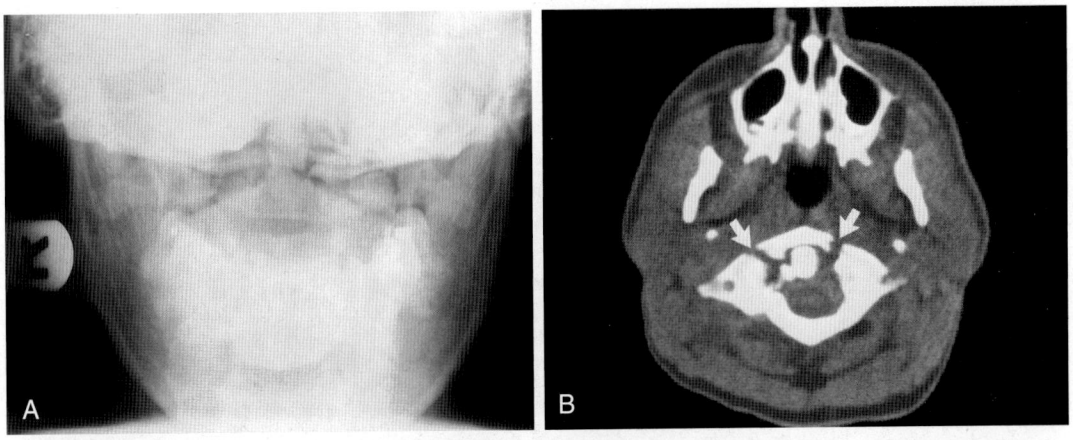

FIG. 5.5 **Jefferson Fracture.** An anteroposterior (AP) open-mouth odontoid view (A) is suspicious for the lateral masses of C-1 being laterally displaced. However, because of overlying structures, this displacement is difficult to appreciate. Therefore a computed tomography (CT) examination (B) was obtained, which shows multiple fracture sites in the C-1 ring *(arrows)*. This is called a Jefferson fracture. CT is routinely used in spinal trauma because of the obvious shortcomings of plain films.

their liking. Get used to viewing lateral spine films (lateral chest films, too) in either anterior left or right orientation, or you will find yourself disadvantaged in many situations.

Examples of Fractures, Dislocations, and Other Abnormalities

A blow to the top of the head, such as when an object falls directly on the apex of the skull, can cause the lateral masses of C-1 to slide apart, splitting the bony ring of C-1. This is called a *Jefferson fracture* (Fig. 5.5). It nicely illustrates how a bony ring will not break in just one place, but must break in several places. This rule is seldom violated. All of the vertebral rings, when fractured, must fracture in two or more places. The bony rings of the pelvis behave the same way. If you see only one fracture on the radiograph, you're certainly missing at least one more. CT is excellent at demonstrating the complete bony ring of C-1, and shows the fractures, as well as any associated soft tissue mass, much better than plain films. In diagnosing a Jefferson fracture on plain film, the lateral masses of C-1 must extend beyond the margins of the C-2 body (Fig. 5.5A). Just seeing asymmetry of the spaces on either side of the dens is not enough to make the diagnosis, as these spaces can be normally asymmetric with rotation.

A relatively innocuous injury is a fracture of the C-6 or C-7 spinous process, called a *clay-shoveler fracture*. Supposedly workers shoveling sticky clay in Australia (I've also read England and North Carolina—this is a vital distinction, and some future researcher can perhaps straighten out this confusion) would toss the shovelfuls of clay over their shoulders; once in a while, the clay would stick to the shovel, causing the ligaments attached to the spinous processes (supraspinous ligaments) to undergo a tremendous force, pulling on the spinous process and avulsing it. This fracture can occur at any of the lower cervical spinous processes (Fig. 5.6).

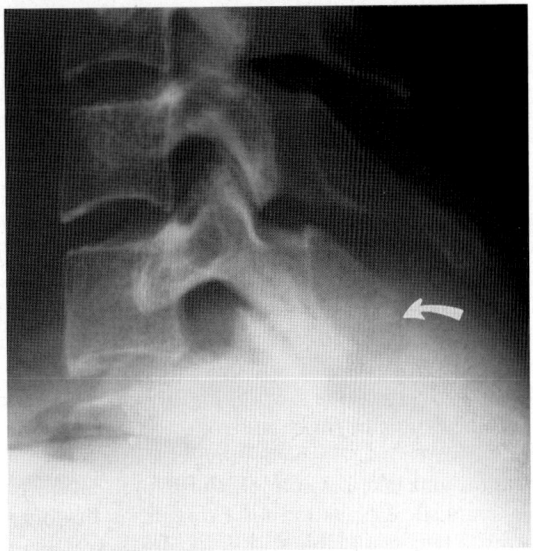

FIG. 5.6 **Clay-Shoveler Fracture.** A nondisplaced fracture of the C-7 spinous process *(arrow)* is noted, which is diagnostic of a clay-shoveler fracture.

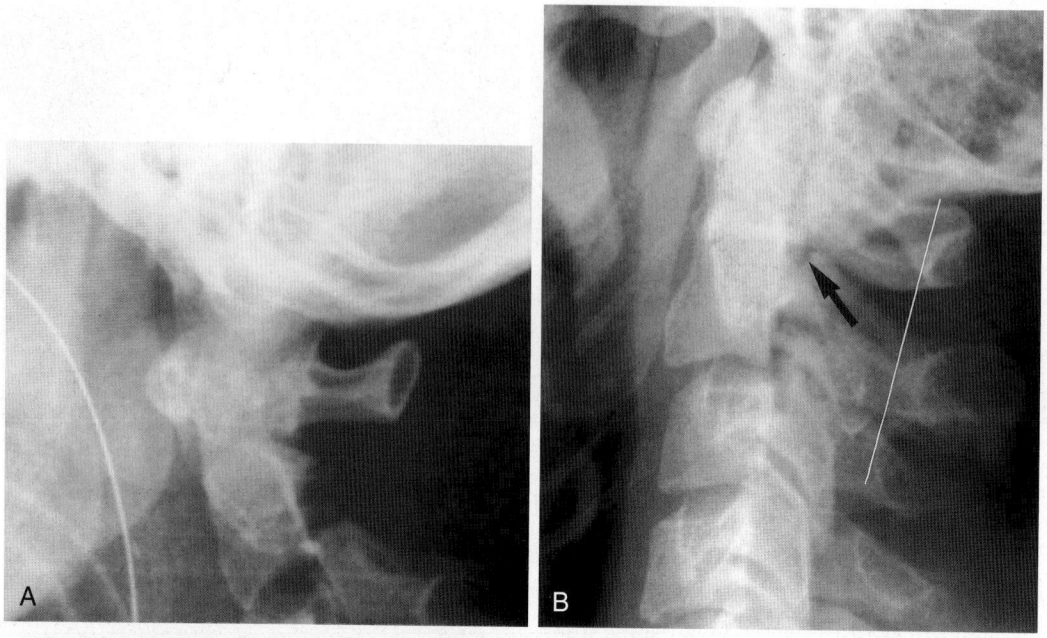

FIG. 5.7 **Hangman's Fracture.** (A) A lateral film of a patient with a hangman's fracture shows an obvious example of the posterior elements of the C-2 vertebral body fractured and displaced inferiorly. (B) The film of another patient shows a subtle fracture through the posterior elements of C-2 *(arrow)*. A line drawn through the spinolaminal lines of the posterior elements shows the C-2 spinolaminal line to be offset in this example.

A *hangman's fracture* is an unstable, serious fracture of the upper C-spine that is caused by hyperextension and distraction (such as hitting one's head on a dashboard). This is a fracture of the posterior elements of C-2 and, usually, displacement of the C-2 body anterior to C-3 (Fig. 5.7). Patients with this type of fracture actually do better than one might think. They often escape neurologic impairment because of the fractured posterior elements of C-2, which, in effect, cause a decompression and take pressure off the injured area. This is a simplistic explanation for a complex entity, but it seems to be a reasonable answer to why these patients often fare well.

Severe flexion of the C-spine can cause a disruption of the posterior ligaments and anterior compression of a vertebral body. This is called a *flexion "teardrop" fracture* (Fig. 5.8). A teardrop fracture is usually associated with spinal cord injury, often from the posterior portion of the vertebral body being displaced into the central canal.

If severe enough, and if associated with some rotation, the apophyseal joint ligaments will rupture and the facet joints dislocate and then override. This can result in locking of the facets in an overriding position, which in effect causes some stabilization to protect against further injury. This condition is called *unilateral locked facets* (Fig. 5.9), but occasionally it occurs bilaterally.

A "seat belt injury" is seen secondary to hyperflexion at the waist (as occurs in a car accident while the person is restrained by a lap belt). This causes distraction of the posterior elements and ligaments, and anterior compression of the vertebral body. It usually involves the L-1 or L-2 level. Several variations of this injury can occur: a fracture of the posterior body is called a *Smith fracture*, and a fracture through the spinous process is called a *Chance fracture*. Horizontal fractures of the pedicles, laminae, and transverse processes can also occur (Fig. 5.10).

A spinal abnormality that may or may not be caused by trauma is spondylolysis. *Spondylolysis* is a break or defect in the pars interarticularis portion of the lamina (Fig. 5.11). It can be seen in about 5.10% of asymptomatic individuals. On oblique views, the posterior elements form the figure of a Scottie dog, with the transverse process being the nose, the

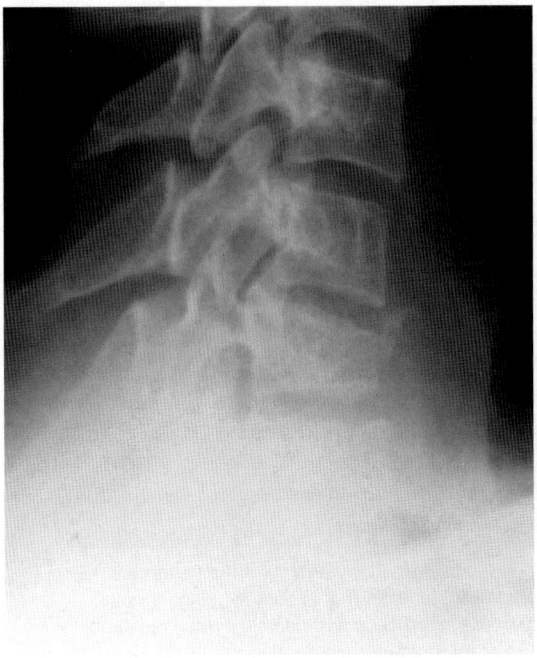

FIG. 5.8 **Flexion Teardrop Fracture.** This patient suffered hyperflexion in a car accident and came to the emergency department with severe neurologic deficits. A lateral radiograph of the lower cervical spine shows wedging anteriorly of the C-7 vertebral body with some displacement of the posterior vertebral line of C-7 into the central canal. A small avulsion fracture off the anterior body is also noted.

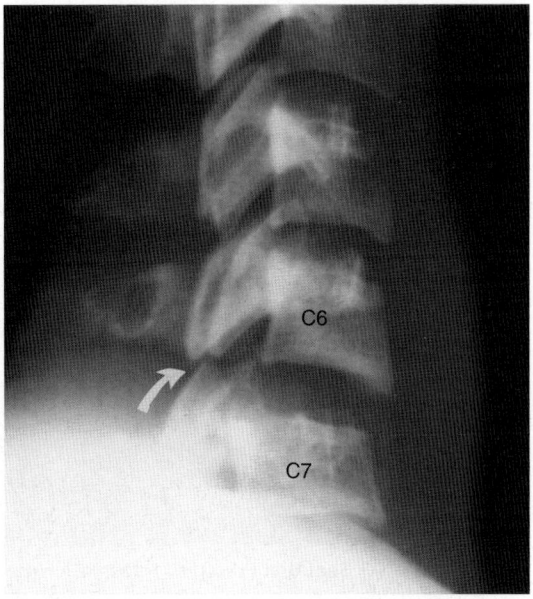

FIG. 5.9 **Unilateral Locked Facets.** The C-6–C-7 disc space is abnormally widened, and the C-7 vertebral body is posteriorly located in relation to C-6. Also note the C-7 facets, which are dislocated and locked on the C-6 facets *(arrow)*. When the facets are perched in this manner, the condition is termed locked facets, which in this example is unilateral.

pedicle forming the eye, the inferior articular facet being the front leg, the superior articular facet representing the ear, and the pars interarticularis (which means the portion of the lamina that lies between the facets) equaling the dog's neck. If a spondylolysis is present, the pars interarticularis, or the neck of the dog, will have a defect or break. It often looks as if the Scottie dog has a collar around its neck. Although often difficult to visualize with MR, spondylolysis should be easily seen on CT (see Chapter 11). The cause of a spondylolysis is said by some investigators to be congenital and by others to be posttraumatic. Many believe that this is a stress-related injury from infancy that develops when toddlers try to walk and repeatedly fall on their buttocks, sending stress to their lower lumbar spine. The significance of spondylolysis is just as controversial as its cause. More and more clinicians are coming to the viewpoint that a spondylolysis is an incidental finding with no clinical significance in most cases. Certainly some patients have pain related to a spondylolysis and get relief after surgical stabilization, but such cases are uncommon.

If a spondylolysis is bilateral and the vertebral body in the more cephalad position slips forward on the more caudal body, spondylolisthesis is said to be present (Fig. 5.12). *Spondylolisthesis* may or may not be symptomatic and by itself has no clinical significance. If severe, it can cause neuroforaminal stenosis and can impinge on the nerve roots in the central spinal canal. If it is symptomatic, it can be surgically stabilized.

Anterior wedge compression fractures of the spine are commonly seen (Fig. 5.13), especially at the thoraco–lumbar junction, due to an old injury; they are often passed off by the radiologist, if they are mentioned at all, as incidental findings. The problem with this is you cannot tell from a plain film if the fracture is old or new, even if degenerative changes are present (which are often not related to the fracture). If acute and left unprotected, a wedge compression fracture can proceed to delayed further collapse with resulting severe

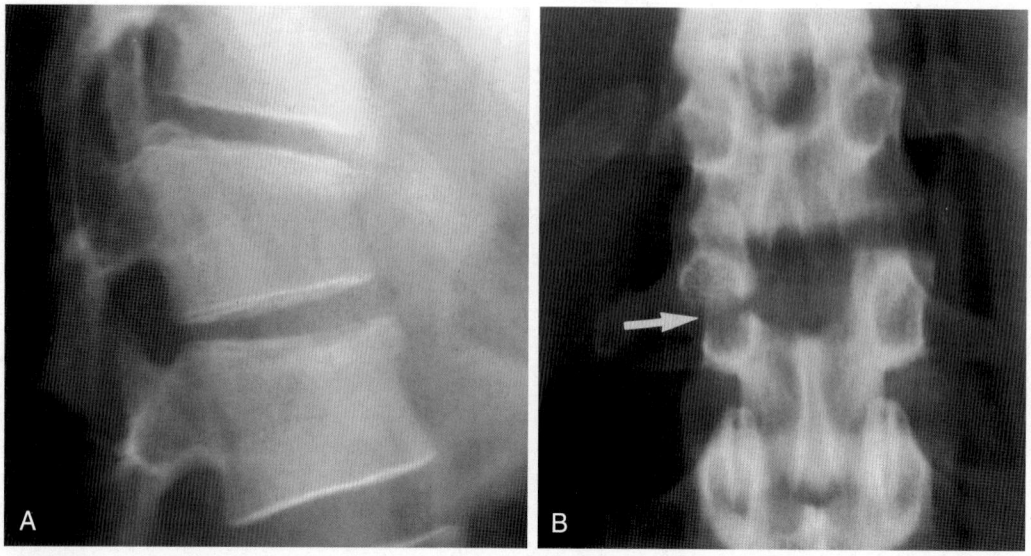

FIG. 5.10 **Seat Belt Fracture.** Hyperflexion at the waist can cause anterior wedging of the vertebral body in the lower thoracic or upper lumbar region, as shown in (A). By itself, that is somewhat innocuous; however, (B) shows a horizontal fracture through the right transverse process and pedicle *(arrow)* resulting from extreme traction during the flexion injury. When fracture of the posterior elements occurs, this injury is considered to be unstable and potentially debilitating. Any anterior wedging injury to a vertebral body should have the posterior elements of that level closely inspected for interpedicular space widening.

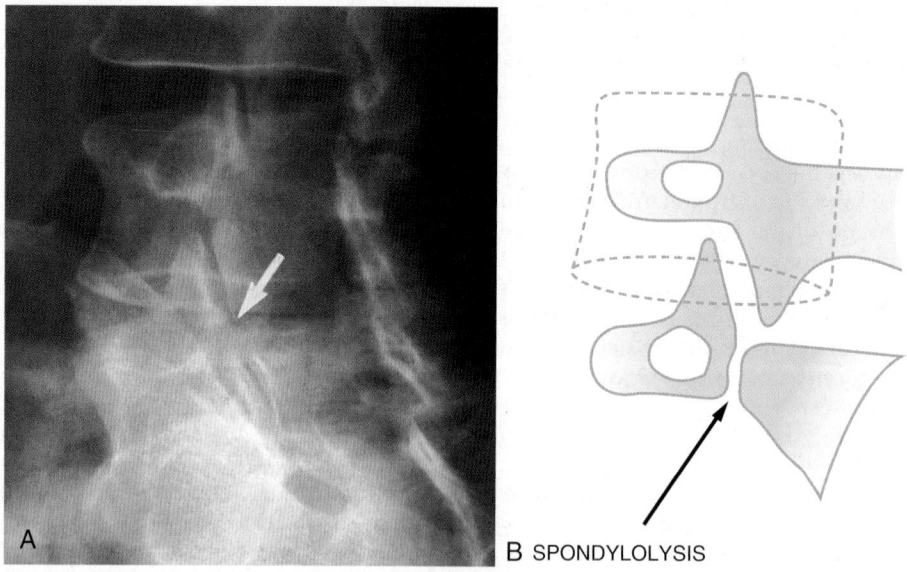

FIG. 5.11 **Spondylolysis.** An oblique film of the lumbar spine (A) shows a defect in the neck of the Scottie dog at L-5 *(arrow)*, which is diagnostic of a spondylolysis. The drawing (B) shows the findings more clearly. This has been described as a collar around the Scottie dog's neck.

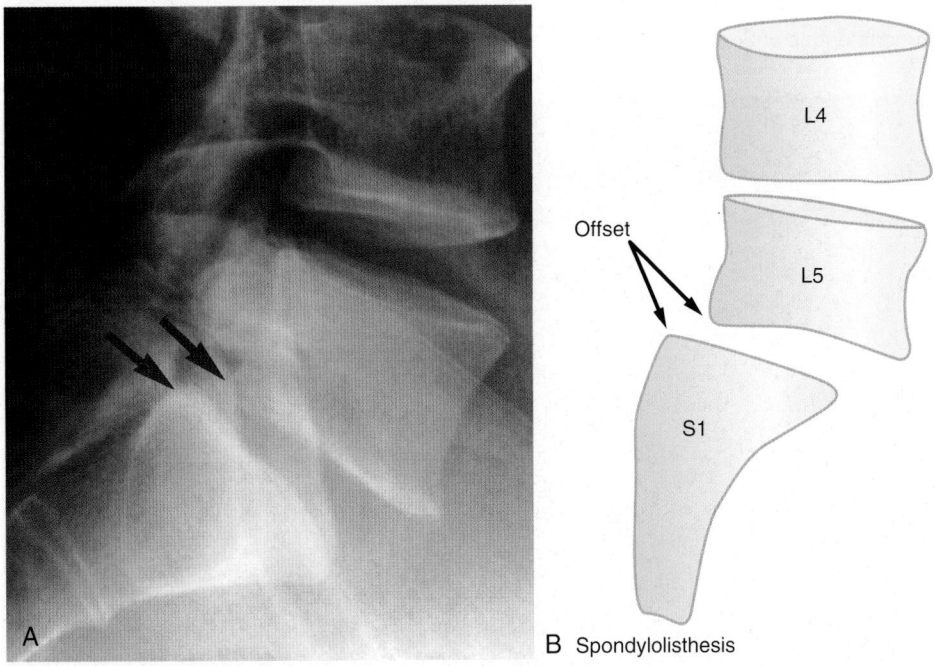

FIG. 5.12 **Spondylolisthesis.** A lateral film of the lumbar spine (A) shows the L-5 vertebral body is slightly anteriorly offset on the S-1 body as noted by the posterior margins *(arrows)*. The drawing (B) shows the findings more clearly. Because the offset is less than 25% as measured by the length of the S-1 end-plate, it is termed a grade 1 spondylolisthesis. A grade 2 offset is more than 25% but less than 50% of the length of the S-1 end plate.

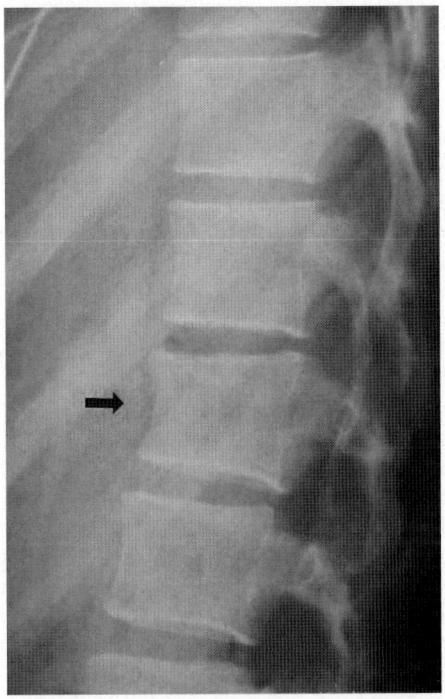

FIG. 5.13 **Anterior Wedge Compression Fracture.** Anterior compression of this lower T-spine vertebral body *(arrow)* is present, which may or may not be acute. If the patient has pain in this area, it is most likely acute and must be protected with a back brace until the symptoms abate.

neurologic deficits (Fig. 5.14). This is called Kummell disease and typically occurs 1–2 weeks after the initial trauma. I have seen over a dozen lawsuits against radiologists who failed to mention minor anterior wedging of a vertebral body, which went on to further collapse with associated paraplegia. All that needs to be mentioned is that a fracture is present that is of indeterminate age and requires clinical correlation. If the patient has pain in that location, a back brace needs to be worn until they are pain-free. Old films can help determine if it is an old fracture. If no pain is present on physical exam, it can be safely assumed to be an old fracture. It is not necessary to obtain a CT or magnetic resonance imaging (MRI) even if pain is present because the treatment will be the same regardless of what the CT or MRI reveal. No spine surgeon will operate on a stable spine fracture without kyphosis or neurologic deficits, so the CT or MRI add nothing but time and expense.

Patients who have fusion of their spine from ankylosing spondylitis and, to a lesser extent, from DISH (diffuse idiopathic skeletal hyperostosis—see Chapter 6), are at a very high risk of spinal fractures from even relatively minor trauma. Patients with ankylosing spondylitis typically have marked osteopososis, which further magnifies their risk of fracture. A fused spine is more likely to fracture than a normal spine in a manner similar to a long glass pipette breaking more easily than a short one because it has a long lever arm. A small force at one end

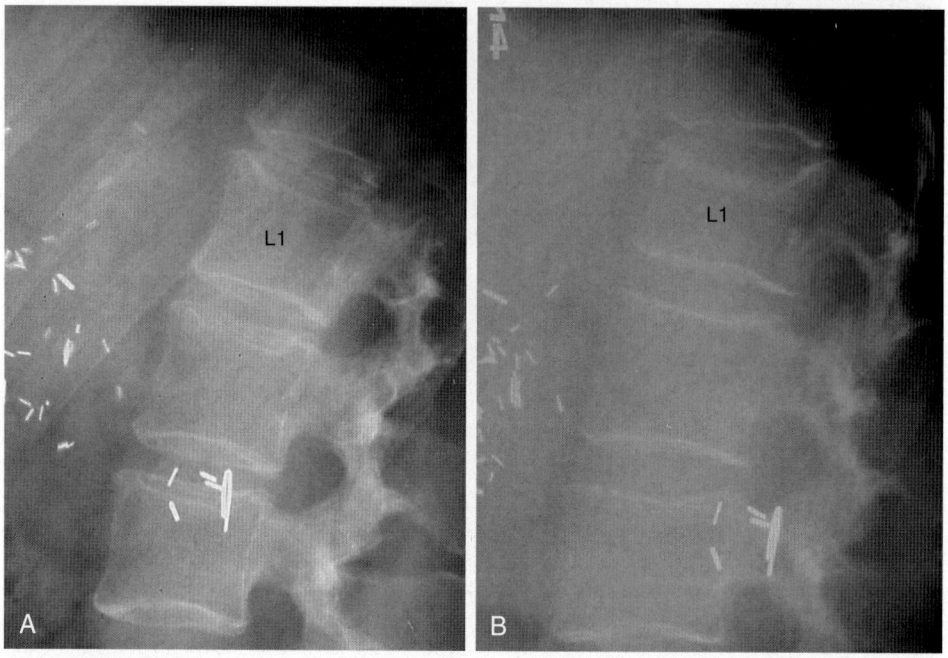

FIG. 5.14 **Kummel Disease.** (A) Very minimal anterior wedging of the L1 vertebral body is noted by comparing the height of the anterior body versus the posterior height. This patient had been in an auto accident and complained of back pain. No treatment for his back was given. (B) After several weeks of continuing pain, he presents with leg weakness, which proceeded to paraplegia. A spine film now shows progression of the vertebral body collapse of L1. This almost certainly could have been avoided with simple bracing of the spine after the initial injury.

is greatly magnified farther down the lever arm. For that reason, a patient with ankylosing spondylitis should be treated as though a spinal fracture is present if they have back pain following trauma. CT and/or MRI are mandatory if plain films are negative (Fig. 5.15).

HAND AND WRIST

Several seemingly innocuous fractures in the hand require surgical fixation rather than just casting and, therefore should be recognized by the radiologist as serious injuries. One such fracture is a fracture at the base of the thumb into the carpometacarpal joint, or a *Bennett fracture* (Fig. 5.16). Because of the insertion of the strong thumb adductors at the base of the thumb, it is almost impossible to keep the metacarpal from sliding off its proper alignment. It almost always requires internal fixation. The radiologist occasionally has to remind a nonorthopedic practitioner of this, as well as closely examine the alignment of a Bennett fracture in plaster that has not been internally fixed with pins.

A comminuted fracture of the base of the thumb that extends into the joint has been termed a *Rolando fracture* (Fig. 5.17), and a fracture of the base of the thumb that does not involve the joint has been called a pseudo-Bennett fracture.

A *mallet finger* or *baseball finger* is an avulsion injury at the base of the distal phalanx (Fig. 5.18) where the extensor digitorum tendon inserts. With the extensor tendon inoperative, the distal phalanx flexes without opposition. If not properly treated, this can result in a flexion deformity and inability to extend the distal phalanx.

Another innocent-appearing fracture that often requires internal fixation is an avulsion on the ulnar aspect of the first metacarpophalangeal joint (Fig. 5.19), which is where the ulnar collateral ligament of the thumb inserts. If the ulnar collateral ligament is torn, the function of the thumb can be impaired; therefore this fracture can have a serious result if not properly treated. This injury is called a *gamekeeper's thumb* because of the propensity of old English game wardens to acquire it from breaking rabbits' necks between their thumbs and forefingers. A more current scenario is falling on a ski pole and having the pole jam into the webbing between the thumb and index finger. Kayakers occasionally suffer a gamekeeper's thumb when their paddles hit a rock.

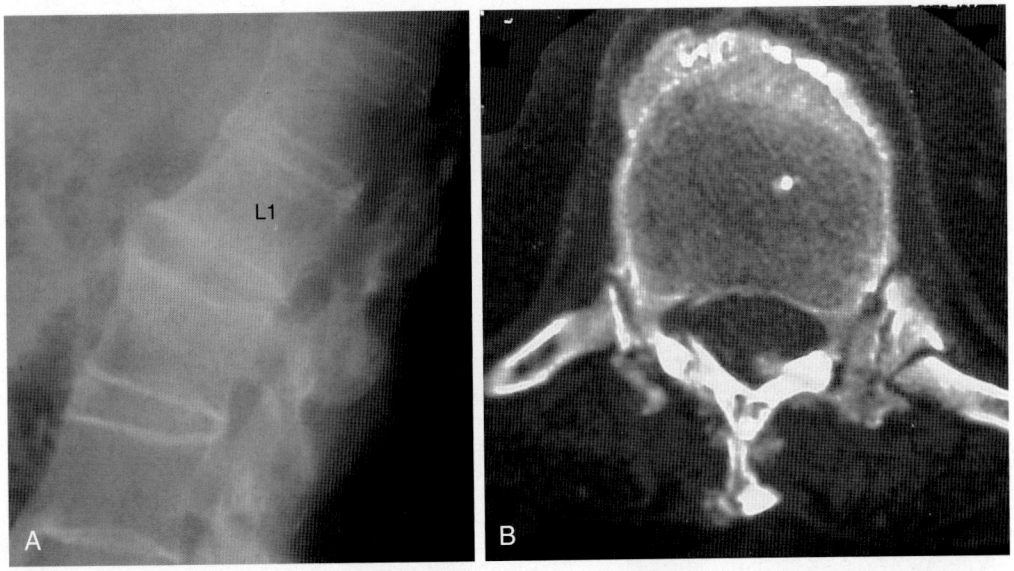

FIG. 5.15 **Spine Fracture in Ankylosing Spondylitis.** (A) A lateral spine plain film following trauma shows fusion of the spine anteriorly, which was secondary to ankylosing spondylitis. Minimal anterior wedging of the L1 vertebral body is present, which was overlooked. (B) Two weeks later, a computed tomography (CT) of the spine was performed because of the sudden onset of paralysis. This axial image through L1 shows a fracture of the posterior elements, which was undoubtedly present on the initial visit to the emergency room. Patients with ankylosing spondylitis need to be examined closely for any back pain following trauma and imaged with CT or magnetic resonance imaging (MRI) if any pain is present.

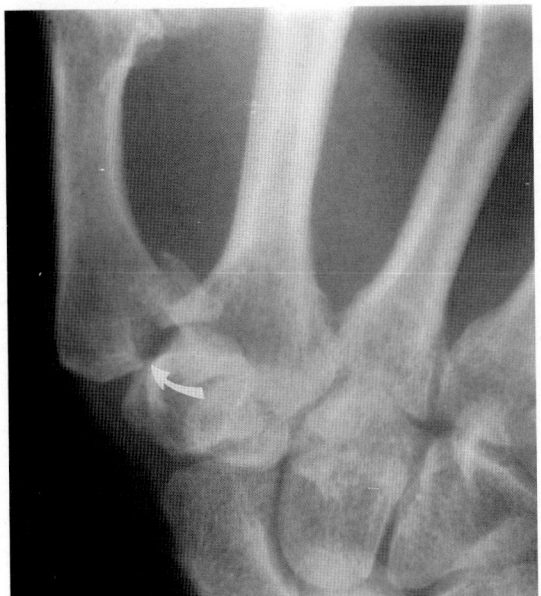

FIG. 5.16 **Bennett Fracture.** A small corner fracture of the base of the thumb is noted that, at first glance, appears minor; however, it involves the articular surface of the base of the thumb *(arrow)*, which makes this a serious injury that almost always requires internal fixation.

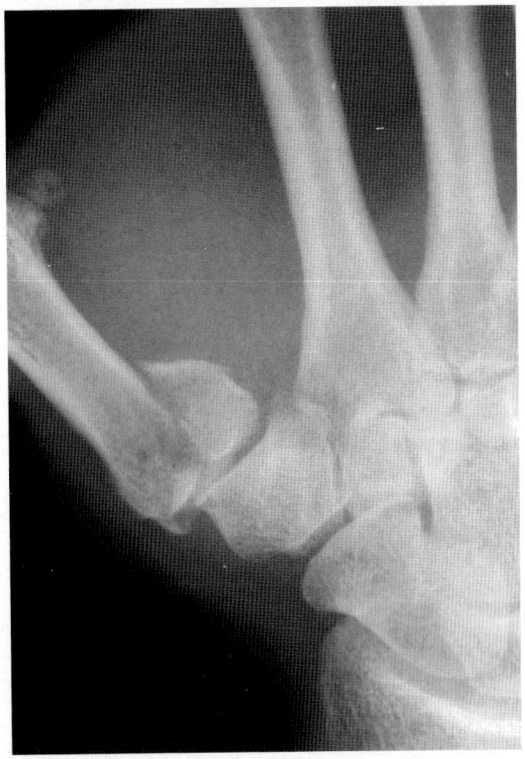

FIG. 5.17 **Rolando Fracture.** A comminuted fracture of the base of the thumb that extends into the articular surface is a more serious type of Bennett fracture and has been termed a Rolando fracture.

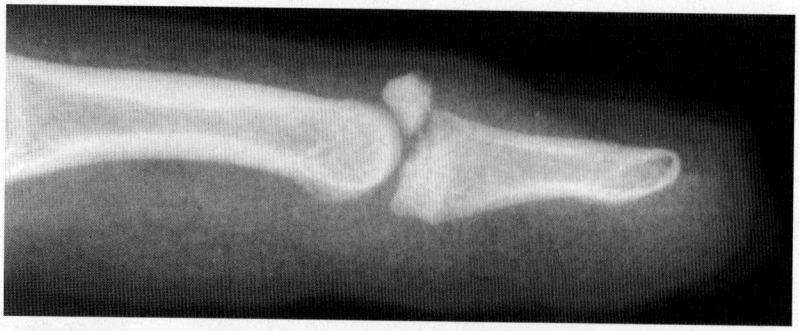

FIG. 5.18 **Mallet Finger.** A small avulsion injury is noted at the base of the distal phalanx, which is where the extensor digitorum tendon inserts. This injury is termed a mallet finger or baseball finger. It is often caused by a baseball striking the distal phalanx, causing the avulsion.

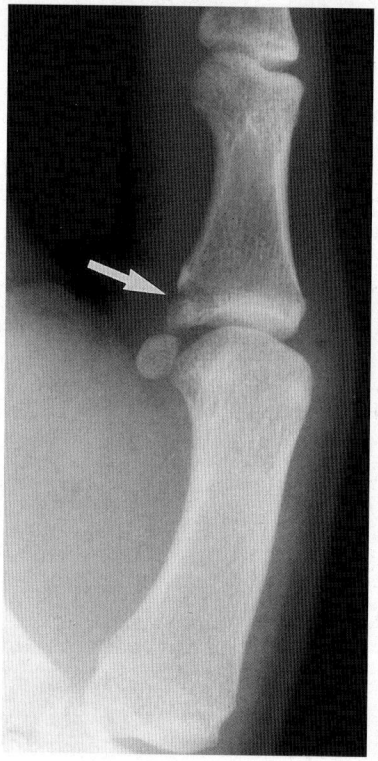

FIG. 5.19 **Gamekeeper's Thumb.** A small avulsion injury on the ulnar aspect of the first metacarpophalangeal joint *(arrow)* is diagnostic of a gamekeeper's thumb. This is the insertion site for the ulnar collateral ligament and usually requires internal fixation.

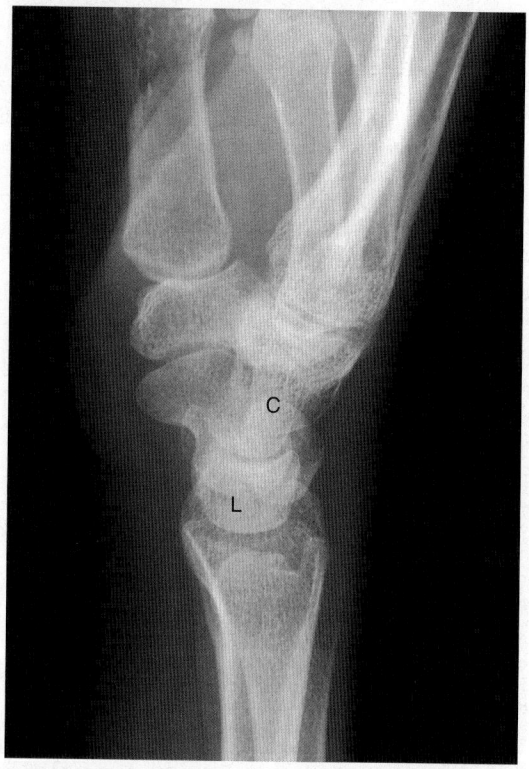

FIG. 5.20 **Normal Lateral Radiograph of theWrist.** The normal lateral view should show the lunate (*L*) seated in the distal radius and the capitate (*C*) in turn seated in the lunate. A line drawn through the radius should connect all three structures. Compare this radiograph with the drawing in Fig. 5.21A.

This avulsion injury usually requires pinning to securely fix the ligament.

A fall on an outstretched arm can result in any number of wrist fractures and dislocations. One serious such injury is the *lunate/perilunate dislocation*. This dislocation occurs when the ligaments between the capitate and the lunate are disrupted, allowing the capitate to dislocate from the cup-shaped articulation of the lunate. This is best seen on the lateral view. Ordinarily, on the lateral view, the capitate should be seen seated in the cup-shaped lunate (Figs. 5.20 and 5.21A. In a *dorsal perilunate*

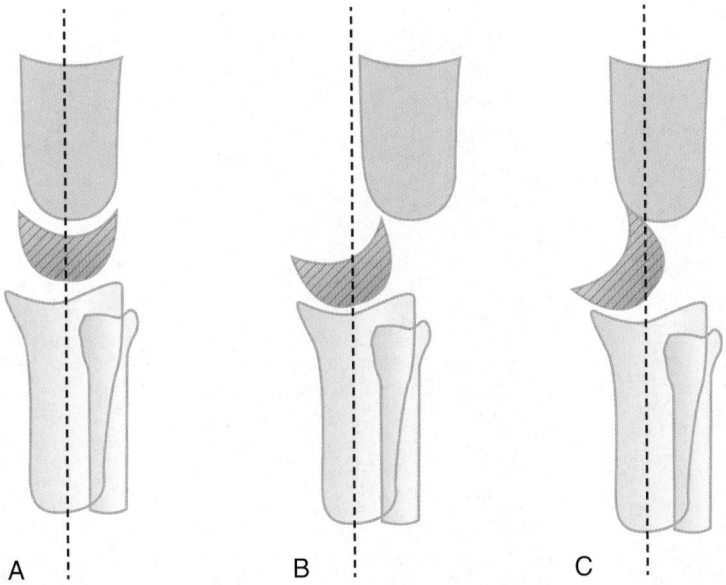

FIG. 5.21 Schematic depiction of normal lateral wrist (A), perilunate dislocation (B), and lunate dislocation (C). (The dark shaded bone is the lunate; the cross-hatched filled bone is the capitate. Ventral is to the left.)

dislocation (occasionally the capitate dislocates volarly, but this is uncommon), the capitate and all of its surrounding bones, including the metacarpals, come to lie dorsal to a line drawn up through the radius and the lunate (Figs. 5.21B and 5.22). If the capitate then pushes the lunate volarly and tips it over, the line drawn up through the radius shows the lunate volarly displaced, and the line goes through the capitate. This has been termed a lunate dislocation (Figs. 5.21C and 5.23). The normal, perilunate, and lunate dislocations are shown schematically in Fig. 5.21. Often it is difficult to tell whether the lunate or the capitate is displaced merely by drawing a line up the radius because it can lie between the lunate and the capitate. In such cases, the designation of lunate or perilunate is difficult or even impossible. In reality, these are all perilunate-type dislocations, and additional trauma or manipulation of the wrist can cause the so-called lunate dislocation. It is certainly possible to turn a perilunate dislocation into a lunate dislocation merely by manipulating the wrist. Therefore strict classification of these entities is not recommended by everyone. For many surgeons, it is a moot point—they want rapid reduction of the capitate–lunate dislocation and don't really care which one happens to be more volarly or dorsally displaced. Failure to diagnose and treat this disorder can result in permanent impairment of the median nerve if it gets impinged on by the lunate.

I strongly recommend that every radiolgist get in the habit of looking at the alignment of the lunate and the

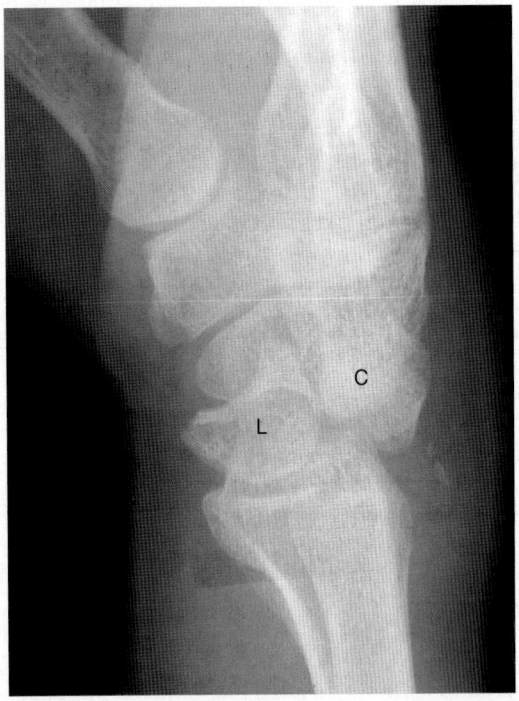

FIG. 5.22 **Perilunate Dislocation.** Although the lunate (*L*) is normal in relation to the distal radius, the capitate (*C*) and the remainder of the wrist are dorsally displaced in relation to the lunate. Compare this radiograph with the drawing in Fig. 5.21B.

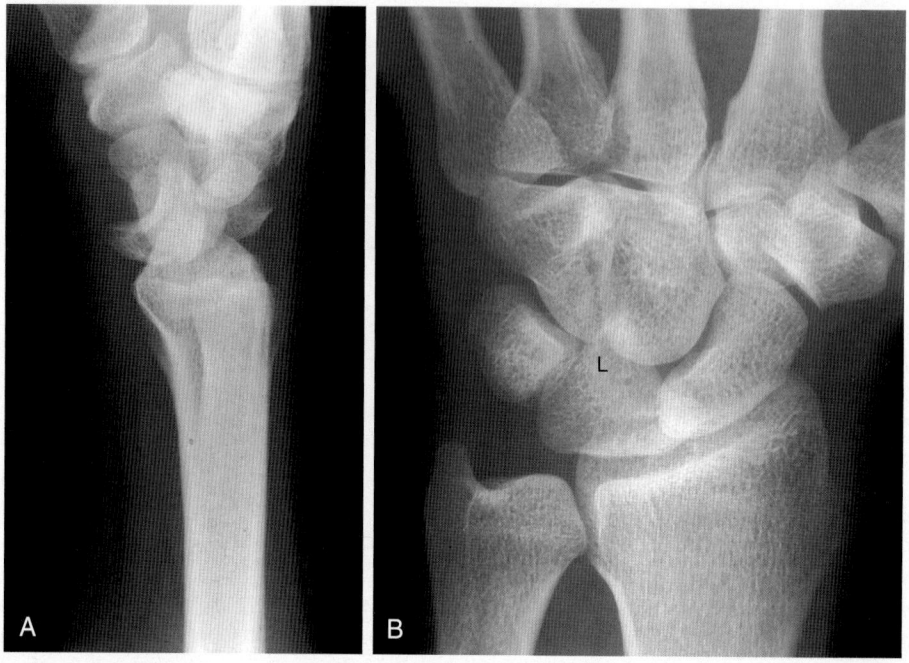

FIG. 5.23 **Lunate Dislocation.** The lateral radiograph of the wrist (A) shows the lunate tipped off the distal radius, whereas the capitate seems to be normally aligned in relation to the radius yet is dislocated from the lunate. Compare this with the drawing in Fig. 5.21C. The anteroposterior (AP) view (B) shows a pie-shaped lunate rather than a lunate with a more rhomboid shape. A pie-shaped lunate (*L*) can be seen in a perilunate or lunate dislocation.

capitate on every lateral wrist film. There's not a whole lot else to look for on the lateral view anyway. I see a missed perilunate dislocation every few years, which usually ends up in litigation.

A lunate or perilunate dislocation can be diagnosed on an AP view of the wrist by noting a triangular or pie-shaped lunate (Fig. 5.23B). Ordinarily the lunate has a rhomboid shape on the AP view, with the upper and lower borders parallel.

Several fractures are known to be associated with a perilunate dislocation, the most common of which is a transscaphoid fracture. The capitate, radial styloid, and triquetrum are also known to frequently fracture when a perilunate dislocation occurs. On occasion, the fractures are identified and treated, while the dislocation is overlooked.

One of the most difficult wrist fractures to identify on plain films is a *fracture of the hook of the hamate*. A special view, the carpal tunnel view, should be obtained when trying to see the hook of the hamate. This view is obtained with the wrist (palm down) flat on a radiograph plate and the fingers and palm pulled dorsally. The x-ray beam is angled about 45 degrees, parallel to the palm, so the carpal tunnel is in profile. The hook of the hamate is seen as a bony protuberance off the hamate on the ulnar aspect of the carpal tunnel. A fractured hook of the hamate can be seen with the carpal tunnel view (Fig. 5.24) but is often difficult to pick up. A CT scan will often show an obvious fracture that the

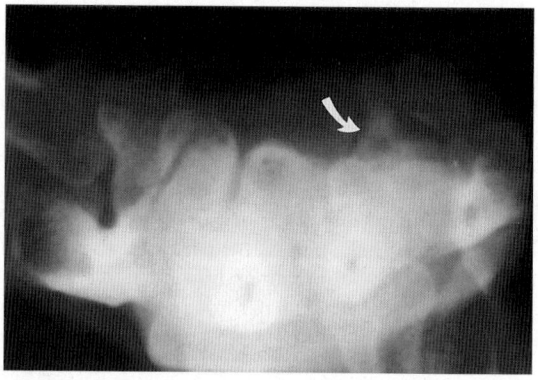

FIG. 5.24 **Fracture of the Hook of the Hamate.** The hook of the hamate is seen on a carpal tunnel view in this patient, as well as an area of sclerosis with a faint cortical break *(arrow)*. This represents a fracture at the base of the hook of the hamate.

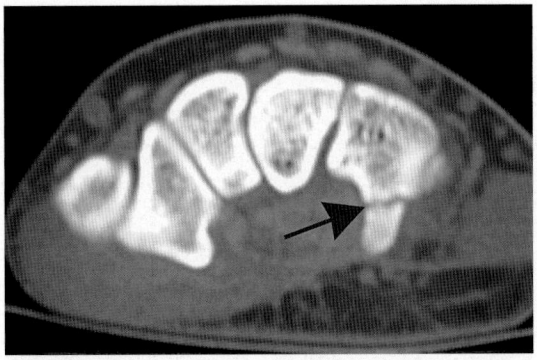

FIG. 5.25 **Computed Tomography (CT) of a fractured hook of the hamate.** A CT scan through the wrist in this patient shows a lucency in the hook of the hamate *(arrow)*, which represents a fracture. This could not be seen in the plain films, even in retrospect.

plain film does not (Fig. 5.25) and should be considered in any possible carpal fracture when plain films are not diagnostic.

A fracture of the hook of the hamate most commonly occurs from a fall on the outstretched hand. A clinical setting that has gained attention in radiology and sports medicine circles is that of a professional athlete who participates in an activity in which the butt of a club, bat, or racket is held in the palm. Overswinging can result in the butt of the club levering off the hook of the hamate. This has been seen in professional baseball players, tennis players, and golfers. Why professionals? Amateurs usually are not strong enough to exert enough force to lever the hook off and, if they do, will usually terminate that activity, allowing healing. Professionals, however, continue their participation, which can lead to a nonunion of the fracture.

Another wrist injury that is seen after a fall onto the outstretched hand is *rotatory subluxation of the scaphoid*. This results from rupture of the scapholunate ligaments, which allows the scaphoid (navicular) to rotate dorsally. On an AP wrist radiograph, a space is seen between the scaphoid and the lunate (Fig. 5.26) when ordinarily they are closely opposed. This space has been called the "Terry Thomas" sign, after a famous British actor from the 1950s and 1960s with a gap between his two front teeth. The latest generation of radiologists is too young to have heard of Terry Thomas, therefore I prefer to call it the "David Letterman" sign.

A *fracture of the scaphoid* is a potentially serious injury because of the high rate of avascular necrosis that occurs with this injury. When avascular necrosis occurs, usually surgical intervention and bone grafting

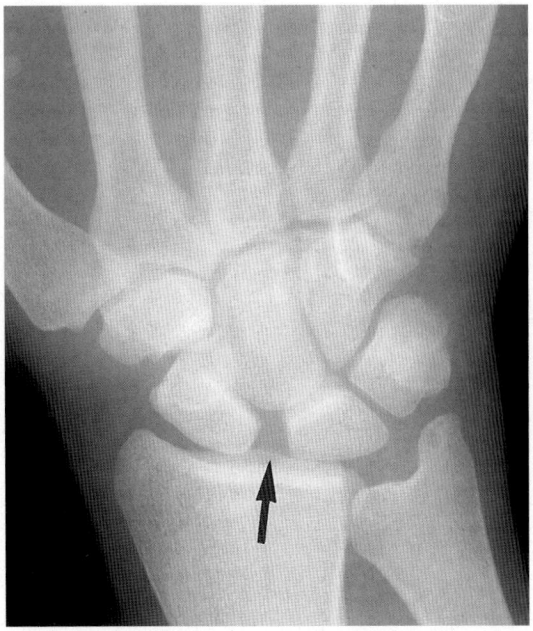

FIG. 5.26 **Rotatory Subluxation of the Scaphoid.** An anteroposterior (AP) view of the wrist shows a gap or space between the scaphoid and the lunate *(arrow)*. This is abnormal and represents the "Terry Thomas" sign, which means that the ligaments between the lunate and the scaphoid are ruptured. This is diagnostic of a rotatory subluxation of the scaphoid.

are required in order to obtain healing. This fracture can be difficult to detect initially; therefore whenever a fracture of the scaphoid is clinically suspect (trauma with pain over the snuffbox of the wrist), the wrist should be casted and repeat radiographs obtained in 1 week. Often the fracture is then visualized owing to the disuse osteoporosis and hyperemia around the fracture site. Thus in the acute setting, a negative film does not exclude a fractured scaphoid. Instead of casting the wrist and repeating the films in a week, many patients now get immediate MRI to determine if a fracture is present (Fig. 5.27). This has been shown to be less expensive overall than having the patient casted and reexamined in a week.[4]

If avascular necrosis develops, it is the proximal fragment that undergoes aseptic necrosis because the blood supply to the scaphoid begins distally and runs proximally. A fracture with disruption of the blood supply thus leaves the proximal pole without a vascular supply; hence it dies. Avascular necrosis is diagnosed by noting increased density of the proximal pole of the scaphoid as compared with the remainder of the carpal bones (Fig. 5.28).

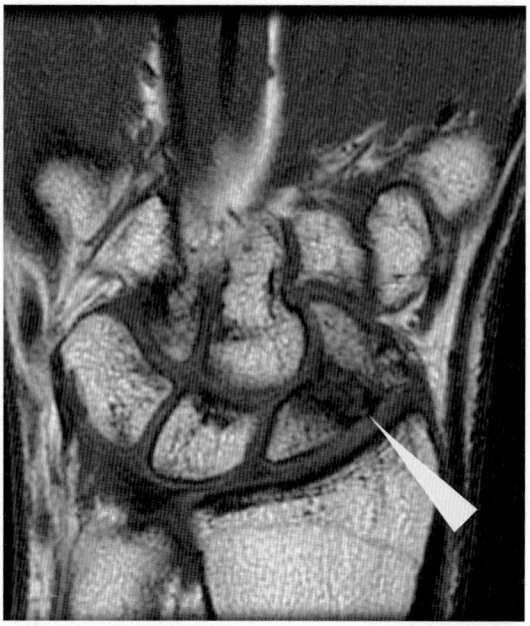

FIG. 5.27 **Scaphoid Fracture.** A coronal T1-weighted image of the wrist in a patient with snuffbox tenderness and a normal plain film shows a fracture of the mid-waist of the scaphoid *(arrow)*.

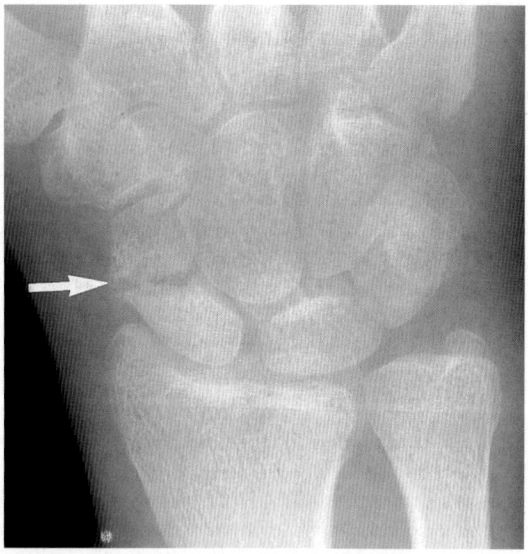

FIG. 5.28 **Avascular Necrosis of the Scaphoid.** An anteroposterior (AP) view of the wrist shows a fracture through the waist of the scaphoid *(arrow)*. The proximal half of the scaphoid is slightly sclerotic in relation to the remainder of the carpal bones, which indicates avascular necrosis of the proximal half.

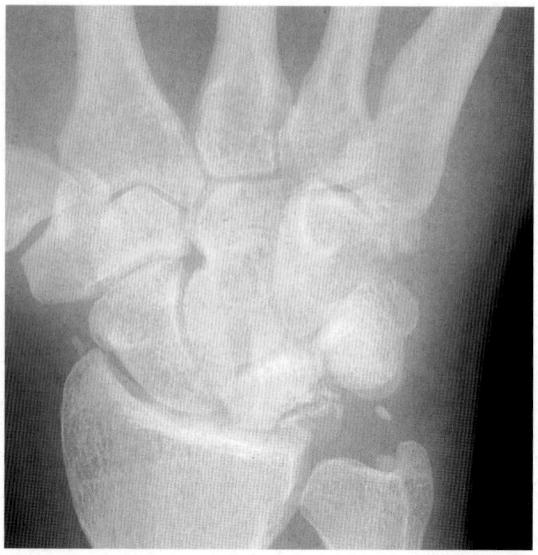

FIG. 5.29 **Kienböck's Malacia.** An anteroposterior (AP) view of the wrist reveals the lunate to be sclerotic and abnormal in shape. The lunate has collapsed owing to aseptic necrosis. This is known as Kienböck malacia. Note that the ulna is shorter than the radius—negative ulnar variance—which is said to be related to an increased incidence of Kienböck malacia.

Avascular necrosis can occur in other carpal bones, most commonly the lunate. This is called *Kienböck malacia* and is most often caused by trauma, although some investigators claim it is idiopathic. The disease is diagnosed by noting increased density of the lunate bone, which may or may not go on to collapse and fragment (Fig. 5.29). It often requires surgical bone grafting and occasionally removal, or proximal carpal row fusion. Kienböck malacia is said to have an increased incidence in patients who have shortening of the ulna in relation to the radius called negative ulnar variance. Positive ulnar variance (the ulna is longer than the radius) is associated with anincreased incidence of triangular fibrocartilage tears.

An avulsion fracture that is frequently seen is a *triquetral fracture*. The fracture is best seen on the lateral film, which shows a small chip of bone on the dorsum of the wrist (Fig. 5.30). This is virtually pathognomonic of avulsion off the triquetrum.

ARM

One of the most common fractures of the forearm is a fracture of the distal radius and ulna after a fall on the outstretched arm. This results in dorsal angulation of

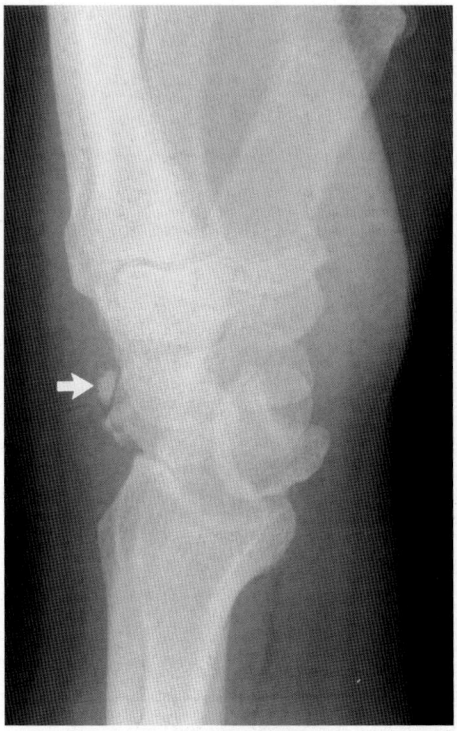

FIG. 5.30 **Triquetral Fracture and Perilunate Dislocation.** A perilunate or lunate dislocation is present (it is difficult to classify exactly which has occurred, since both the lunate and the capitate are out of their normal positions). Compare this radiograph with the drawing in Fig. 5.21A. A small avulsion is seen on the dorsum of the wrist *(arrow)*, which is virtually diagnostic of an avulsion off the triquetrum. It is often associated with a lunate or perilunate dislocation.

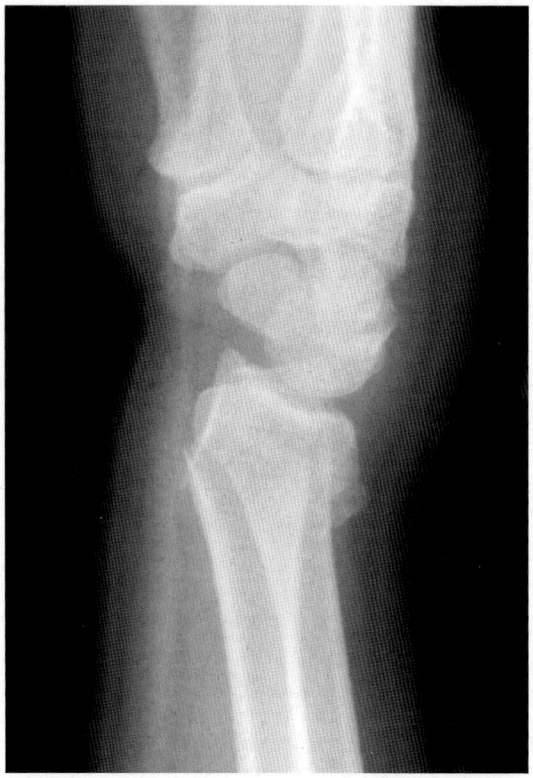

FIG. 5.31 **Colles Fracture.** A fracture of the distal radius with dorsal angulation is noted, which has been termed a Colles fracture (volar is to the left).

the distal forearm and wrist and is called a *Colles fracture* (Fig. 5.31). When the fracture angulates volarly, it is called a *Smith fracture* (Fig. 5.32). A Smith fracture is a much less common occurrence than a Colles fracture. Sometimes the radius and ulna suffer a traumatic insult, and the force on the bones causes bending instead of a frank fracture. This has been termed *plastic bowing deformity of the forearm* (Fig. 5.33) and is often treated by breaking the bones (under anesthesia, of course) and resetting them. Left untreated, a plastic bowing deformity can result in reduced supination and pronation.

The forearm is a two-bone system that has some of the same properties as a bony ring. For example, a solid ring cannot break in only a single place; it must break in at least two points (try to break a pretzel—not a soft New York pretzel—in only one place). Likewise, the rings in the spine or pelvis always break in at least two places. In the forearm, a fracture of one bone should be accompanied by a fracture of the other. If the second fracture is not present, a dislocation of the nonfractured bone usually occurs. The most common example of this is a fracture of the ulna with a dislocation of the proximal radius (Fig. 5.34). This is called a *Monteggia fracture*. [In prior editions of this book, I termed this a "nightstick injury" from the policeman hitting someone with a nightstick (who hasn't had that happen!)—the person being hit instinctively raises an arm for protection, and the nightstick falls on the ulna, fracturing it and dislocating the radial head. Lee Rogers called me and informed me that a nightstick fracture is a different entity than a Monteggia fracture. He's right, of course, but the mechanism I described is correct.] The dislocated radial head can be missed clinically and go on to aseptic necrosis with subsequent elbow dysfunction. Therefore anytime the ulna is fractured, the elbow must be examined to exclude a dislocation.

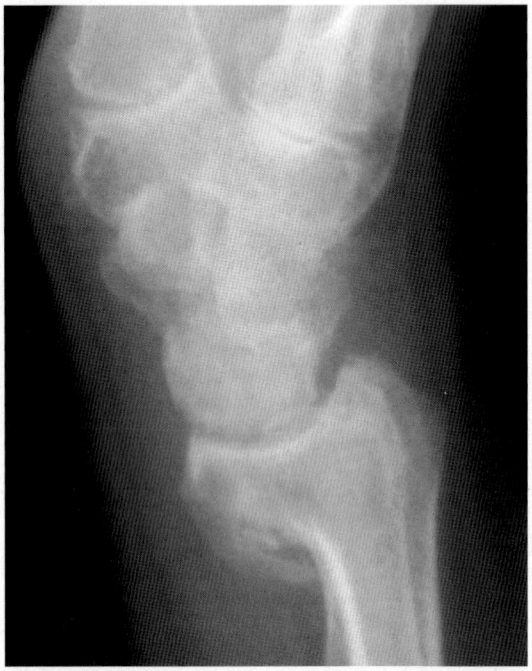

FIG. 5.32 **Smith Fracture.** A fracture of the distal radius with volar angulation such as this is called a Smith fracture. This injury is much less common than the Colles fracture shown in Fig. 5.31 (volar is to the left).

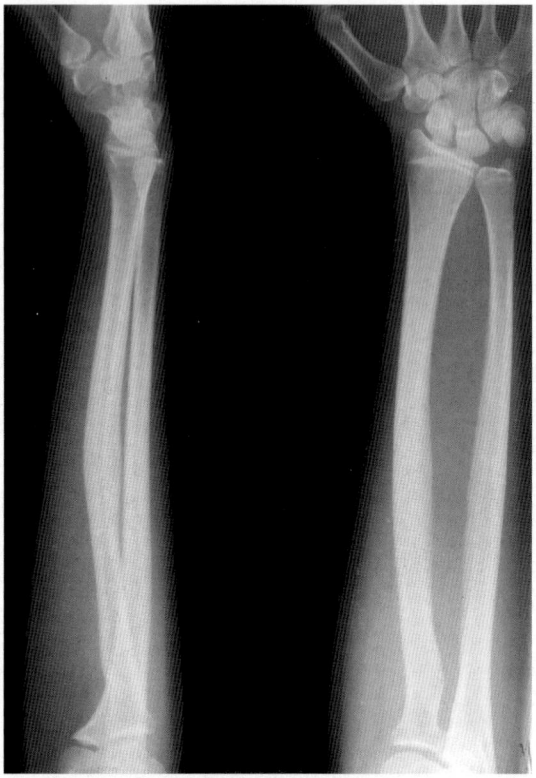

FIG. 5.33 **Plastic Bowing Deformity of the Forearm.** These anteroposterior (AP) and lateral views of a child's forearm show the radius to be abnormally bowed. This condition has been termed a plastic bowing deformity of the forearm, and occurs only in children.

A fracture of the radius with dislocation of the distal ulna is called a *Galeazzi fracture* (Fig. 5.35). This is much less common than a Monteggia fracture.

A helpful indicator of a fracture about the elbow is a displaced posterior fat pad. Ordinarily the posterior fat pad is not visible on a lateral view of the elbow because it is tucked away in the olecranon fossa of the distal humerus. When the joint becomes distended with blood secondary to a fracture, the posterior fat pad is displaced out of the olecranon fossa and is visible on the lateral view (Fig. 5.36). Therefore in the setting of trauma, a visible posterior fat pad indicates a fracture. In an adult (epiphyses closed), the fracture site is almost always the radial head (Fig. 5.36B). In a child (epiphyses open), it is usually indicative of a supracondylar fracture (Fig. 5.37). Often the fracture itself is not visualized, and heroic steps are taken by clinicians and radiologists alike to demonstrate the fracture. These steps include oblique views, special radial head views, tomograms, and even CT scans and MRI. These are costly and unnecessary attempts to document pathology that will be treated identically whether or not it is radiographically recorded. So long as there is no obvious deformity or loose body, it does not matter if the fracture is definitely identified or not in a patient with a posttraumatic painful elbow and a visible posterior fat pad.

Couldn't an infection cause a joint effusion and a displaced posterior fat pad? Of course, but the clinical setting would not be to rule out a fracture. In fact, any elbow effusion will cause a posterior fat pad to be visible.

The anterior fat pad also gets displaced with a joint effusion. Ordinarily it is visible as a small triangle just anterior to the distal humeral diaphysis on a lateral film (Fig. 5.38). With an effusion, it gets displaced superiorly and outward from the humerus and has been called a "sail" sign because it resembles a spinnaker sail (Figs. 5.36 and 5.37). I have seen only one example of a displaced anterior fat pad

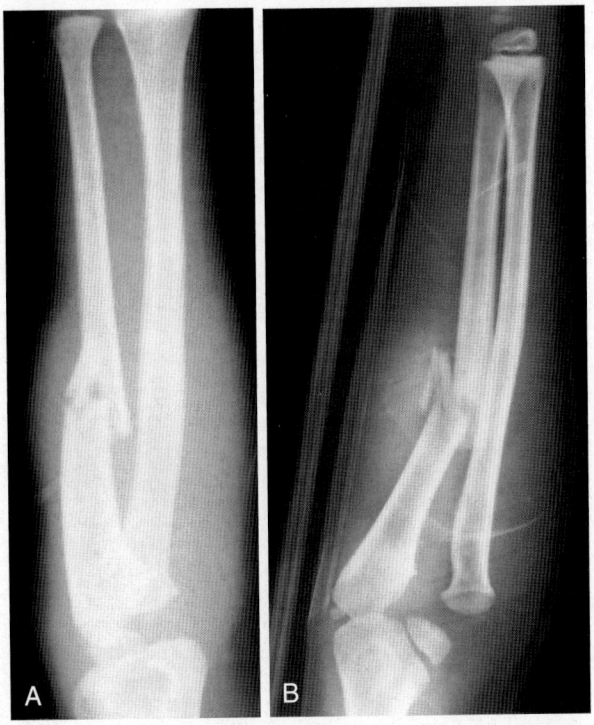

FIG. 5.34 **Monteggia Fracture.** A blow to the forearm, such as with a policeman's nightstick, can result in a fracture of the ulna. Although the head of the radius appears normally placed on the AP view (A), the lateral examination (B) reveals the head of the radius to be displaced. Failure to recognize this abnormality can result in death of the radial head with subsequent elbow dysfunction. This illustrates the importance of always obtaining two views of a bone in an injury.

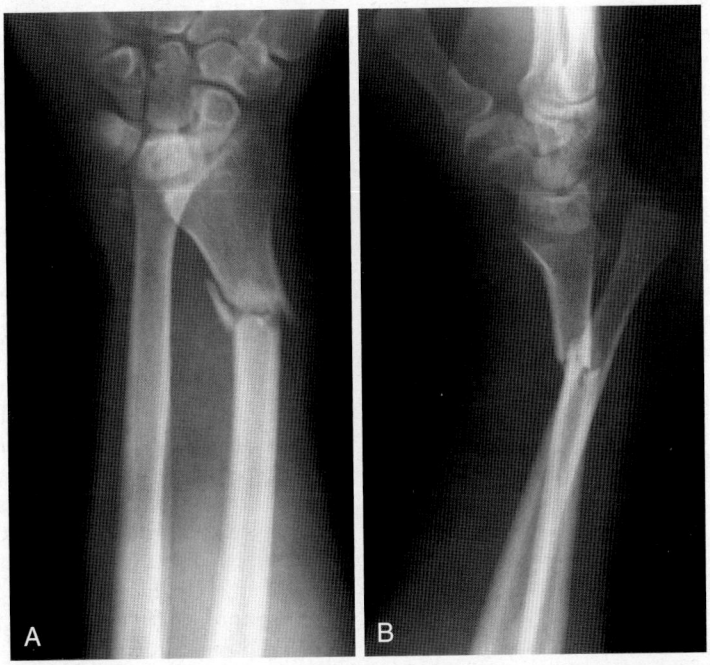

FIG. 5.35 **Galeazzi Fracture.** A fracture of the distal radius in this patient is seen on the anteroposterior (AP) view (A) without a definite fracture of the ulna. The lateral view (B) shows an obvious dislocation of the distal ulna, which would almost certainly not be missed clinically. This has been termed a Galeazzi fracture and is much less common than a Monteggia fracture.

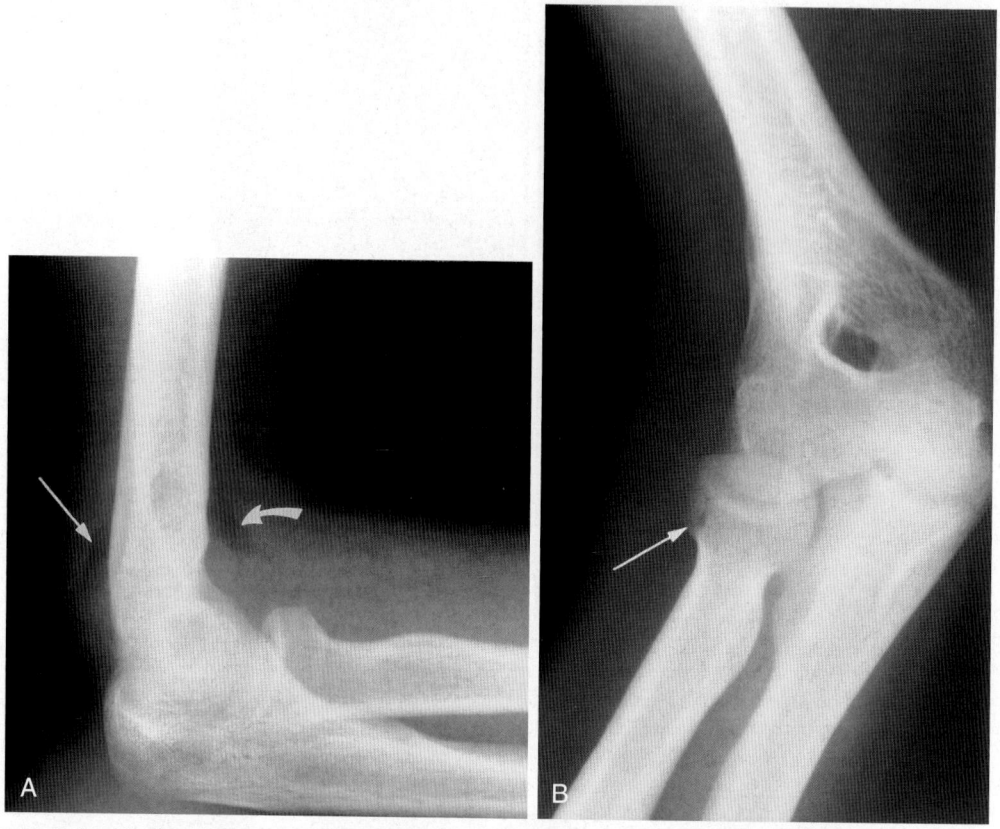

FIG. 5.36 **Displaced Fat Pads About the Elbow.** On the lateral view of the elbow in this patient (A), the posterior fat pad is visible *(arrow)*, and the anterior fat pad is elevated and anteriorly displaced (curved arrow). These findings indicate a fracture about the elbow, which in an adult should be in the radial head. An oblique view in this patient (B) shows the fracture of the radial head *(arrow)*. Even without definitely seeing the fracture on the radiographs it should be surmised to be present when the posterior fat pad is visualized in the setting of trauma. The elevated and displaced anterior fat pad has been termed a "sail" sign because it resembles a spinnaker sail.

without a visible posterior fat pad, and that was in a patient with a prior elbow fracture who probably scarred down the joint posteriorly, preventing it from distending enough to push the fat pad out of the fossa. Therefore I usually don't care what the anterior fat pad looks like, and find it easier to concentrate on the presence or absence of the posterior fat pad. Keep things as simple as possible. Why be concerned over the appearance of two fat pads when one will do quite nicely?

Shoulder dislocations are generally easily diagnosed, both clinically and radiographically. The most common shoulder dislocation is the anterior dislocation. It is at least 10 times more common than the posterior dislocation. For all practical purposes, these are the only two types of shoulder dislocations to be concerned about.

An anterior dislocation occurs when the arm is forcibly externally rotated and abducted. This is commonly seen when football players "arm tackle," when kayakers "brace" with the paddle above their heads and allow their arms to get too far posterior, when skiers plant their uphill pole and get it stuck, and as a result of similar athletic positions. Radiographically, the diagnosis is easily made on an AP shoulder film: the humeral head is seen to lie inferiorly and medial to the glenoid (Fig. 5.39). The humeral head often impacts against the inferior lip of the glenoid, causing an indentation on the posterosuperior portion of the humeral head called a *Hill–Sachs deformity*. A Hill–Sachs deformity

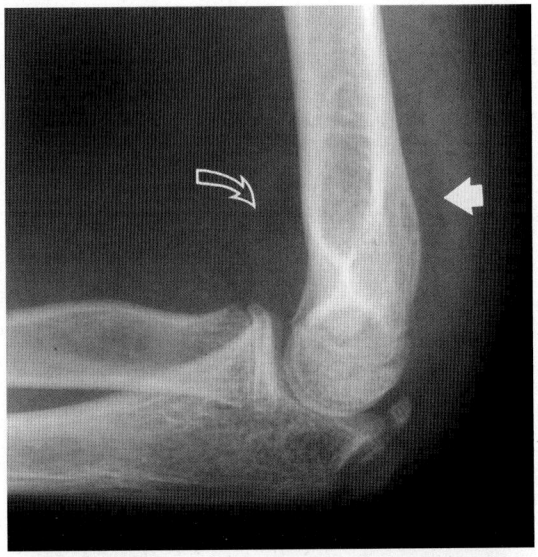

FIG. 5.37 **Displaced Elbow Fat Pads.** A lateral view of the elbow in this patient shows a posterior fat pad *(arrow)* and a "sail" sign anteriorly *(curved arrow)*. This is indicative of a fracture about the elbow, which, in a child (the epiphyses are open), usually means a supracondylar fracture.

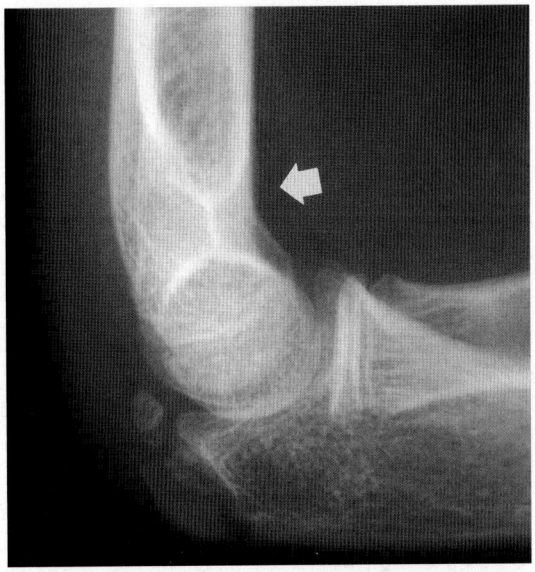

FIG. 5.38 **Normal Anterior Fat Pad of the Elbow.** Note the lucency just anterior to the humerus of this normal elbow *(arrow)*, and compare this with the "sail" sign of the anterior fat pads in Figs. 5.38 and 5.39.

is said to indicate a greater likelihood of recurrent dislocation, and some surgeons use it as an indicator to surgically intervene so as to prevent a recurrence. A bony irregularity or fragment off the inferior glenoid, which occurs from the same mechanism as does the Hill–Sachs deformity, is called a bony *Bankhart deformity* (see Chapter 10).

A posterior dislocation can be a difficult diagnosis to make, both clinically and radiographically. An AP view may look normal, or nearly so. On the AP view of a normal shoulder, the humeral head should slightly overlap the glenoid (Fig. 5.40), forming a "crescent sign." In a patient with a posterior dislocation, this crescent of bony overlap is often absent, and a small space is seen between the glenoid and the humeral head (Fig. 5.41).

The best way to unequivocally diagnose a dislocated shoulder is to obtain a transscapular view. An axillary view will show basically the same thing but requires the patient to move his arm and shoulder, which can be painful and can even redislocate the shoulder if it has already been reduced. The transscapular view is obtained by angling the x-ray beam across the shoulder in the same plane as the blade of the scapula. This gives an *en face* view of the glenoid, and the humeral head can easily be related to it as either normal, anterior

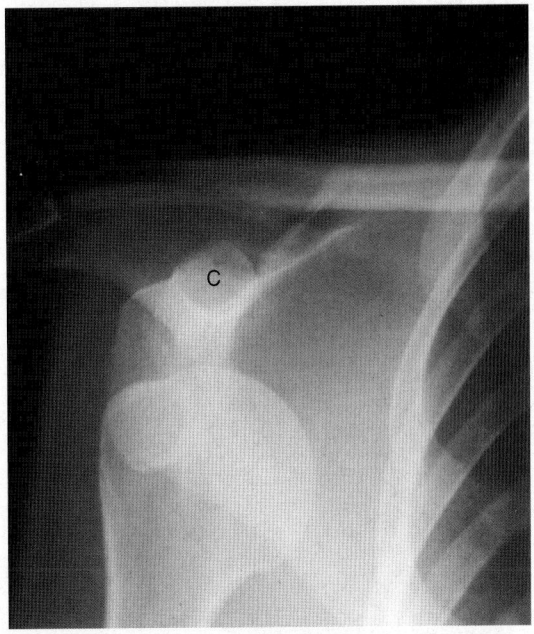

FIG. 5.39 **Anterior Dislocation of the Shoulder.** An anteroposterior (AP) view of the right shoulder shows the humeral head to lie medial to the glenoid and inferior to the coracoid process (*C*). This is diagnostic of an anterior dislocation of the shoulder.

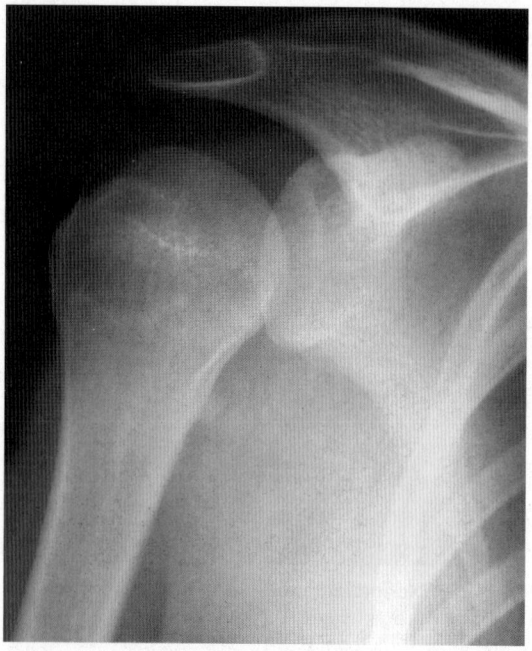

FIG. 5.40 **Normal Anteroposterior (AP) View of the Shoulder.** Note on this example of a normal shoulder that the humeral head slightly overlaps the glenoid. This has been termed the "crescent sign."

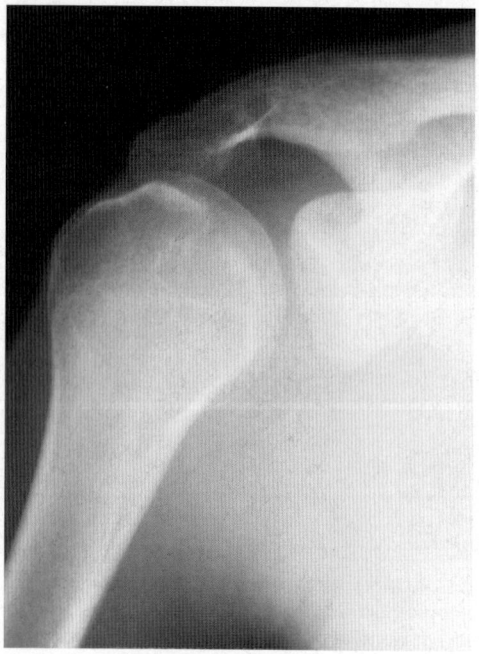

FIG. 5.41 **Posterior Dislocation of the Shoulder.** Note that the humeral head in this patient is slightly displaced from the glenoid on the anteroposterior (AP) view. This is termed absence of the "crescent sign" and is often seen with a posterior dislocation. Compare this with Fig. 5.40.

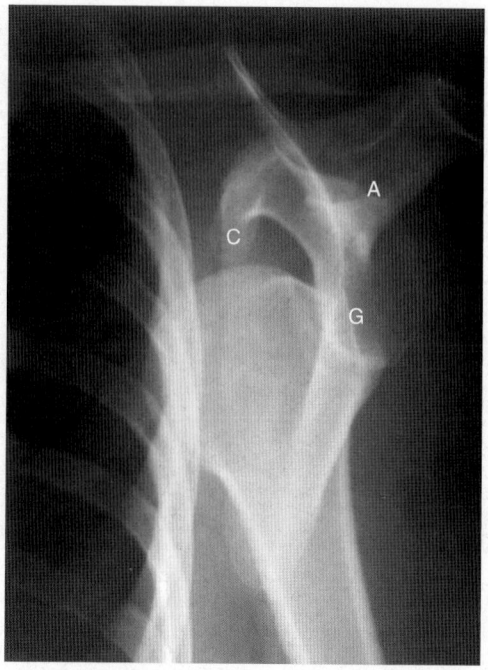

FIG. 5.42 **Transscapular View of an Anterior Dislocation.** This transscapular view of the shoulder is obtained by aiming the x-ray beam parallel to the shoulder blade. The coracoid process (*C*) can be seen anteriorly, and the spine of the acromion (*A*) can be seen posteriorly. Both of these structures extend inwardly and meet at the glenoid (*G*). In this example, the humeral head is seen to lie outside of the glenoid in an anterior direction.

(Fig. 5.42), or posterior (Fig. 5.43). Because of overlapping ribs and clavicles, the exact anatomy is often difficult to discern on the transscapular view. To find the glenoid, one has to find the coracoid, the spine of the acromion, and the blade of the scapula. These three structures all lead to the glenoid and form a *Y* around it. All one has to do to find the center of the glenoid is to find two of those bony landmarks—usually the coracoid and the blade of the scapula. The humeral head can then be found and its position determined.

I was once involved in a court case where an ER doc and a radiologist both missed a posterior dislocation in a patient who fell and had shoulder pain. The patient had the diagnosis made 2 weeks later and needed surgery—he was left with some permanent shoulder disability. The radiologist's lawyer argued that a community hospital radiologist should not be expected to diagnose such a rare disorder, even though the "university radiologist" (me) said it should be routinely identified. You certainly cannot expect to pass boards if you miss a posterior dislocation on your exam—this is bread and butter radiology.

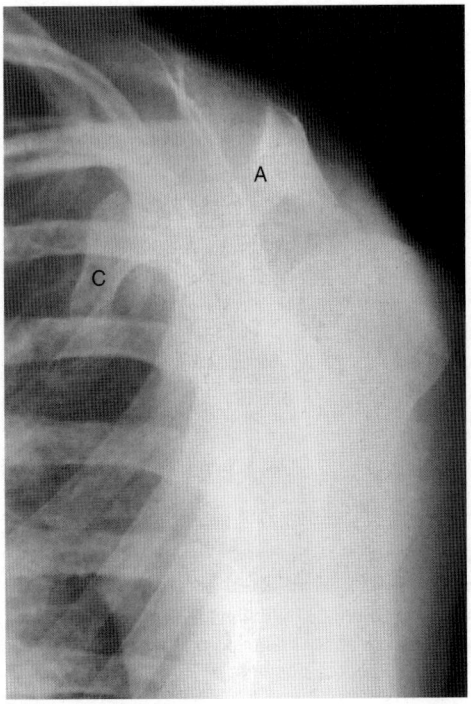

FIG. 5.43 **Transscapular View of a Posterior Dislocation.** The transscapular view in this patient is more difficult to appreciate; however, the coracoid process (*C*) and the acromion (*A*) can still be identified, and the position of the glenoid can be extrapolated. The humeral head is seen to lie posterior to where the glenoid lies.

An entity that can be mistaken for a dislocated shoulder is a traumatic hemarthrosis that displaces the humeral head inferolaterally on the AP film. Because the anterior dislocation displaces inferomedially, it should not be confused with this. The posterior dislocation will easily be excluded by looking at a transscapular view. This is termed a pseudodislocation (see Chapter 4).

If a fracture about the shoulder is suspected and the plain films are negative or equivocal, a CT scan should be performed. Any complex joint, such as the shoulder or hip, is best examined with CT scanning when the full extent of the fracture needs to be identified (Fig. 5.44).

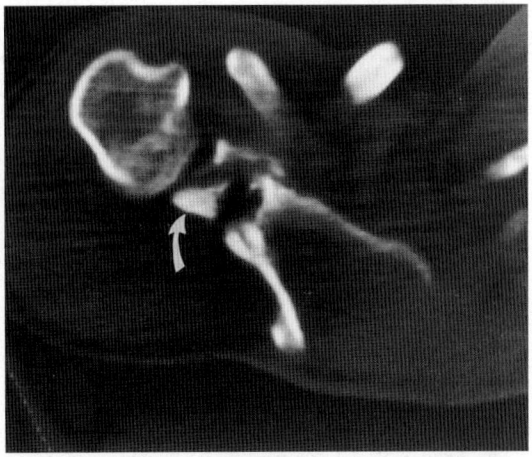

FIG. 5.44 **Fracture of the Glenoid.** A computed tomography (CT) of the shoulder in this patient who had a fracture identified on a plain film shows extension into the articular portion with a possible loose fragment *(arrow)*. The plain film did not show the fracture extending into the joint.

PELVIS

Fractures of the pelvis, and especially those involving the acetabulum, can be difficult to evaluate completely with plain films alone. Because plain films often do not show free fragments and subtle fractures, CT scanning should be considered in almost all acetabular fractures (Fig. 5.45).

Sacral fractures are said to occur in half of the cases that have pelvic fractures, yet radiologists see a lot of pelvic fractures without seeing very many sacral fractures. Why is this? Simple—we miss a lot of sacral fractures. They can be difficult to see on even the best of films because the sacrum is often hidden by bowel gas. In looking for sacral fractures, one should examine the arcuate lines of the sacrum bilaterally to see if they are intact. Fractures often interrupt these lines and, because of the side-to-side asymmetry, can be identified (Fig. 5.46).

Sacral insufficiency fractures occur commonly in patients who are osteoporotic or who have undergone radiation therapy. These present as patchy or linear sclerosis in the sacral ala that may or may not show cortical disruption (Fig. 5.47). They should be differentiated from metastatic disease because of their characteristic location, appearance, osteoporosis or history of prior radiation, and by the presence of a cortical break. These are often bilateral and then have a pathognomonic appearance on bone scan called a "Honda sign" (Fig. 5.48). They also have a characteristic MR appearance with geographic involvement of one or both sacral alae with low signal on T1WI, which may or may not have high signal on T2WI (Fig. 5.49).

Avulsion injuries affect the pelvis quite often and should be easily recognized by radiologists. On occasion, an avulsion can appear somewhat "aggressive," and if it is not diagnosed radiographically, a biopsy might be performed. This action can be calamitous, as avulsion injuries have been known to mimic malignant

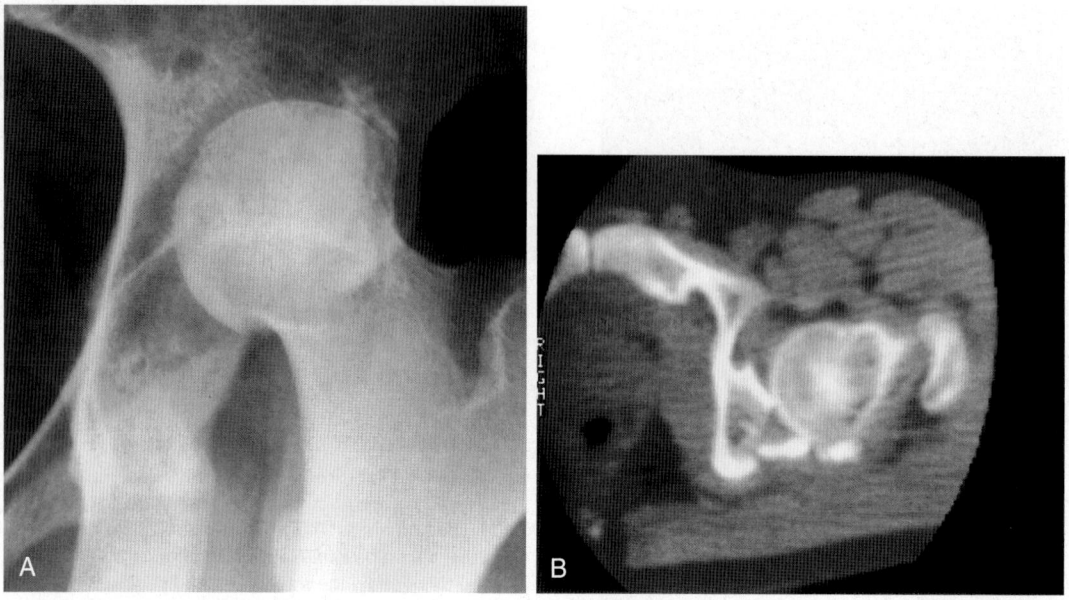

FIG. 5.45 **Dislocation of the Hip.** (A) An anteroposterior (AP) plain film of the left hip shows dislocation of the femoral head, which lies superior to the acetabulum. Fractures are easily identified on the computed tomography (CT) scan (B). A cortical break through the articular surface of the posterior acetabulum, as well as the dislocation, is identified.

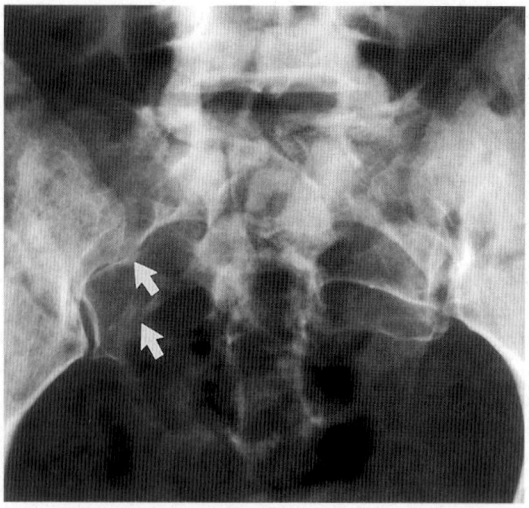

FIG. 5.46 **Fracture of the Sacrum.** An anteroposterior (AP) view of the sacrum in this patient shows normal arcuate lines on the left side of the sacrum that are interrupted on the right side *(arrows)*. Interruption of these lines indicates a fracture through this portion of the sacrum.

lesions histologically, with a misdiagnosis leading to radical treatment (Fig. 5.50). Therefore when an avulsion injury is a consideration, it becomes a "don't touch" lesion (see Chapter 4). Common sites for pelvic avulsion include the ischium, the superior and inferior anterior iliac spines (Fig. 5.51), and the iliac crest. Such injuries are fairly common in long jumpers, sprinters, hurdlers, gymnasts, and cheerleaders.

The symphysis pubis is another area in the pelvis that can demonstrate radiologic findings as a result of stress. In ultramarathoners, marathon cross-country skiers, and soccer players, the symphysis often undergoes degenerative changes (Figs. 5.52 and 5.53). The hallmarks of degenerative disease (osteoarthritis) are sclerosis, joint space narrowing, and osteophytosis. In certain joints, however, erosions occur as a result of degenerative joint disease. These joints include the temporomandibular joint (TMJ), the acromioclavicular (AC) joint, and the sacroiliac (SI) joint. These are easy to remember because they are the "letter joints"—the TMJ, the AC, and the SI. The symphysis pubis also behaves in this manner. Ordinarily when erosions are a feature of an articular process, osteoarthritis (degenerative joint disease) is not in the differential diagnosis. It should be if the TMJ, the AC joint, the SI joint, or the symphysis is involved, however.

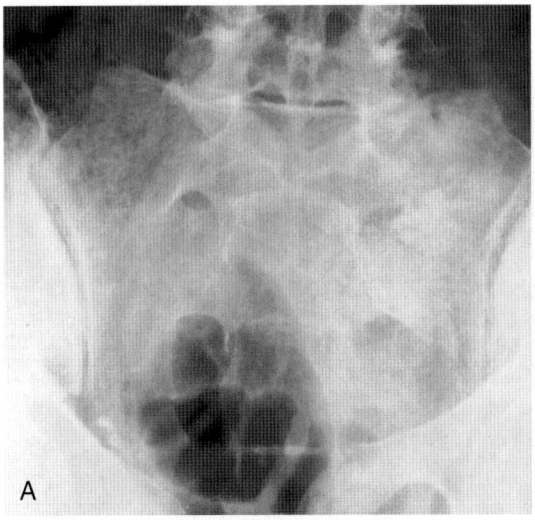

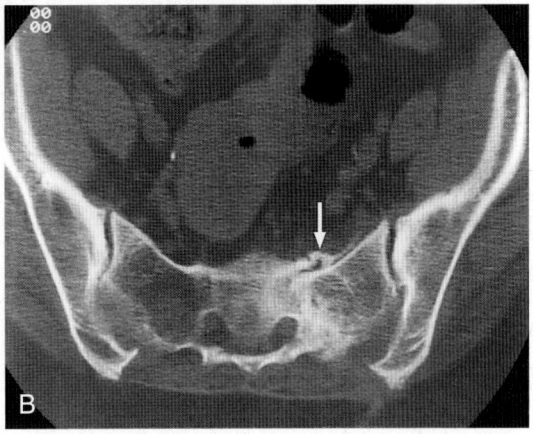

FIG. 5.47 **Insufficiency Fracture of the Sacrum.** (A) Faint sclerosis is noted in the left part of the sacrum as compared with the right in this patient complaining of pelvic pain. A radionuclide bone scan showed increased isotope uptake on the left half of the sacrum, and metastatic disease was postulated. A CT scan through this region (B) demonstrates a cortical disruption *(arrow)* indicative of a fracture. This is a characteristic plain film and computed tomography (CT) appearance of an insufficiency fracture of the sacrum.

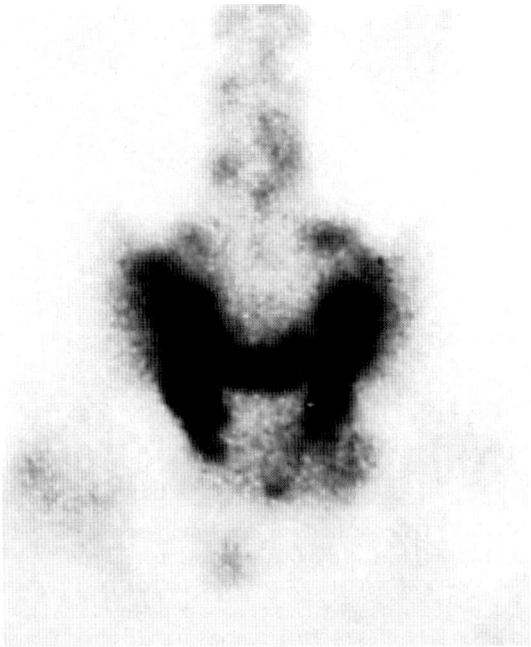

FIG. 5.48 **"Honda Sign."** A radionuclide bone scan in a patient with bilateral sacral insuffiency (or stress) fractures shows increased uptake in the sacrum corresponding to an *H*, which has been termed a "Honda sign." This finding is virtually pathognomonic for sacral insufficiency fractures.

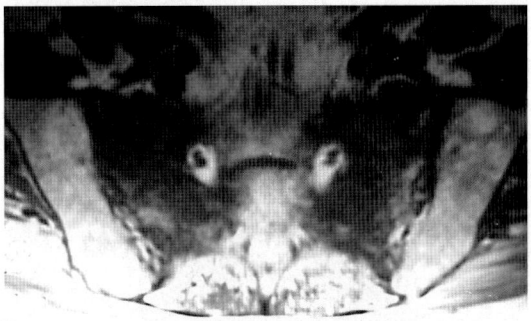

FIG. 5.49 **Magnetic Resonance Imaging (MRI) of Sacral Insufficiency Fracture.** A T1-weighted coronal MR through the sacrum in the patient with the bone scan shown in Fig. 5.48 reveals areas of low signal corresponding to the edema and reactive bone around the sacral fractures. Much of the area of low signal will get increased in signal on a T2-weighted sequence. Why get an MR if the bone scan is pathognomonic? A good question. The MR is certainly not necessary if the bone scan had been performed already, and the bone scan would not be needed if the MR were the first study.

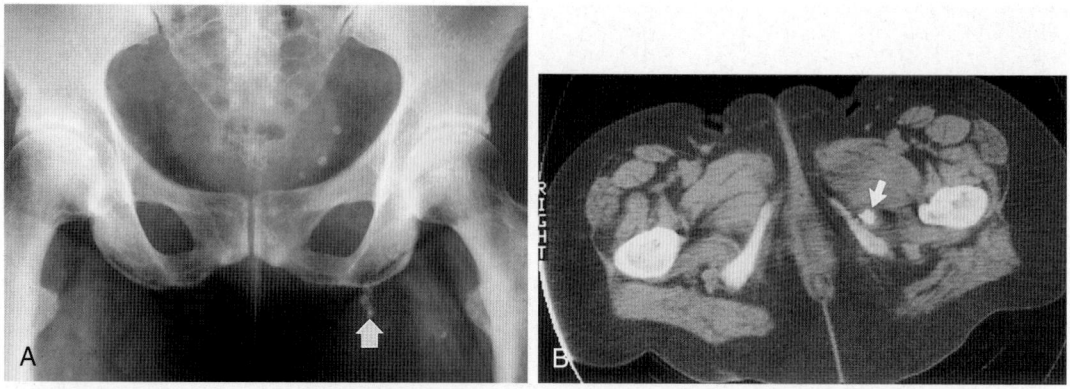

FIG. 5.50 **Avulsion off the Ischium.** (A) An AP view of the pelvis shows calcification extending off the left ischium *(arrow)* in a patient complaining of pain at this site. Note the irregular cortical surface, suggesting periostitis. (B) The computed tomography (CT) scan shows dense calcification adjacent to the ischium *(arrow)*. These findings are characteristic for an ischial avulsion, and a biopsy should not be done.

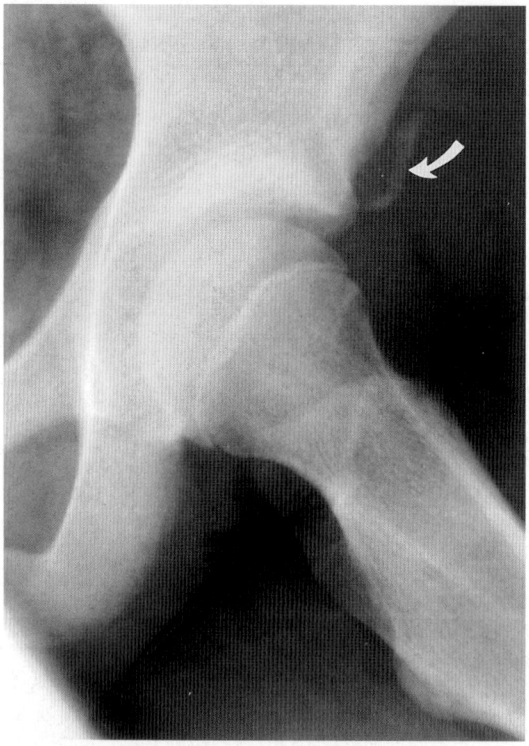

FIG. 5.51 **Avulsion From Anterior Inferior Iliac Spine.** A plain film of the pelvis shows a calcific density near the anterior inferior iliac spine *(arrow)*, which is typical for an avulsion of the rectus femoris muscle.

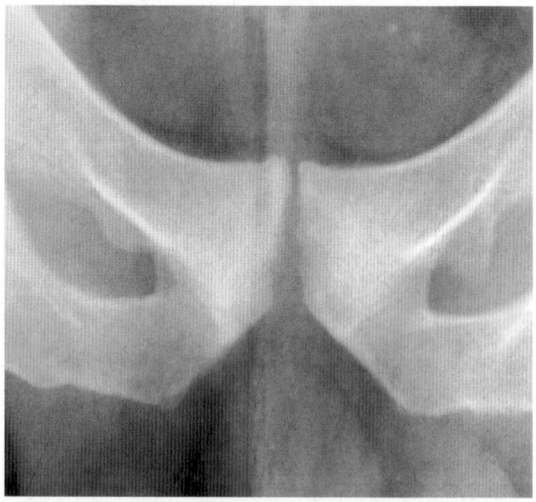

FIG. 5.52 **Osteoarthritis of the Symphysis Pubis.** Sclerosis with erosion is noted at the symphysis in this ultramarathoner complaining of severe pubic pain. This is characteristic of degenerative disease or osteoarthritis at this site in an overuse setting, such as in an ultramarathoner. Erosions are ordinarily not seen in degenerative disease except in certain joints, such as the symphysis pubis, the sacroiliac (SI) joints, and the acromioclavicular (AC) joints.

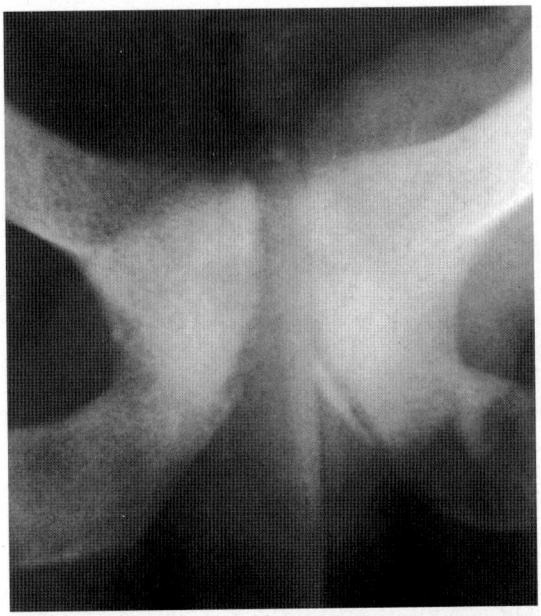

FIG. 5.53 **Osteoarthritis of the Symphysis Pubis.** This is another example of sclerosis and erosive changes at the symphysis pubis in an ultramarathoner.

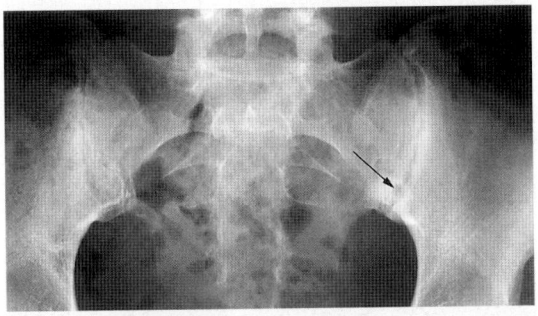

FIG. 5.54 **Osteoarthritis of the Sacroiliac Joint.** Sclerosis and erosions *(arrow)* are seen in the left sacroiliac (SI) joint in this young professional dancer. Although this finding has the appearance of an inflammatory arthritis, it is also seen in degenerative disease or osteoarthritis secondary to overuse.

When the SI joints are involved with degenerative joint disease, the condition can closely resemble an HLA-B27 spondyloarthropathy (Fig. 5.54) and lead to erroneous diagnosis and treatment. Large osteophytes can develop across the SI joints and mimic sclerosis (Fig. 5.55) or even a tumor (Fig. 5.56).

LEG

Overt fractures in the femur and lower leg are, for the most part, straightforward, and deserve no special radiologic treatment for fear of missing subtle abnormalities. Stress fractures, however, need to be considered in anyone with hip or leg pain, as overlooking the diagnosis can lead to catastrophe. The most serious stress fracture—and fortunately one of the rarest—is the femoral neck stress fracture. It has been divided into three types by orthopedic surgeons: type 1: sclerosis without a fracture line evident (Fig. 5.57); type 2: a lucent fracture line without displacement (Fig. 5.58); type 3: a displaced fracture is evident. The prognosis is best for a type 1 and worst for a type 3 fracture. Many surgeons believe that type 2 and type 3 fractures require internal fixation, whereas a type 1 fracture requires nonweight bearing for at least 3 to 4 weeks. Many type 1 fractures progress to complete fractures with displacement (type 3) with continued weight bearing; therefore these are considered very serious lesions. If a femoral stress fracture is a clinical concern and plain films are normal, an MRI should be obtained.

Stress fractures also occur in the distal diaphysis of the femur and in the proximal, middle, and distal thirds of the tibia. All of these stress fractures need to be treated with the utmost caution, since complete fractures are not uncommon with continued stress (Figs. 5.59 and 5.60). Sclerosis in a weight-bearing bone that has a horizontal or oblique linear pattern should be considered a stress fracture until proved otherwise. Occasionally a stress fracture will appear somewhat aggressive, with aggressive periostitis and no definite linearity to the sclerosis (Fig. 5.61). If the fracture is mistaken for a tumor and a biopsy is performed, it can be confused with a malignancy, with subsequent radical therapy. Therefore in such cases, a biopsy should not be done under any circumstances. If the clinical presentation is unusual for a stress fracture and the plain films are not diagnostic, take additional films 1 or 2 weeks later. Sometimes CT and MRI will better delineate the lesion. Stress fractures can be difficult to diagnose radiologically early on but should be straightforward after several weeks. A history of repetitive stress is not always obtained, so the diagnosis should not depend solely on the history.

An unusual stress fracture is a fibular stress fracture (Fig. 5.62). The fibula is ordinarily not thought of as a weight-bearing bone, but in certain people, it must serve as such.

One final stress fracture that deserves mention because it is frequently misdiagnosed clinically and overlooked radiographically is the calcaneal stress fracture (Fig. 5.63). It is often misdiagnosed clinically as a "heel spur," or plantar fasciitis, and can be a subtle

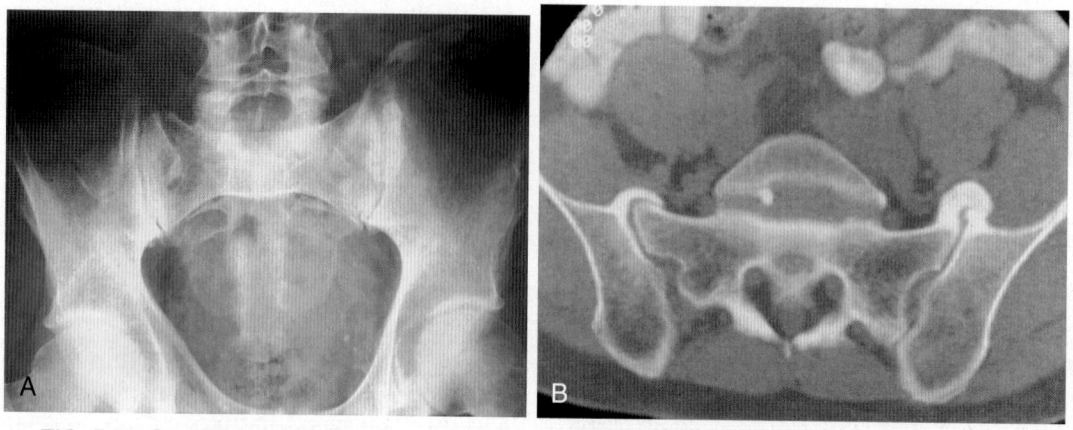

FIG. 5.55 **Sacroiliac Osteophytes.** An anteroposterior (AP) view of the pelvis (A) in this marathoner shows dense sclerosis over both sacroiliac (SI) joints. A computed tomography (CT) scan through this area (B) demonstrates dense, bridging osteophytes characteristic of degenerative disease.

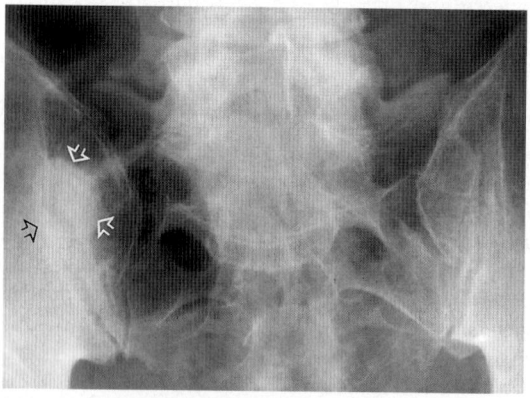

FIG. 5.56 **Sacroiliac Osteophytosis.** A focal area of sclerosis is seen overlying the right sacroiliac (SI) joint *(arrows)* in this elderly patient. A metastatic process was a diagnostic consideration. This is characteristic, however, of a sacroiliac osteophyte seen in degenerative disease of the SI joints.

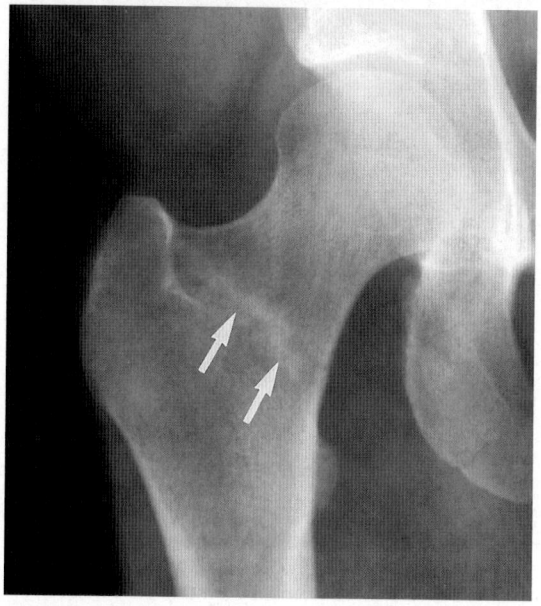

FIG. 5.57 **Femoral Stress Fracture.** An area of linear sclerosis *(arrows)* is seen at the base of the femoral neck in a neophyte runner with hip pain. This finding is diagnostic of a stress fracture of the femur.

radiographic finding. MRI can be helpful in cases in which plain films are negative (Fig. 5.64).

Overt fractures in the lower extremity are uncommonly missed on radiographs; however, a few exceptions should be noted. Hip fractures in the elderly population can be difficult to detect (Fig. 5.65), and a high index of suspicion should be maintained. A negative plain film in an elderly patient with hip pain after trauma (even relatively mild trauma) does not exclude a femoral neck fracture. An immediate MRI should be obtained to exclude a fracture. MRI has proved to be very useful in diagnosing hip fractures when plain films are negative (Fig. 5.66) and, even though expensive, can actually reduce the overall costs by ensuring that no fractures are missed.[5]

Another fracture that can be difficult to exclude on routine plain films is a tibial plateau fracture (Fig. 5.67). Many emergency rooms routinely take a cross-table lateral view of the knee to look for a fat/fluid level in the suprapatellar recess. This finding indicates that a fracture has occurred and allowed fatty marrow

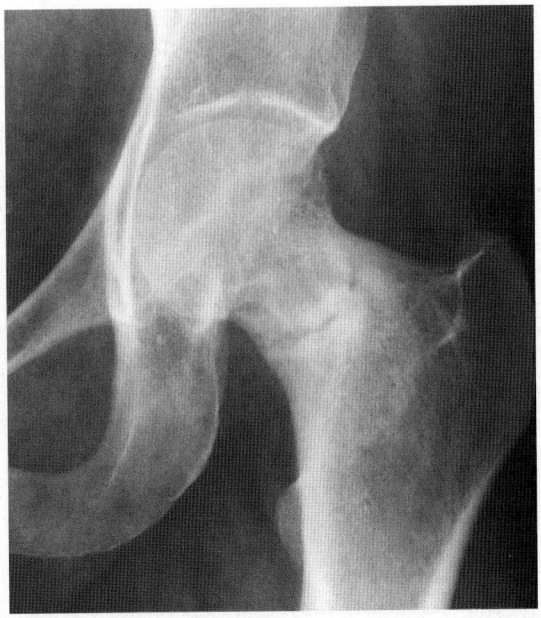

FIG. 5.58 **Stress Fracture of the Femoral Neck.** A linear lucency with surrounding sclerosis is seen in the femoral neck in this jogger with hip pain. This is a severe femoral neck stress fracture.

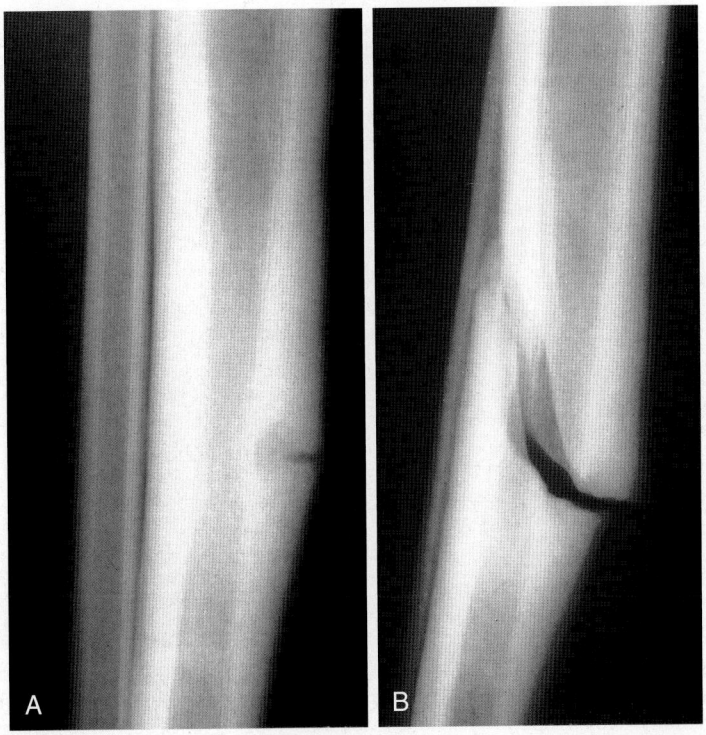

FIG. 5.59 **Stress Fracture With Completion.** (A) A linear lucency is seen in the anterior cortex of the tibia in this runner, which is diagnostic for a stress fracture. (B) This radiograph shows the result of continued exercise. The stress fracture went on to a complete fracture, which illustrates why any stress fracture of a long bone should be protected.

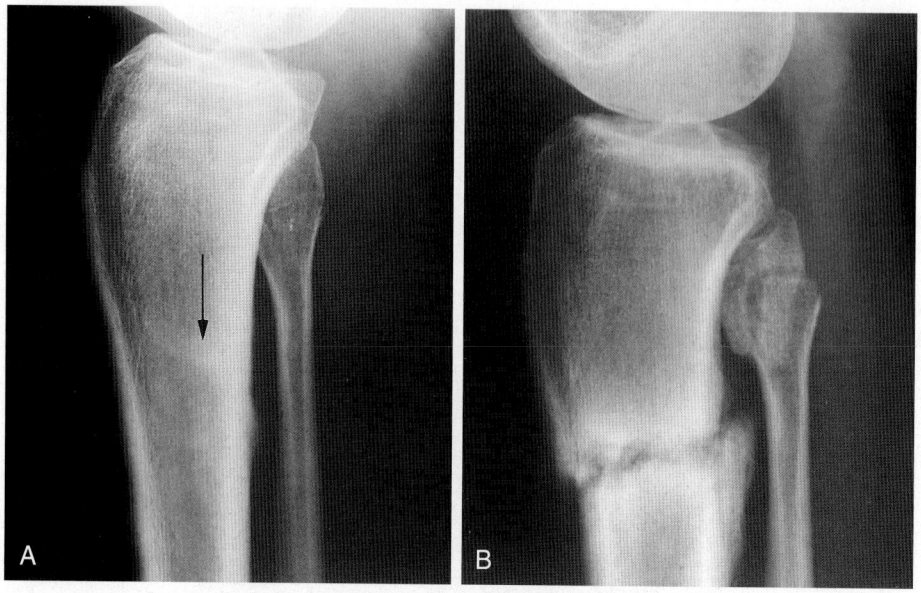

FIG. 5.60 **Stress Fracture With Completion.** (A) A faint linear sclerotic area *(arrow)* is seen, which is characteristic for a stress fracture of the proximal tibia. (B) This radiograph shows the result of continued exercise in this patient: a complete fracture of the tibia and of the proximal fibula.

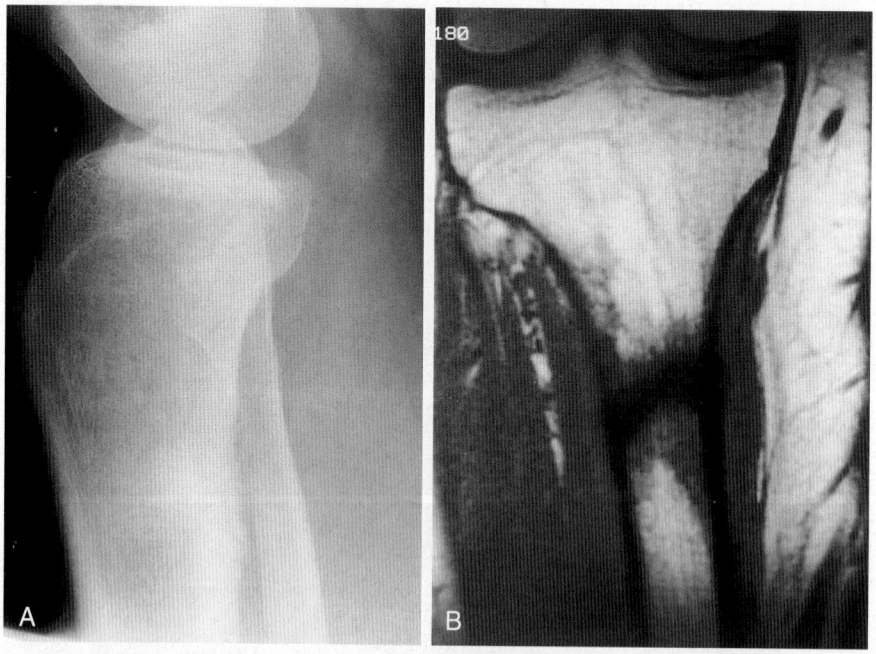

FIG. 5.61 **Stress Fracture of the Tibia.** (A) An irregular focus of sclerosis is seen in the posterior proximal tibia with adjacent periostitis. There was concern that this might represent a primary bone tumor, and the surgeons recommended a biopsy. A magnetic resonance imaging (MRI) scan was performed (B), however, showing a linear low-signal area running obliquely across the tibia, which is characteristic of a stress fracture. No soft tissue mass was found. The patient's recent history included an increase in his jogging, and a stress fracture was diagnosed based on these images.

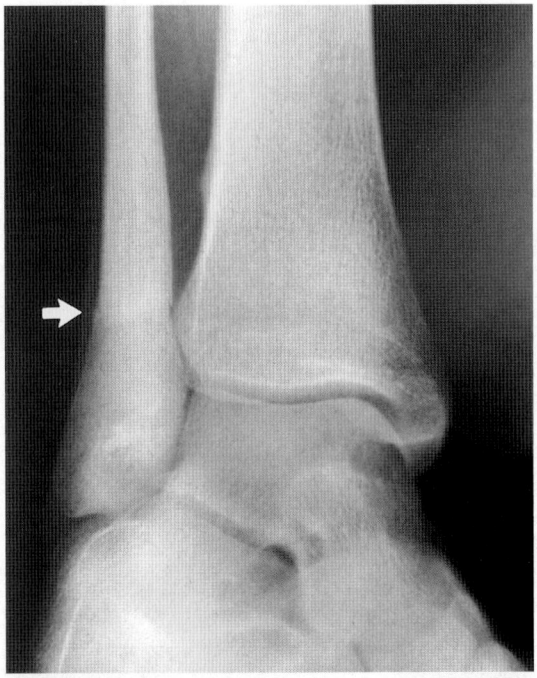

FIG. 5.62 **Fibular Stress Fracture.** A linear band of sclerosis with adjacent periostitis *(arrow)* is seen in the distal fibula in this young woman jogger. This is diagnostic for a stress fracture of the fibula.

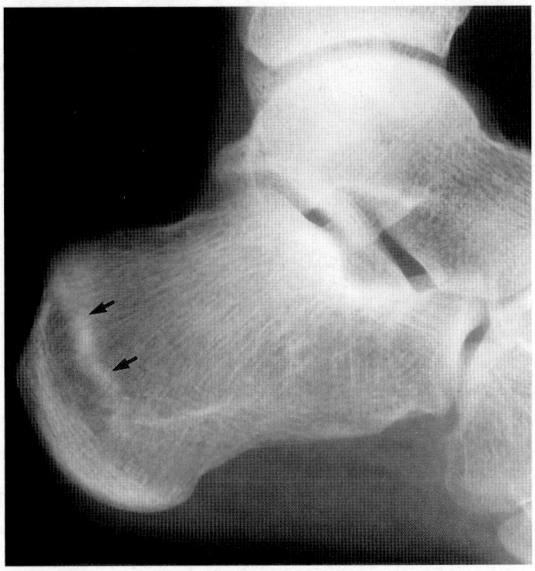

FIG. 5.63 **Calcaneal Stress Fracture.** A linear band of sclerosis is seen in the posterior calcaneus *(arrows)*, which is diagnostic for a stress fracture of the calcaneus.

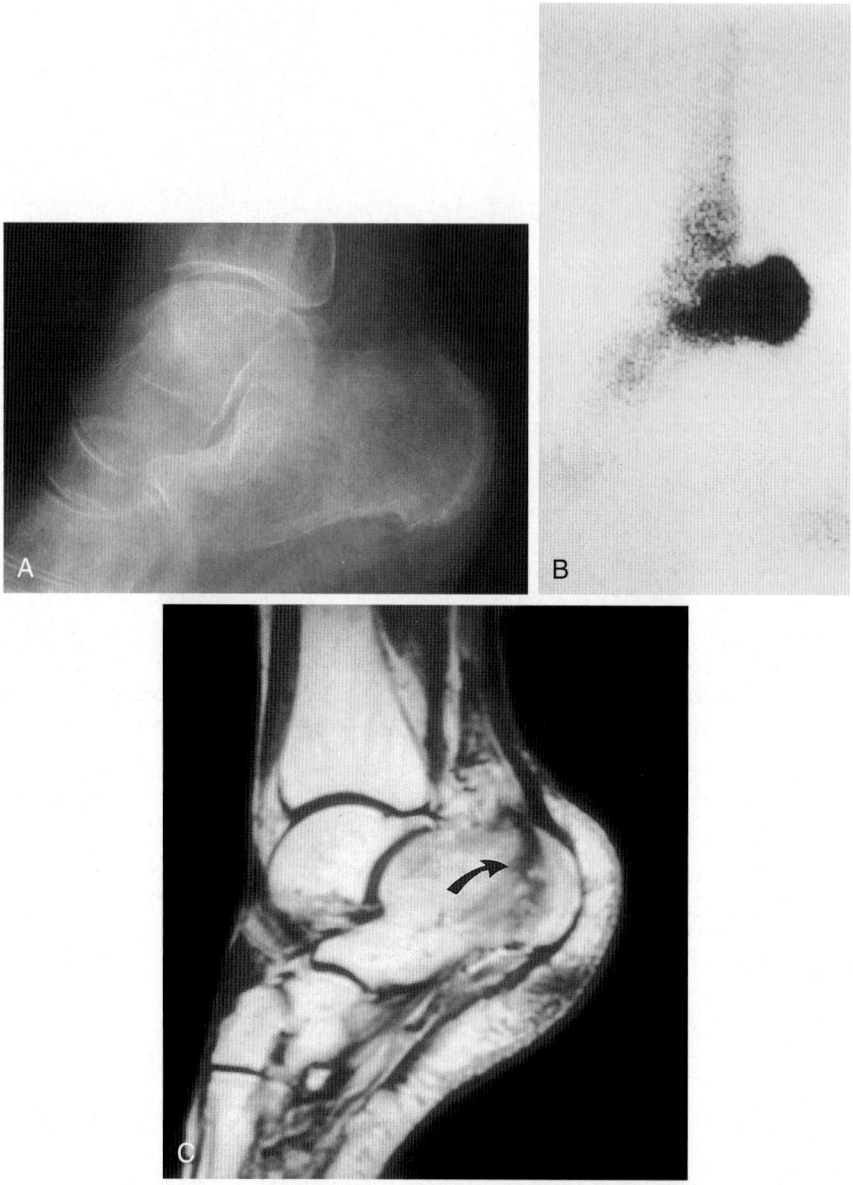

FIG. 5.64 **Magnetic Resonance Imaging (MRI) of Calcaneal Stress Fracture.** (A) A lateral plain film of the calcaneus in an elderly woman with heel pain and a history of lung carcinoma shows only osteoporosis. (B) A radionuclide bone scan reveals diffuse increased uptake throughout the calcaneus. The question of whether to treat the calcaneus with radiation for metastatic lung carcinoma or to do a biopsy first was a dilemma. (C) An MR was obtained to get a better idea of where the met might be. This sagittal T1-weighted image shows a linear low signal area *(arrow)*, which is characteristic for a stress fracture. Obviously, no biopsy or radiation was necessary.

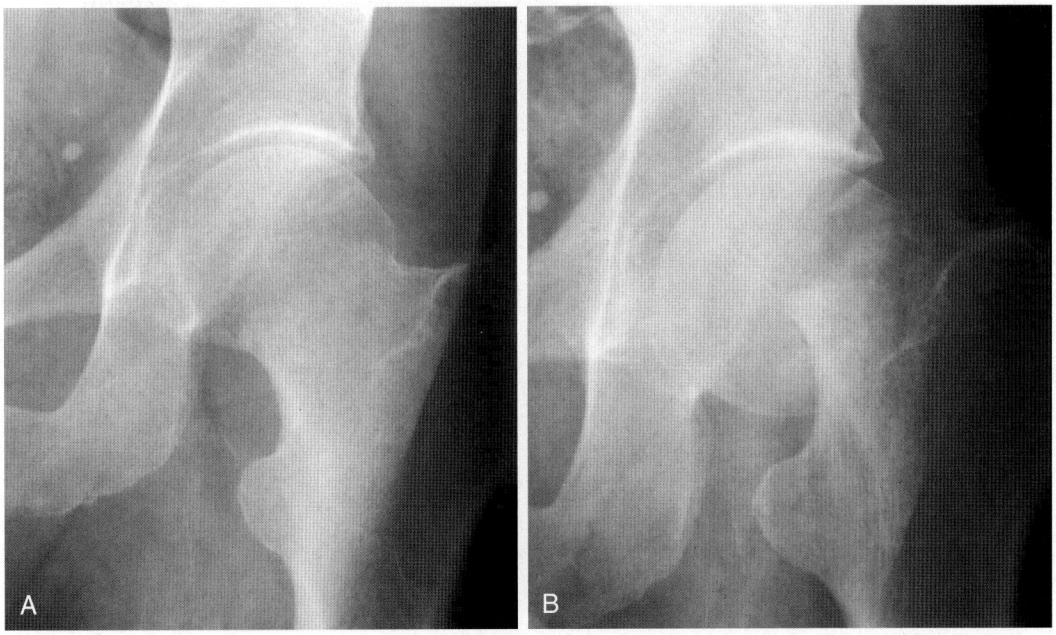

FIG. 5.65 **Fracture of the Hip.** (A) An anteroposterior (AP) view of the hip was obtained in an elderly man after he had fallen. It was interpreted as normal, and the patient was dismissed from the emergency department. Two weeks later, the patient returned to the emergency department because he was unable to walk. Another radiograph was obtained (B), and this shows a complete fracture through the femoral neck. In retrospect the fracture can be faintly seen in (A) and should have been picked up initially. Fractures of the hip in the elderly can be difficult to see and should be diligently searched for with additional views when the clinical setting is appropriate.

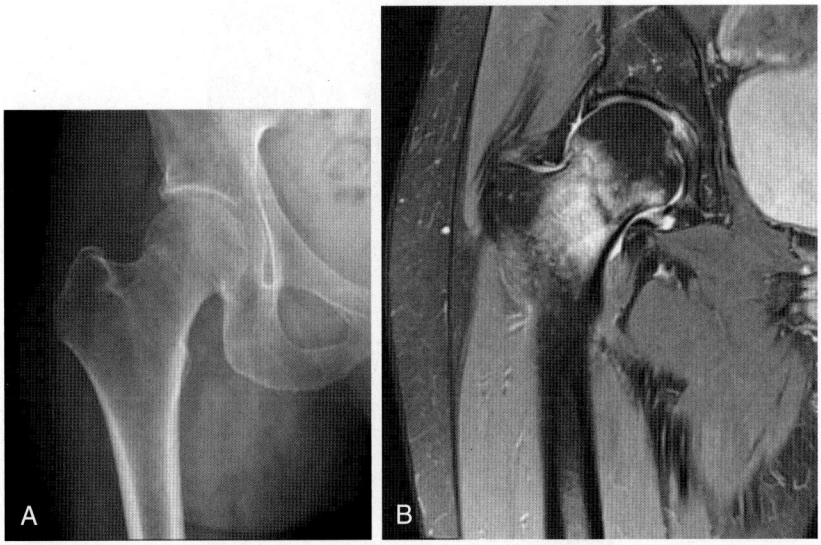

FIG. 5.66 **Magnetic Resonance Imaging (MRI) of Hip Fracture.** (A) A plain film of the hip in this elderly patient who has hip pain following a fall does not show a fracture. (B) A T2-weighted MR shows linear low signal and edema in the intertrochanteric region, which is diagnostic for a hip fracture.

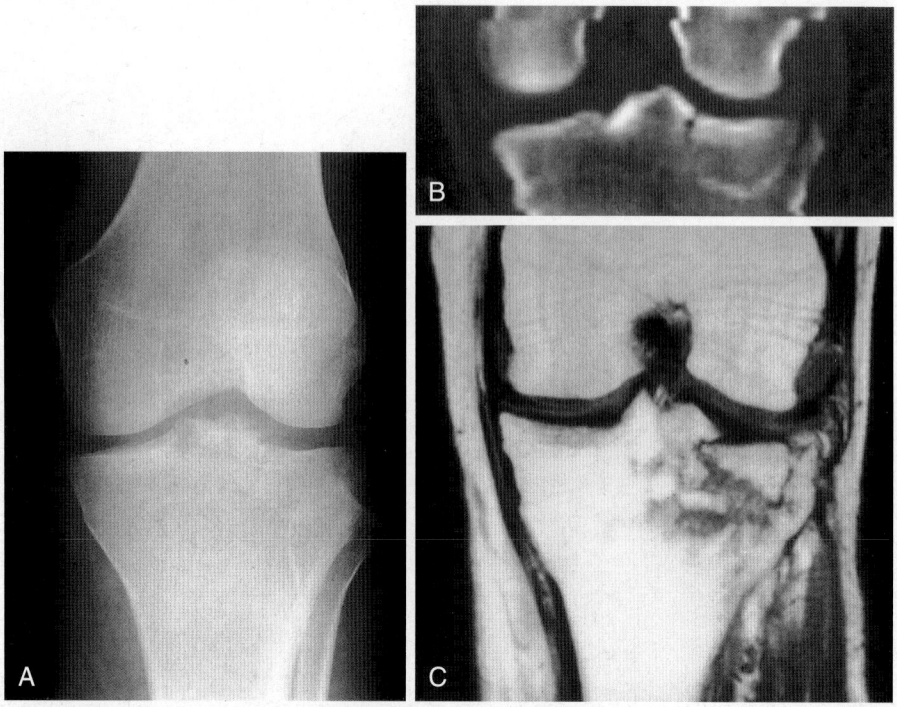

FIG. 5.67 **Tibial Plateau Fracture.** (A) An anteroposterior (AP) view of the knee shows no obvious abnormalities at first glance. However, a computed tomography (CT) scan with reformations of the knee (B) demonstrates a plateau fracture of the lateral tibia. Note the rounded sclerosis, which in retrospect can be barely appreciated in A. (C) A T1 coronal MR shows a tibial plateau fracture which was barely discernable on plain films. MR is an excellent imaging choice for subtle fractures. Tibial plateau fractures are probably the most commonly missed fractures about the knee.

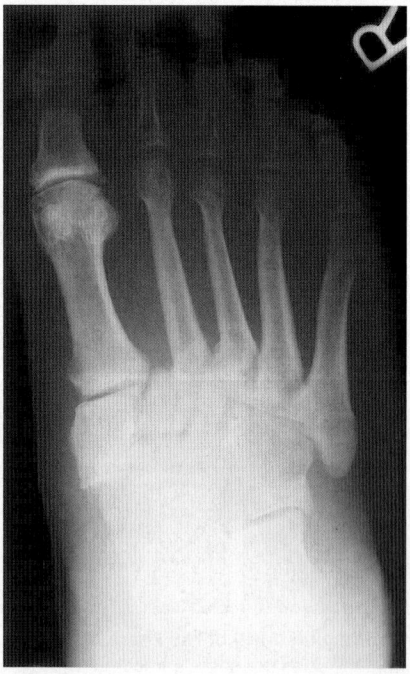

FIG. 5.68 **Lisfranc Fracture.** An anteroposterior (AP) view of the foot in this patient shows a space between the first and second metatarsals with the base of the second metatarsal displaced off the second cuneiform. This is indicative of a Lisfranc fracture–dislocation.

to enter the joint; it has a high correlation with a tibial plateau fracture. In the appropriate clinical setting, CT or MRI may be necessary to make the diagnosis.

A serious fracture in the foot that can be missed radiographically when little or no displacement occurs is the so-called Lisfranc fracture (Fig. 5.68). It is named after a famous surgeon in Napoleon's army who would do forefoot amputations in patients with gangrenous toes after frostbite. The Lisfranc fracture is a fracture–dislocation of the tarsometatarsals. If the dislocation is minimal, it can be easily overlooked. A key to normal alignment is that the medial border of the second metatarsal should always line up with the medial border of the second cuneiform, and the medial border of the fourth metatarsal should line up with the medial border of the cuboid. If they do not, a Lisfranc fracture–dislocation should be suspected. This fracture is seen most commonly as a result of catching the forefoot in something such as a hole in the ground, or in a horseback rider falling and hanging by the forefoot in the stirrups. It is not uncommonly seen as a neurotropic or Charcot joint in diabetics. As with many fractures, MRI can be very helpful in finding or excluding fractures when the clinical exam and the plain films are discordant.

A fracture of the calcaneus can be difficult to appreciate on routine radiographs. Boehler's angle is a normal anatomical landmark that should be looked for in every foot film when trauma has occurred (Fig. 5.69). If the angle is narrower than 20 degrees, a compression of the calcaneus is indicated, such as is seen with jumping injuries (Fig. 5.70). This fracture has been termed a "lover's fracture" for the propensity of lovers to jump out of windows when discovered in compromising surroundings by apparently larger or armed jealous suitors.

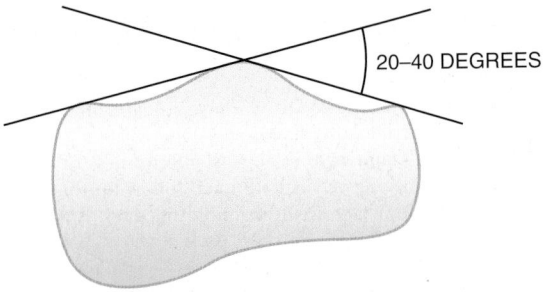

FIG. 5.69 **Boehler's Angle in a Normal Calcaneus.** This drawing shows the normal calcaneus with a line across the anterior process extending to the apex of the calcaneus, intersecting with a line from the posterior portion of the calcaneus to the apex. This is termed Boehler's angle, and when it becomes flattened or less than 20 degrees, a calcaneal fracture should be diagnosed.

A fracture that is easily overlooked by untrained or inexperienced physicians is one that involves the base of the fifth metatarsal. It frequently occurs in conjunction with a sprained ankle; hence the distracting element of the ankle pain from the injured ligaments can lead this fracture to be overlooked clinically as well. On lateral plain films, the fracture line can resmble an articular surface and be somewhat inconspicuous (Fig. 5.71). In addition, the base of the fifth metatarsal has an apophysis that, prior to its closure, can resemble a fracture; however, the apophysis has its physeal line parallel to the metatarsal shaft (Fig. 5.72), whereas a fracture of the base of the fifth is perpendicular to the metatarsal shaft.

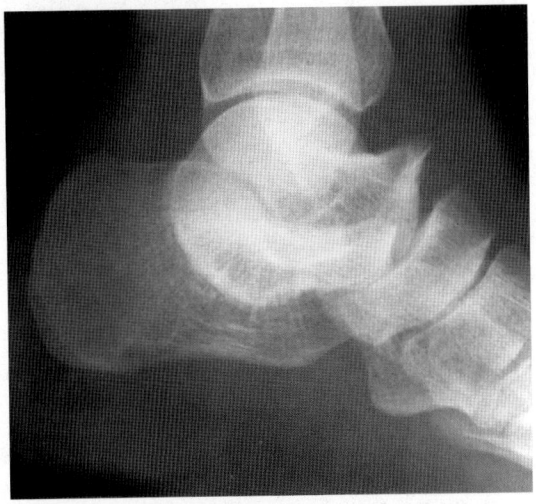

FIG. 5.70 **Calcaneal Fracture.** Boehler's angle in this calcaneus is less than 20 degrees, which is indicative of a fracture of the calcaneus.

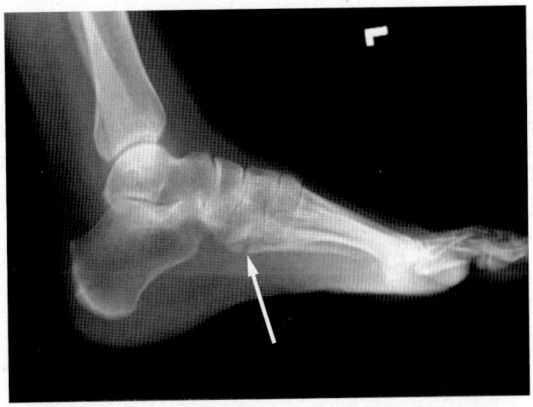

FIG. 5.71 **Fracture of the Base of the Fifth Metatarsal.** This lateral plain film in a woman who sprained her ankle shows the classic appearance of a fracture of the base of the fifth metatarsal *(arrow)*.

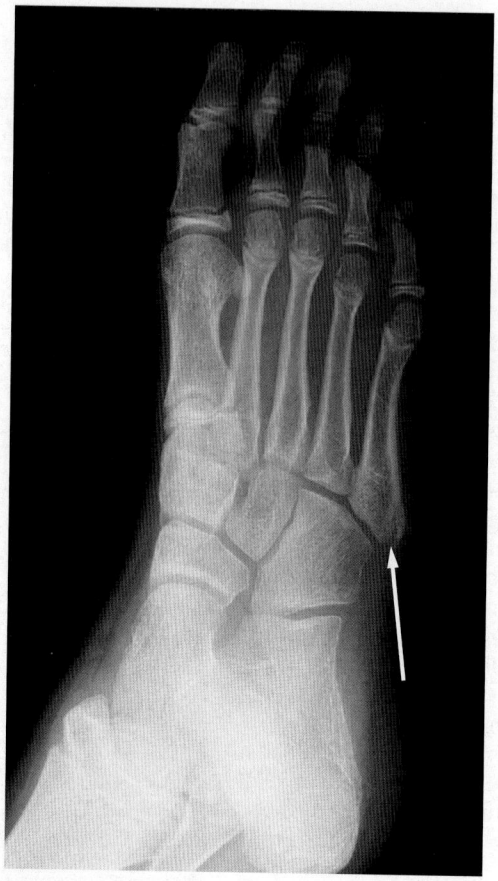

FIG. 5.72 **Normal Apophysis at the Base of the Fifth Metatarsal.** This anteroposterior (AP) film of the foot shows a normal fifth metatarsal apophysis. This 12-year-old boy sprained his ankle, and this was thought to be a fracture by the emergency room physician, even though it was nontender to palpation. Unfortunately, he was treated for several weeks in a walking boot and missed the remainder of his basketball season unnecessarily (case courtesy of Jennifer Stenner.)

This fairly simplified overview of some commonly overlooked fractures and dislocations should in no way be interpreted as a substitute for the more complete texts listed in the bibliography. For most residents and medical students, it can serve as a starting point, however, and perhaps stimulate reading in more depth on some of the topics.

REFERENCES

1. Rogers LF. *Radiology of Skeletal Trauma*. 2nd ed. New York: Churchill Livingstone; 2002.
2. Harris Jr JH, Harris WH. *The Radiology of Emergency Medicine*. 4th ed. Baltimore: Lippincott Williams & Wilkins; 2000.
3. Rockwood Jr CA, Green DP. *Fractures in Adults*. 5th ed. Philadelphia: Lippincott Williams and Wilkins; 2001.
4. Dorsay TA, Major NM, et al. Cost-effectiveness of immediate MR imaging versus traditional follow-up for revealing radiographically occult scaphoid fractures. *AJR*. 2001; 177(6):1257–1263.
5. Deutsch AL, Mink JH, Waxman AD. Occult fractures of the proximal femur: MR imaging. *Radiology*. 1989;170: 113–116.

CHAPTER 6

Arthritis

The radiologic study of arthritis can be extremely difficult for the inexperienced because of the wide variety of patterns of disease, which produces a tremendous amount of overlap among the various diseases. What at first seems to be simple characterization of disease entities is found by the more experienced observer to be broad generalizations that may or may not fit into any one category of disease.

This chapter gives an overview of radiologic evaluation of arthritis with the caveat that it is, by necessity, a simplified version and in no way complete. If one is interested in greater detail or more accuracy, I would urge reading either Debbie Forrester's excellent monograph[1] on the subject or Anne Brower's superb book.[2] The definitive work on this subject is Don Resnick's six-volume tome,[3] but most can't read even the arthritis portion during a 4-year residency—it's best used as a reference.

The majority of arthritides are most easily examined and categorized by looking at their effect on the hands. Forrester recommends a search pattern that she calls the ABCs, with the *A* indicating alignment, *B* standing for bone mineralization, *C* standing for cartilage and including a search for erosions, and the *S* standing for soft tissues. I would add to this search pattern by making it the ABCDs, with the *D* indicating distribution of the pathology. Although this is implied in Forrester's search pattern, I feel that it cannot be overemphasized.

In general, if the distribution of the arthropathy can be determined, the differential diagnosis becomes very short (Table 6.1). Although on paper this sounds quite nice, it can, on occasion, be difficult to accurately determine the distribution of the arthropathy. The distribution of the arthropathy is difficult to determine when it is not clearly distal or proximal but is more general, such as occurs with gout and sarcoid. It can also be difficult to accurately determine the distribution when advanced disease is present, such as occurs with severe rheumatoid arthritis. With severe rheumatoid arthritis, the proximal nature of the pathology is not so apparent because of involvement with the metacarpophalangeal joints and even the phalangeal joints. In a similar manner, when psoriatic disease, Reiter syndrome, or osteoarthritis are severely advanced, they can involve the more proximal portion of the hand and wrist, although this is unusual.

Side-to-side symmetry of the arthropathy is occasionally helpful in selecting a differential diagnosis (Box 6.1). Primary osteoarthritis and rheumatoid arthritis are classically described as bilaterally symmetric. Exceptions occur quite frequently, however, so that bilateral symmetry in these disorders is probably only on the order of 80% to 90%. Rheumatoid arthritis is a common offender of the bilateral symmetry rule, and one should not be surprised if rheumatoid arthritis is seen to be asymmetric in up to 20% of cases.

Involvement of joints other than the hand and wrist is not a common feature with most of the arthritides. In general, when a large joint such as the shoulder, hip, or knee is involved with arthritis, only a few entities need to be considered (Table 6.2). Although it must be emphasized that almost any arthritis can affect almost any joint, the diseases listed in Table 6.2 probably will account for 90% or more of the large joint arthropathies.

Involvement of certain joints can often give a clue as to the underlying disease process. For example, if the sacroiliac (SI) joints are involved, the differential diagnosis is as listed in Table 6.3. Again, almost any arthritis can affect any joint, but if the SI joint is involved, using Table 6.3 for the differential diagnosis will give a 95% or better chance of having the right answer.

The abovementioned differential diagnoses are to be considered generalizations and are, for the most part (except when mentioned), probably not more than 75% to 85% accurate. They are a nice starting point, however, for developing the differential diagnosis. I cannot overemphasize that the exceptions are exceedingly common. There are probably more missed diagnoses in the field of arthritis than in almost any other area of radiology. The remainder of this chapter gives a brief overview of arthritides with which most radiologists should be familiar. Rather than provide an in-depth description of each process—which can be obtained in any of the major radiology texts—I give salient discriminating points that might make it easier to differentiate one process from another.

TABLE 6.1
Arthropathy Distribution in Hands and Wrists

Distal	Proximal
Psoriasis	Rheumatoid arthritis
Reiter syndrome	Calcium pyrophosphate dihydrate crystal deposition disease
Osteoarthritis	(CPPD)

BOX 6.1
Bilateral Symmetry of Arthropathy

Primary osteoarthritis
Rheumatoid arthritis

TABLE 6.2
Large Joint Involvement

Osteoarthritis (degenerative joint disease)	Ankylosing spondylitis
Rheumatoid arthritis	Pigmented villonodular synovitis
Calcium pyrophosphate dihydrate crystal deposition disease (CPPD)	Synovial osteochondromatosis
	Infection

TABLE 6.3
Sacroiliac Joint Involvement

Ankylosing spondylitis	Osteoarthritis (degenerative joint disease)
Inflammatory bowel disease	Infection
Psoriasis	Gout
Reiter syndrome	

OSTEOARTHRITIS

The most common arthritis seen by radiologists is osteoarthritis, or degenerative joint disease (DJD). It is felt to be caused by trauma—either overt or as an accumulation of microtrauma over the years. The hallmarks of DJD are joint space narrowing, sclerosis, and osteophytosis (Box 6.2) (Fig. 6.1). If all three of these findings are not present on the radiograph, another diagnosis should be considered.

BOX 6.2
Hallmarks of Degenerative Joint Disease

Sclerosis
Osteophytes
Joint space narrowing

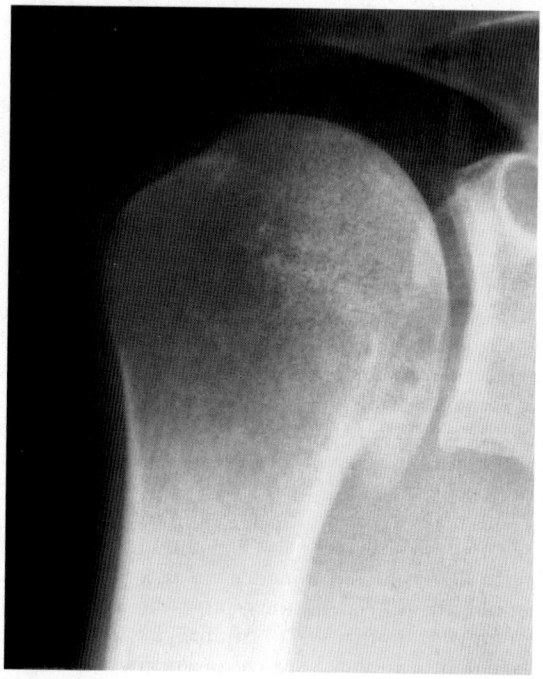

FIG. 6.1 **Degenerative Joint Disease of the Shoulder.** This former professional baseball pitcher with long-standing shoulder pain has joint space narrowing, subchondral sclerosis, and osteophytosis, which are hallmarks of degenerative joint disease (DJD).

Joint space narrowing is the least specific finding of the three, yet it is virtually always present in DJD. Unfortunately, it is also seen in almost every other joint abnormality, so by itself it means little.

Sclerosis should be present in varying amounts in all cases of DJD unless severe osteoporosis is present. Osteoporosis causes the sclerosis to be diminished. For instance, in long-standing rheumatoid arthritis where the cartilage has been destroyed, DJD often occurs with little sclerosis. Osteophytosis will be diminished in the setting of osteoporosis also. Otherwise, sclerosis and osteophytosis should be prominent in DJD.

The only disorder that will cause osteophytes without sclerosis or joint space narrowing is diffuse idiopathic skeletal hyperostosis (DISH). This common

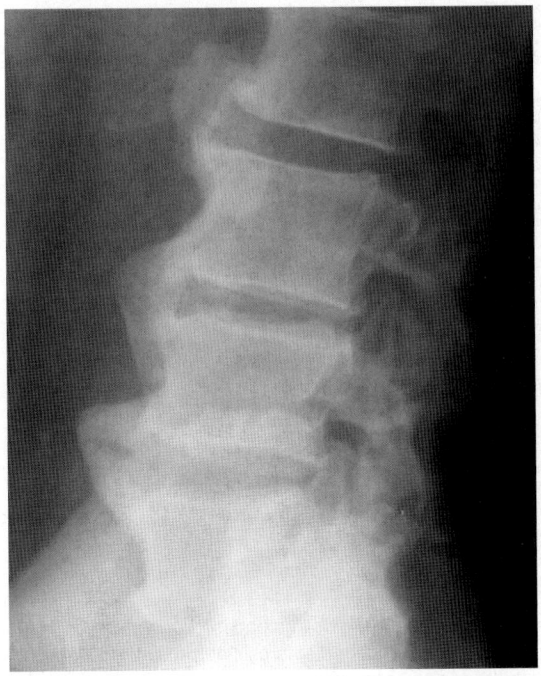

FIG. 6.2 **Diffuse Idiopathic Skeletal Hyperostosis.** A lateral of the lumbar spine shows extensive osteophytosis without significant disc space narrowing or sclerosis. This is a classic picture for diffuse idiopathic skeletal hyperostosis (DISH).

bone-forming disorder is seen primarily in the spine and at first glance resembles DJD except there is no disc space narrowing and there is no sclerosis (Fig. 6.2). DISH is not felt to be caused by trauma or stress, as is DJD, and is not painful or disabling, as DJD can be. Millions of dollars per year are awarded to government employees on retirement for "disability" payments for supposed DJD acquired on their jobs when in fact they have DISH and are misdiagnosed. It is hoped that such errors will be rectified in the future as more radiologists become informed of the difference between DJD and DISH.

Osteoarthritis is divided into two types: primary and secondary. Secondary osteoarthritis is what radiologists refer to when speaking of DJD. It is, as mentioned, secondary to trauma of some sort. It can occur in any joint in the body, but is particularly common in the knees, hips, and spine.

Primary osteoarthritis is a familial arthritis that affects middle-aged females almost exclusively and is seen only in the hands. It affects the distal interphalangeal (DIP) joints, the proximal interphalangeal (PIP) joints, and the base of the thumb in a bilaterally symmetric fashion (Fig. 6.3). If the arthritis is not bilaterally symmetric, the diagnosis of primary osteoarthritis should be questioned (Fig. 6.4).

A type of primary osteoarthritis that can be very painful and debilitating is erosive osteoarthritis. It has the identical distribution as mentioned for primary osteoarthritis but is associated with severe osteoporosis of the hands as well as erosions. It is somewhat uncommon, and radiologists generally see little of this disorder. Residents tend to mention erosive osteoarthritis in every example of joint erosions encountered, whether it is in the hands, knees, hips, or wherever. This is totally inappropriate because erosive osteoarthritis only occurs in the hands, and there it has a characteristic distribution, which should make for an easy diagnosis.

There are a few exceptions to the classic triad of findings seen in DJD (sclerosis, narrowing, and osteophytes). Several joints also exhibit erosions as a manifestation of DJD. I call these joints the "letter joints" because they are all often called by their initials: the TMJ (temporomandibular joint), the AC (acromioclavicular) joint, and the SI (sacroiliac) joints; the symphysis pubis behaves similarly (Table 6.4). When erosions are seen in one of these joints, DJD must be considered, or inappropriate treatment can occur (Fig. 6.5).

Another process that can occasionally be seen in DJD is a subchondral cyst or geode (taken from the geologic term used when a volcanic rock has a gas pocket that leaves a large cavity in the rock). Geodes are cystic formations that occur around joints in a variety of disorders (Table 6.5). Presumably, one method by which they form is synovial fluid being forced into the subchondral bone, causing a cystic collection of joint fluid. They seldom cause problems by themselves but are often misdiagnosed as something more sinister (Fig. 6.6) (see Chapter 4).

RHEUMATOID ARTHRITIS

Rheumatoid arthritis is a connective tissue disorder of unknown cause that can affect any synovial-lined joint in the body. The radiographic hallmarks are soft tissue swelling, osteoporosis, joint space narrowing, and marginal erosions (Table 6.6). In the hands, it is classically a proximal process that is bilaterally symmetrical (Fig. 6.7). There are so many exceptions to these rules, however, that I have come to regard them as no better than 80% accurate. Rheumatoid arthritis has a large variety of appearances and can be difficult to diagnose with any degree of assurance from its radiographic appearance alone.

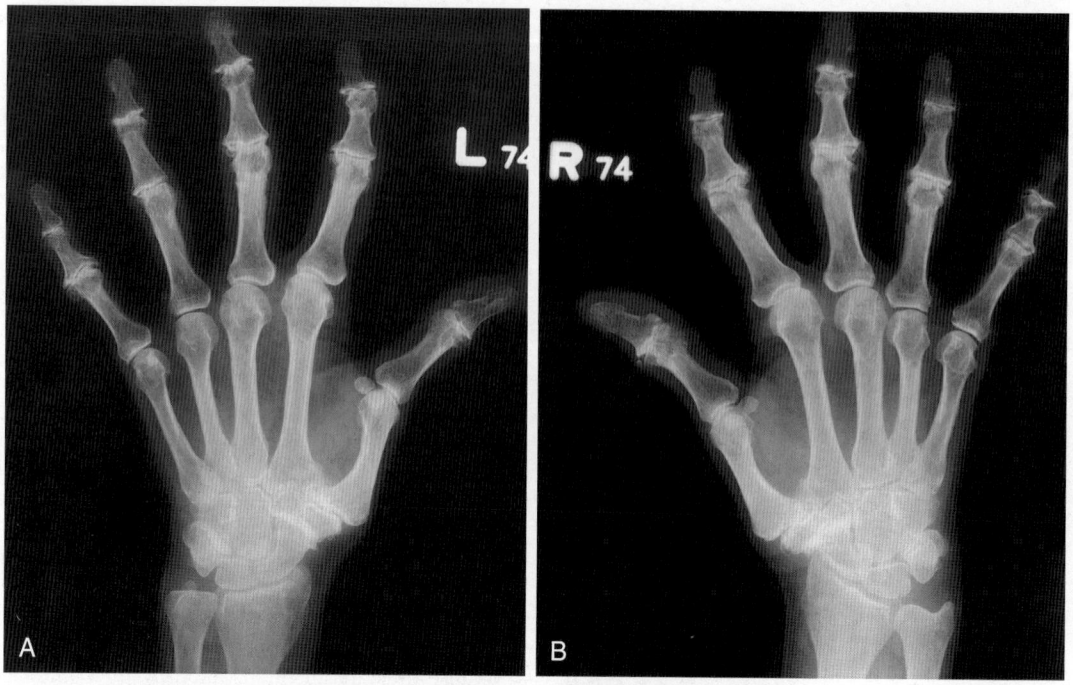

FIG. 6.3 **Primary Osteoarthritis.** A radiograph of the left (A) and right (B) hands in a patient with primary osteoarthritis shows classic findings of osteophytosis, joint space narrowing, and sclerosis at the distal interphalangeal joints, the proximal interphalangeal joints, and the base of the thumb. This was bilaterally symmetric in this patient, which is typical for primary osteoarthritis.

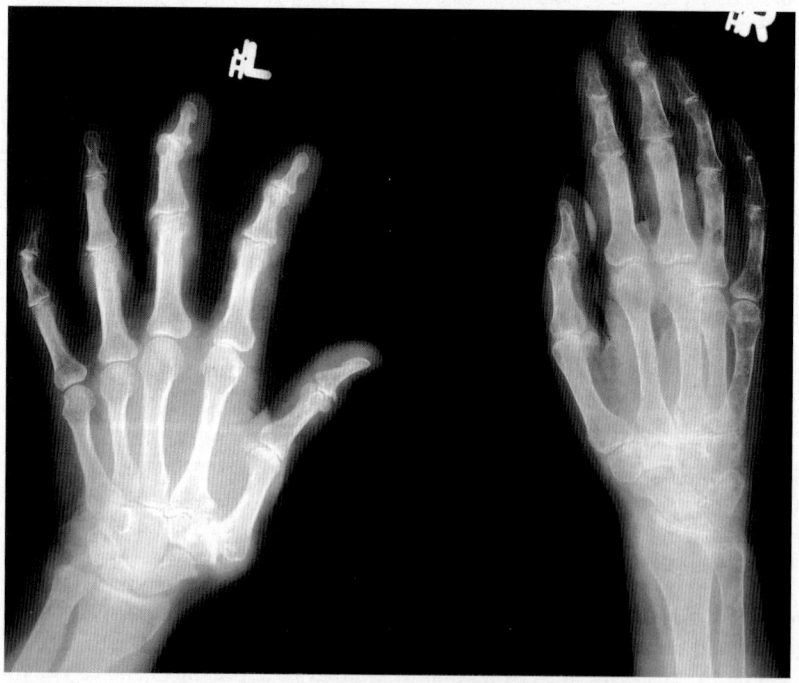

FIG. 6.4 **Lack of Bilateral Symmetry in Primary Osteoarthritis.** This patient has classic radiographic findings of primary osteoarthritis in the left hand; however, the right hand shows only osteoporosis and soft tissue wasting without evidence of osteoarthritis. The reason for the lack of bilaterality is that this patient has long-standing right-sided paralysis, which has blocked the onset of the arthritic changes in the right hand.

TABLE 6.4 Joints that Exhibit Erosions with Osteoarthritis	
Temporomandibular (TMJ)	Acromioclavicular (AC)
Sacroiliac (SI)	Symphysis pubis

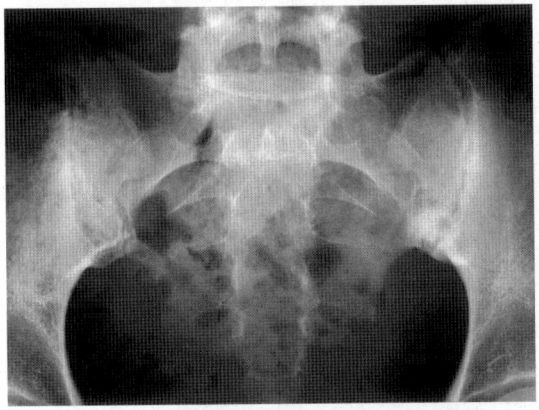

FIG. 6.5 **Osteoarthritis of the Sacroiliac (SI) Joint.** A young woman, who is a professional dancer, complained of left-sided hip pain. This anteroposterior (AP) film of the pelvis demonstrated left SI joint sclerosis, joint irregularity, and erosions. A complete workup to rule out an HLA-B27 spondyloarthropathy was negative, and no laboratory or clinical evidence for infection was found. Her clinical history pointed to this process being completely occupation related, and an aspiration biopsy to rule out infection was therefore not performed. This is not an unusual appearance for DJD of the SI joints.

TABLE 6.5 Diseases that Cause Subchrondral Cysts (Geodes)	
Rheumatoid arthritis	Calcium pyrophosphate dihydrate crystal deposition disease (CPPD)
Degenerative joint disease	Avascular necrosis

Rheumatoid arthritis in large joints is fairly characteristic in that it causes a lot of joint space narrowing and is associated with marked osteoporosis. Erosions may or may not be present and tend to be marginal, that is, away from the weight-bearing portion of the joint. In the hip, the femoral head tends to migrate axially, whereas in osteoarthritis, it tends to migrate superolaterally (Figs. 6.8 and 6.9). In the shoulder, the humeral head

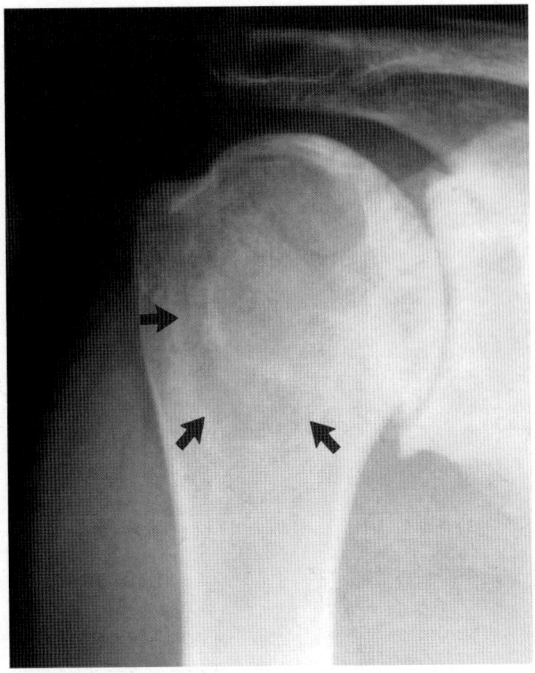

FIG. 6.6 **Subchondral Cyst or Geode of the Shoulder.** This patient has marked DJD of the shoulder with joint space narrowing, sclerosis, and osteophytosis. A large lytic process *(arrows)* seen in the humeral head is a subchondral cyst or geode, which often occurs in association with DJD. Because of the DJD in the shoulder, a biopsy to rule out a more sinister lesion in the humeral head should be avoided.

TABLE 6.6 Hallmarks of Rheumatoid Arthritis	
Proximal and bilaterally symmetric (hands)	Osteoporosis
Soft tissue swelling	Joint space narrowing
	Marginal erosions

tends to be "high-riding" (Fig. 6.10). Other things to think of when confronted with a high-riding shoulder are a torn rotator cuff and calcium pyrophosphate dihydrate crystal deposition disease (CPPD) (Table 6.7).

When rheumatoid arthritis is long-standing, it is not unusual for secondary DJD to superimpose itself on the findings one would expect with rheumatoid. This picture of DJD differs somewhat from that usually seen in that the sclerosis and osteophytes are considerably diminished in severity as compared with the joint space narrowing (Fig. 6.11).

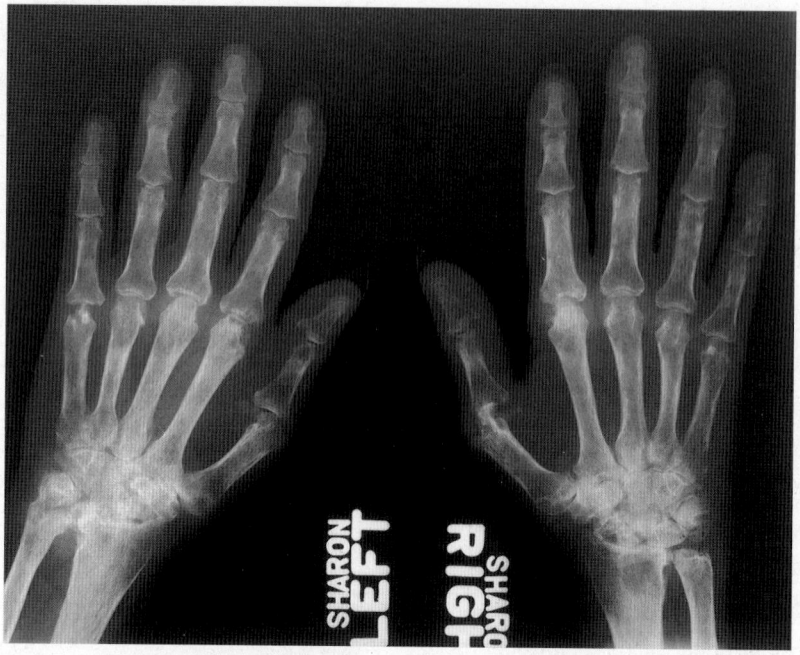

FIG. 6.7 **Rheumatoid Arthritis.** An erosive arthritis that primarily affects the carpal bones and the metacarpophalangeal joints is seen that has osteoporosis and soft tissue swelling (note the soft tissue over the ulnar styloid processes). It is a bilaterally symmetrical process in this patient, which is classic. The marked joint space narrowing in the wrist is known as "carpal crowding" and is characteristically seen in rheumatoid arthritis (RA).

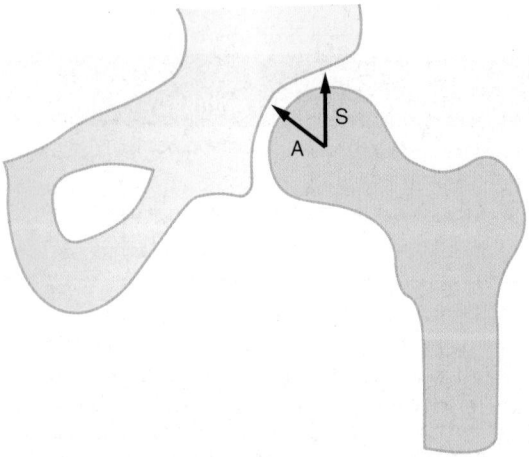

FIG. 6.8 **Routes of Migration of the Femoral Head.** Osteoarthritis of the hip tends to cause superior (*S*) migration of the femoral head in relation to the acetabulum, whereas rheumatoid arthritis tends to cause axial (*A*) migration of the femoral head in relation to the acetabulum.

HLA-B27 SPONDYLOARTHROPATHIES

A group of diseases that was formerly called "rheumatoid variants" is now known as the "seronegative HLA-B27 positive spondyloarthropathies." What was wrong with "rheumatoid variants"? It was short and concise. It has been replaced with a polysyllabic mouthful that is perhaps more descriptively correct, but so what? That is the problem with most academicians—make it sound more erudite and maybe everyone will think we're smarter than we really are. They shouldn't be so insecure. I liked "rheumatoid variants."

These disorders are all linked to the HLA-B27 histocompatibility antigen. Included in this group of diseases are ankylosing spondylitis, inflammatory bowel disease, psoriatic arthritis, and Reiter syndrome. They are characterized by bony ankylosis, proliferative new bone formation, and predominantly axial (spinal) involvement.

One of the more characteristic findings is that of syndesmophytes in the spine. A syndesmophyte is a paravertebral ossification that resembles an osteophyte except that it runs vertically, whereas an osteophyte has its orientation in a horizontal axis. Sometimes deciding

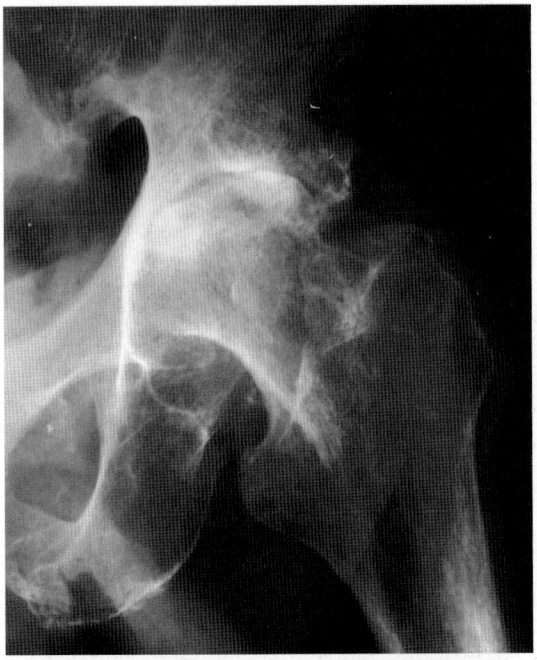

FIG. 6.9 **Rheumatoid Arthritis of the Hip.** Note the severe joint space narrowing in this patient with rheumatoid arthritis. The femoral head has migrated in an axial direction with fairly concentric joint space narrowing. Minimal secondary degenerative changes have occurred, as noted by the sclerosis in the superior portion of the joint; however, these have been diminished somewhat by the osteoporosis that usually accompanies rheumatoid arthritis.

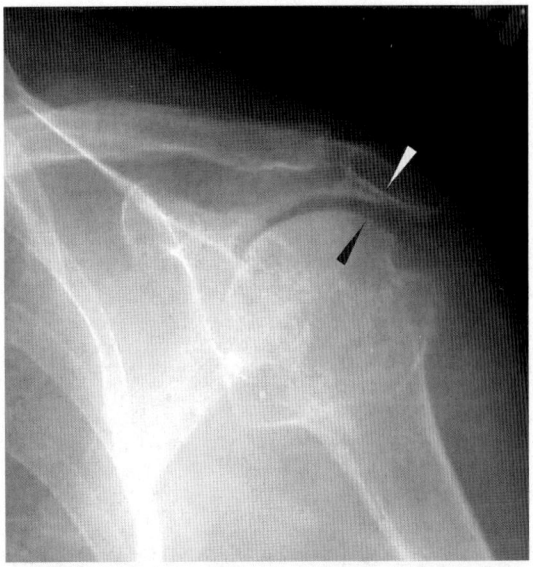

FIG. 6.10 **Rheumatoid Arthritis in the Shoulder.** An anteroposterior (AP) view of the shoulder in this patient with rheumatoid arthritis shows that the distance between the acromion and the humeral head is diminished *(arrows)*. Ordinarily this space is about one fingerbreadth in width to allow the rotator cuff to move freely. This is a common finding in rheumatoid arthritis as well as in calcium pyrophosphate dihydrate crystal deposition disease (CPPD) or with a torn rotator cuff.

TABLE 6.7
Diseases that Cause a High-Riding Shoulder

Calcium pyrophosphate dihydrate crystal deposition disease (CPPD)	Rheumatoid arthritis Torn rotator cuff

whether a particular paravertebral ossification is an osteophyte or a syndesmophyte is difficult based on its orientation alone (Fig. 6.12). Bridging osteophytes and large syndesmophytes can have a similar appearance, with both having an orientation halfway between vertical and horizontal. How should one evaluate those examples? Easy—ignore them. Look at the other vertebral bodies and use the ossifications on them to determine whether you are dealing with osteophytes or syndesmophytes. If no other level is involved, you might just have to make the diagnosis based on something else. In other words, sometimes you just will not be able to tell one from the other. Osteophytes should be accompanied by disc space narrowing (except in DISH), but sometimes narrowing is not obvious.

Syndesmophytes are classified as to whether they are marginal and symmetric or nonmarginal and asymmetric. A marginal syndesmophyte has its origin at the edge or margin of a vertebral body and extends to the margin of the adjacent vertebral body. Marginal syndesmophytes are invariably bilaterally symmetric as viewed on an anteroposterior (AP) spine film. Ankylosing spondylitis classically has marginal, symmetric syndesmophytes (Fig. 6.13). Inflammatory bowel disease has an identical appearance when the spine is involved.

Nonmarginal, asymmetric syndesmophytes are generally large and bulky. They emanate from the vertebral body away from the end plate or margin and are unilateral or asymmetric as viewed on an AP spine film (Figs. 6.12 and 6.14). Psoriatic arthritis and Reiter syndrome classically have this type of syndesmophyte.

Since marginal syndesmophytes are always bilaterally symmetrical and nonmarginal syndesmophytes are always asymmetrical, I find it easier to simply decide if they are bilaterally symmetrical or not. It can often be

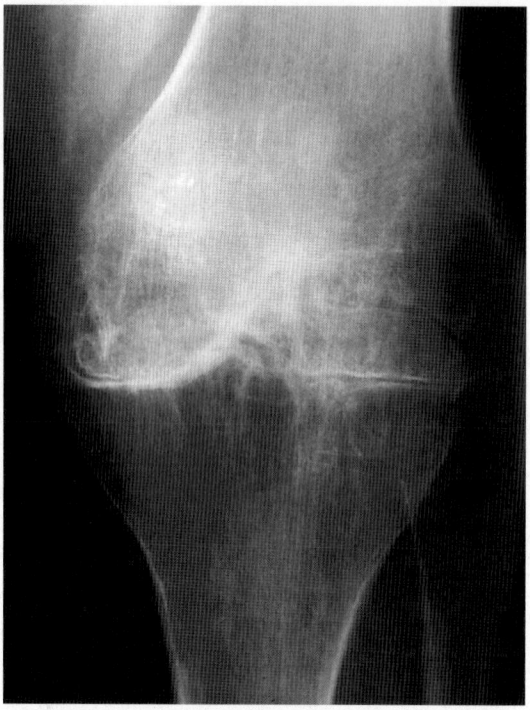

FIG. 6.11 **Secondary Degenerative Disease in the Knee in a Patient with Rheumatoid Arthritis.** This patient has a history of long-standing rheumatoid arthritis. An anteroposterior (AP) view of the knee shows severe osteoporosis and joint space narrowing. Secondary DJD is occurring, as evidenced by the sclerosis and osteophytosis; however, these findings are out of proportion to the severe joint space narrowing. When DJD narrows a joint to this extent, the osteophytosis and sclerosis are invariably much more pronounced.

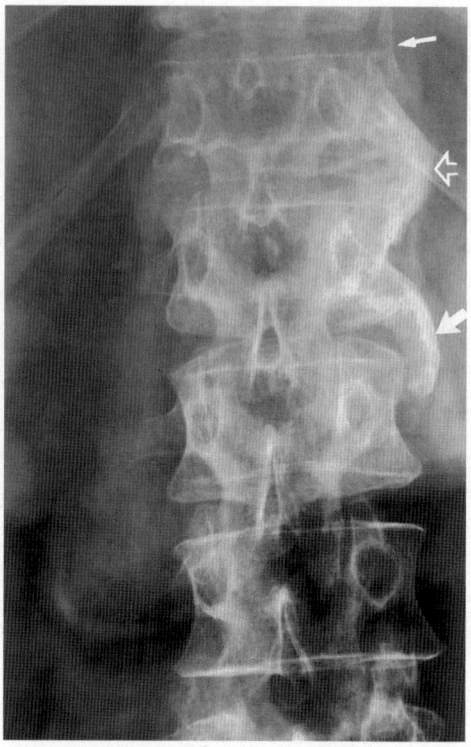

FIG. 6.12 **Psoriasis with Syndesmophytes.** The large paravertebral ossification on the left side of the T12–L1 disc space *(open arrow)* is difficult to differentiate between an osteophyte and a syndesmophyte. Either could have this appearance. However, the paravertebral ossification at the left L1–2 disc space *(solid arrow)* definitely has a vertical rather than a horizontal orientation, as does the faint ossification seen at the T11–12 disc space *(small arrow)*. These definitely represent syndesmophytes. Therefore it makes sense to logically assume that the ossification at the T12–L1 disc space is almost certainly a syndesmophyte as well. This patient has large nonmarginal asymmetric syndesmophytes, which are typical of psoriatic arthritis or Reiter syndrome. This patient indeed has psoriasis.

difficult to discern if the syndesmophyte begins at the margin of the vertebral body or not, but it's easy to tell if they are bilateral or not.

Involvement of the SI joints is common in the HLA-B27 spondyloarthropathies. The patterns of involvement, like the patterns of involvement of the spine, are somewhat typical for each disorder. Ankylosing spondylitis and inflammatory bowel disease typically cause bilaterally symmetric SI joint disease that is initially erosive and progresses to sclerosis and fusion (Figs. 6.15 and 6.16). It is extremely unusual to have asymmetric or unilateral SI joint disease in these two disorders. Another entity that can have bilateral SI joint erosions is hyperparathyroidism. Subperiosteal resorption along the SI joints mimics erosive changes. This is more commonly seen in children.

Reiter syndrome and psoriatic arthritis can exhibit unilateral or bilateral SI joint involvement. It is said that it is bilateral about 50% of the time. It is often asymmetric when it is bilateral, but exact symmetry can be difficult to assess on plain films. Therefore when it is definitely bilateral and not clearly asymmetric, I consider the SI joints to be in the bilateral symmetric category. This means that if I have a case with bilateral, symmetric SI joint disease, it could be caused by any of the four HLA-B27 spondyloarthropathies. If I have a case with unilateral (or clearly asymmetric) SI

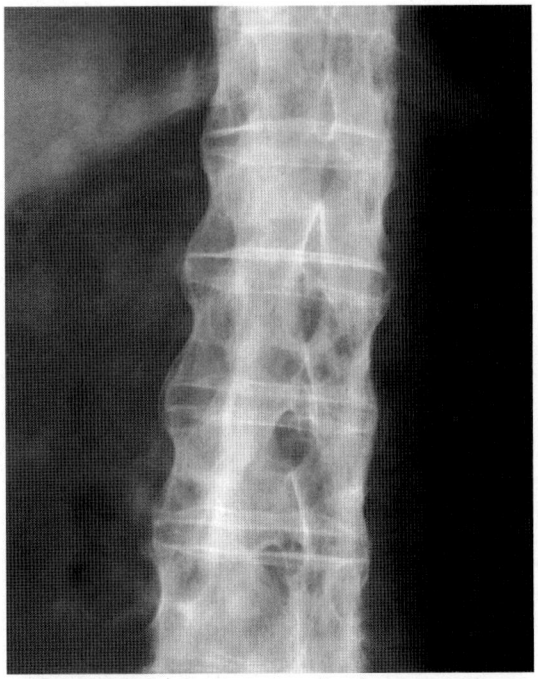

FIG. 6.13 **Marginal Symmetric Syndesmophytes in a Patient with Ankylosing Spondylitis.** Bilateral marginal syndesmophytes are seen bridging the disc spaces throughout the lumbar spine in this patient. This is a "bamboo spine" and is classic for ankylosing spondylitis or inflammatory bowel disease.

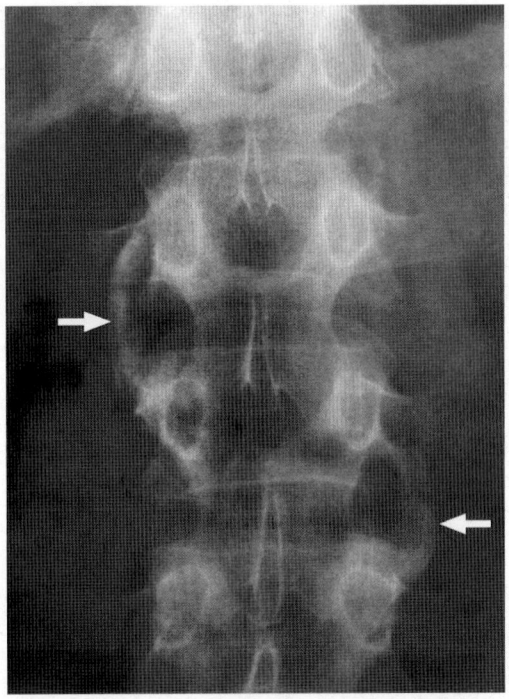

FIG. 6.14 **Syndesmophytes in Psoriatic Arthritis.** Large, bulky, nonmarginal asymmetric syndesmophytes *(arrows)* are seen in this patient with psoriatic arthritis.

joint involvement, I can confidently exclude ankylosing spondylitis and inflammatory bowel disease, and I would consider Reiter syndrome and psoriatic disease. In this example, I would have to also consider infection and DJD (don't forget that DJD can cause erosions in the SI joints) (Figs. 6.5 and 6.17) and, in older patients, gout. Computed tomography (CT) is very helpful in examining the SI joints and is considered by many to be the diagnostic procedure of choice because of the unobstructed view of the entire joint (Fig. 6.18).

That is, in a nutshell, my approach to the SI joints (Table 6.3). Other considerations in the differential are too uncommon for me to worry about for the most part, and you shouldn't either.

Large joint involvement with the HLA-B27 spondyloarthropathies is uncommon (except for ankylosing spondylitis) but occurs often enough to warrant learning about. In general, the arthropathy will resemble rheumatoid arthritis with the typical features thereof (Fig. 6.19). The hips are involved in up to 50% of the patients with ankylosing spondylitis.

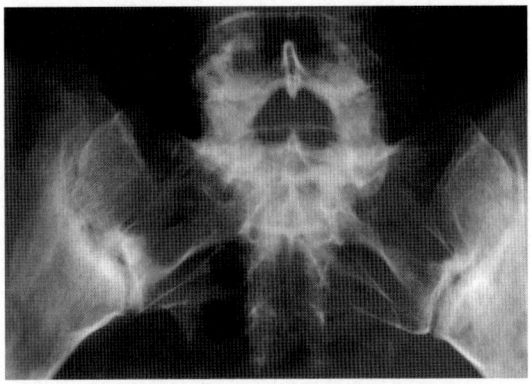

FIG. 6.15 **Ankylosing Spondylitis.** Bilateral, symmetric sacroiliac (SI) joint sclerosis and erosions are seen in this patient with ankylosing spondylitis. Inflammatory bowel disease could have an identical appearance. Although this is classic for these two disorders, it would not be that unusual for psoriatic disease or Reiter syndrome to have this appearance. It would be unlikely for infection or degenerative joint disease (DJD) to be bilateral in this fashion.

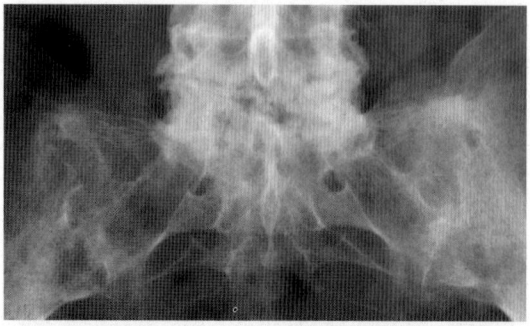

FIG. 6.16 **Fusion of the Sacroiliac (SI) Joints in Ankylosing Spondylitis.** Bilateral complete fusion of the SI joints in this patient with ankylosing spondylitis makes the SI joints totally indistinguishable. Inflammatory bowel disease could have a similar appearance. I have not seen other disease processes affect the SI joints to this extent, with the exception of long-standing paralysis.

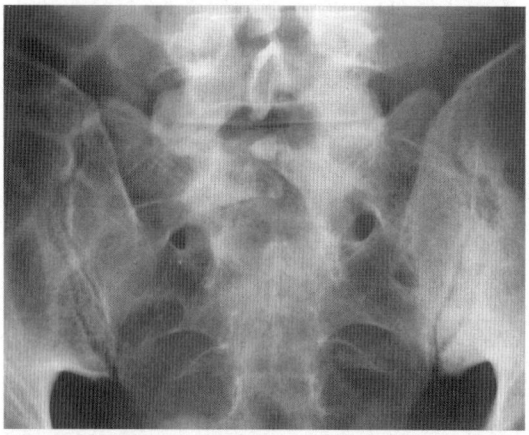

FIG. 6.17 **Psoriasis with Sacroiliac (SI) Joint Disease.** Unilateral SI sclerosis and erosions are seen in this patient with psoriasis. Ankylosing spondylitis and inflammatory bowel disease virtually never have this unilateral distribution.

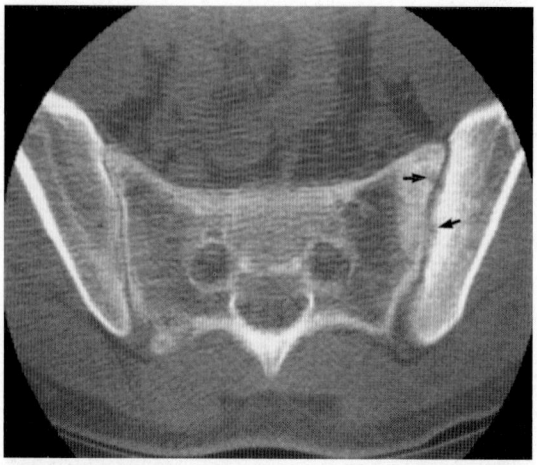

FIG. 6.18 **Computed Tomography (CT) of the Sacroiliac (SI) Joints in Psoriasis.** A CT scan through the SI joints in this patient with psoriasis shows unilateral SI joint sclerosis and erosions *(arrows)* typical for psoriasis or Reiter syndrome. Infection could have a similar appearance.

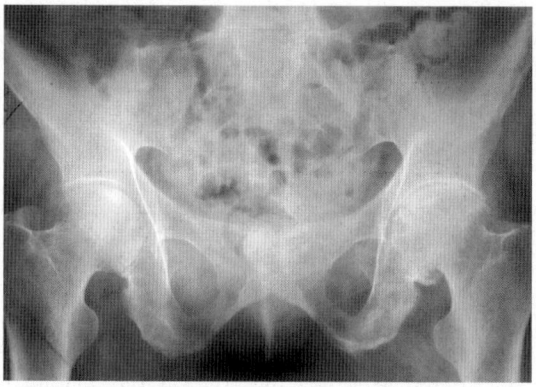

FIG. 6.19 **Ankylosing Spondylitis with Hip Disease.** An anteroposterior (AP) view of the pelvis in this patient with ankylosing spondylitis shows bilateral complete fusion of the sacroiliac (SI) joints. Concentric left hip joint narrowing is present with axial migration of the femoral head. The hip changes would be typical findings in rheumatoid arthritis or, as in this example, ankylosing spondylitis. Note the secondary degenerative joint disease (DJD) changes in the hip.

Small joint involvement, specifically the hands and feet, is not commonly seen in ankylosing spondylitis and inflammatory bowel disease and tends to resemble rheumatoid arthritis. Psoriasis causes a distinctive arthropathy in the hands that is characterized by its distal predominance, proliferative erosions, soft tissue swelling, and periostitis. The erosions are different from the clean-cut, sharply marginated erosions seen in all other erosive arthritides in that they often have fuzzy margins with wisps of periostitis emanating from them (Fig. 6.20A). The severe forms are often associated with bony ankylosis across joints (Fig. 6.20B) and mutilans deformities. A fairly common finding is a calcaneal heel spur that has fuzzy margins as opposed to the well-corticated heel spur seen in DJD (Fig. 6.21).

Reiter syndrome causes changes that are identical in every respect with those of psoriasis with the exception that the hands are not as commonly involved

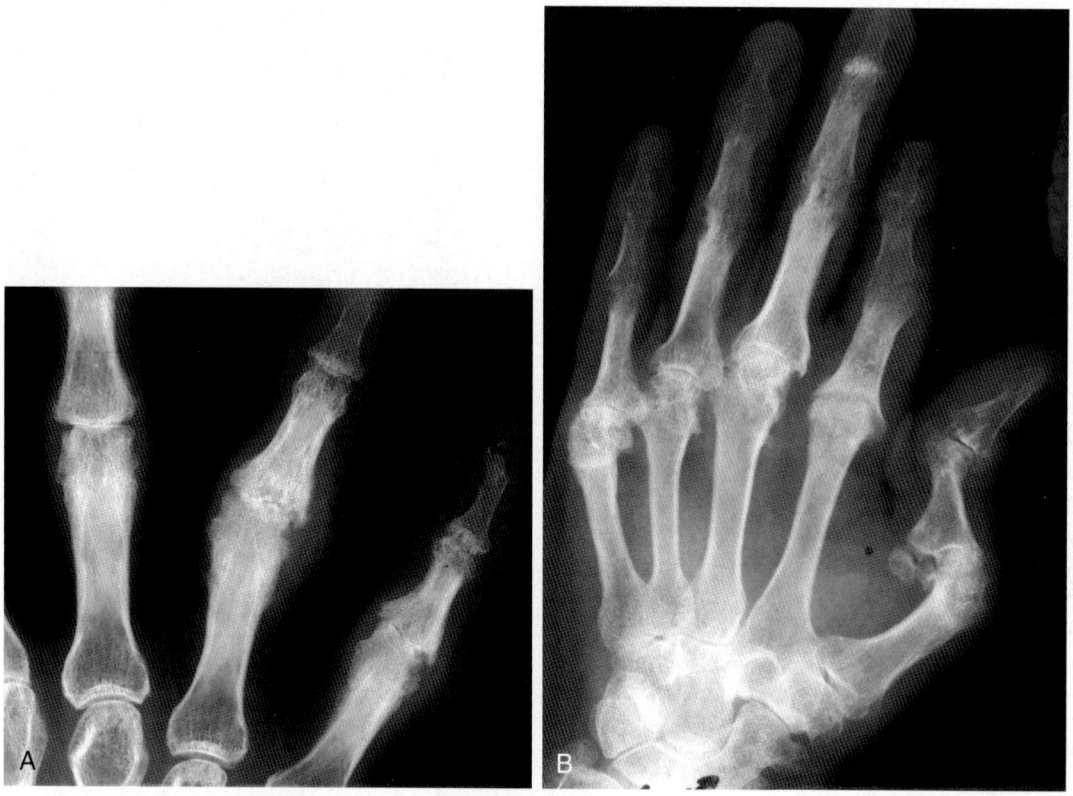

FIG. 6.20 **Psoriatic Arthritis.** (A) Cartilage loss at the proximal interphalangeal joints of the third, fourth, and fifth digits in this hand is apparent, with erosions noted most prominently in the fourth and fifth digits. These erosions are not sharply demarcated but are covered with fluffy new bone, which are termed proliferative erosions. Note also the periostitis along the shafts of each of the proximal phalanges. (B) Advanced psoriatic arthritis. Fusion or ankylosis is apparent across the proximal interphalangeal joints of the second through the fifth digits. Several of the distal interphalangeal joints are also ankylosed. Severe joint space narrowing at the metacarpophalangeal joints is noted. This distal arthritis is typical for psoriatic arthritis.

(Fig. 6.22). Also, Reiter is rare in women. Therefore I recommend storing the findings for psoriasis and Reiter syndrome on a single neuron and saving the other for a phone number or something else.

CRYSTAL-INDUCED ARTHRITIS

The crystal-induced arthritides include gout and pseudogout (CPPD). Ochronosis and a few other arcane crystal deposition diseases are so rare that they don't deserve mention except to say that you will probably never see an example outside of a textbook or teaching file.

Gout

Gout is a metabolic disorder that results in hyperuricemia and leads to monosodium urate crystals being deposited in various sites in the body, especially joint cartilage. The actual causes of the hyperuricemia are myriad, including inherited, and are not germane to this discussion. Gout is found in women only after menopause and typically in men only after the age of 40, although many exceptions occur.

The arthropathy caused by gout is very characteristic radiographically, yet it is not commonly seen. Why is that? Because it takes 4 to 6 years for gout to cause radiographically evident disease, and most patients are successfully treated long before the destructive arthropathy occurs.

The classic radiographic findings are well-defined erosions, often with sclerotic borders or overhanging edges, soft tissue nodules that calcify in the presence of renal failure, and a random distribution in the hands without marked osteoporosis (Fig. 6.23). I know of

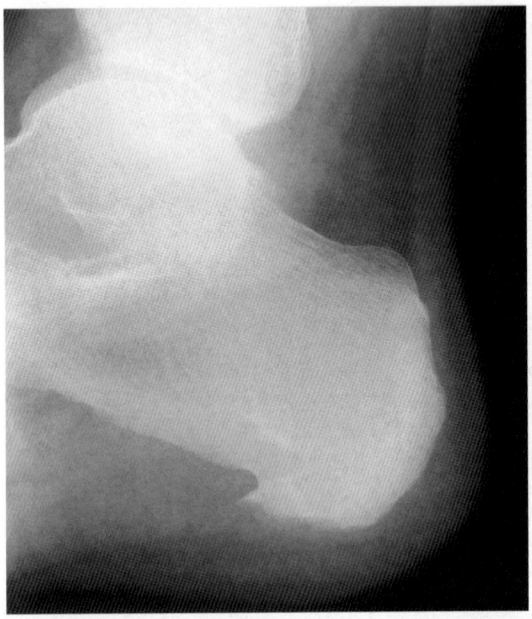

FIG. 6.21 **Reiter Syndrome.** A lateral view of a calcaneus in a patient with Reiter syndrome shows poorly defined new bone on the inferior margin of the calcaneus with a calcaneal spur that is also poorly defined. This is typical of psoriatic arthritis or Reiter syndrome as opposed to the well-formed calcaneal spur in degenerative joint disease (DJD).

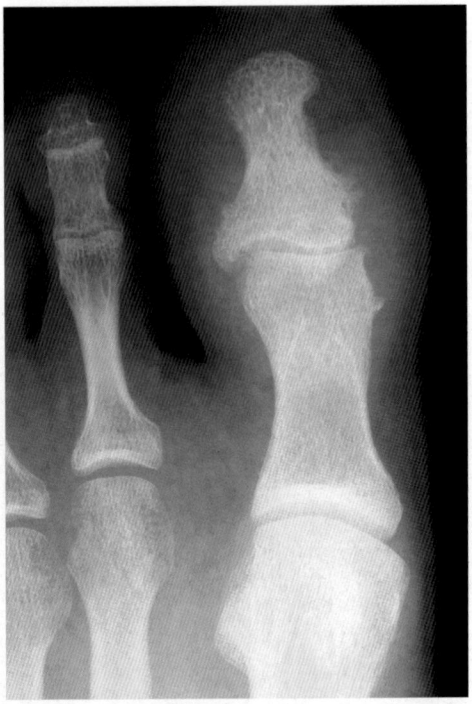

FIG. 6.22 **Reiter Syndrome.** An anteroposterior (AP) view of the great toe in a patient with Reiter syndrome shows fluffy periostitis *(arrow)* in the erosions adjacent to the interphalangeal joint of the great toe. Marked soft tissue swelling is also present throughout the great toe. These changes are typical in appearance and location for Reiter syndrome or psoriasis.

no other disorder that typically has erosions with sclerotic margins; therefore this is a very specific finding for gout. It typically affects the metatarsophalangeal joint of the great toe (called podagra) (Fig. 6.24). In advanced stages, it can be very deforming (Fig. 6.25). Patients with gout often have chondrocalcinosis because they have an increased chance of having pseudogout (CPPD). Up to 40% of the patients with gout concomitantly have CPPD.

It is worth repeating that patients must have clinically evident gout for years before changes will be apparent on a radiograph, and it is getting to be uncommon to find such a case. Also, even though erosions with overhanging edges can occur with gout, they can occur in other disorders as well and are by no means pathognomonic.

Pseudogout (Calcium Pyrophosphate Crystal Deposition Disease)

CPPD causes much confusion among radiologists as well as other specialists. It is actually quite simple if you don't read all the conflicting literature. First, what do you call it? Is it pseudogout or CPPD? Who cares? Call it either, or both. Many academicians say that it should be called pseudogout only when symptoms are present. Do we call lung cancer something else if the patient is asymptomatic? Of course not. For all practical purposes, the terms pseudogout and CPPD are synonymous, and argument over the issue is academic BS.

CPPD occurs almost exclusively in persons over the age of 50 and is extremely common. CPPD has a classic triad: pain, cartilage calcification, and DJD. The patient may have any combination of one or more of this triad at any one time. Each of these signs and symptoms will be dealt with individually in some detail, but note that two of the three are radiographic findings. This disorder is best diagnosed radiographically.

The pain of CPPD is nonspecific. It can mimic that of gout (hence the term pseudogout) or infection or just about any arthritis. It typically is intermittent over

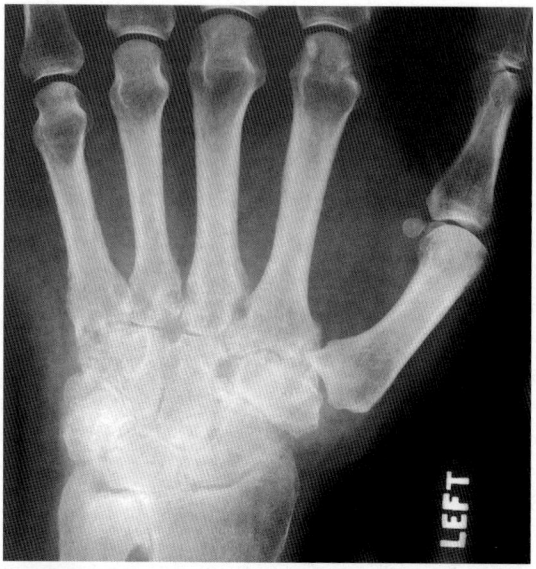

FIG. 6.23 **Gout.** Sharply marginated erosions, some with a sclerotic margin, are noted throughout the carpus and proximal metacarpals. These erosions are classic in gout. Note the absence of marked demineralization.

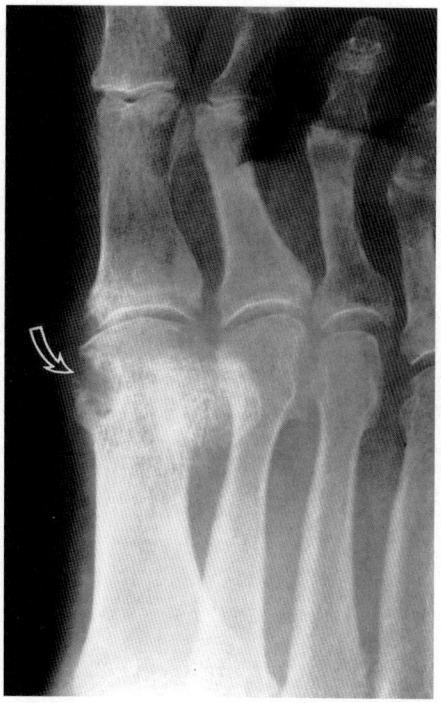

FIG. 6.24 **Gout.** A sharply marginated erosion with an overhanging edge *(arrow)* is seen in the metatarsophalangeal joint in the great toe in this patient with gout. This appearance and location are classic for gout, whereas psoriasis and Reiter syndrome usually involve the interphalangeal joint and do not have erosions that are this sharply marginated.

many years until DJD occurs and becomes the main cause of pain. It is often asymptomatic.

Cartilage calcification, known as chondrocalcinosis, can occur in any joint but tends to affect a few select sites in the overwhelming majority of patients. These are the medial and lateral compartments of the knee (Fig. 6.26), the triangular fibrocartilage of the wrist (Fig. 6.27), and the symphysis pubis. Chondrocalcinosis in any joint is virtually diagnostic of CPPD. When CPPD crystals occur in the soft tissues, such as in the rotator cuff of the shoulder, a radiograph cannot differentiate between CPPD and calcium hydroxyapatite (CHA), which occurs in calcific tendinitis. Some refer to the deposition of CHA crystals in soft tissues as HAD—Hydroxy Apatite Deposition. It is by far the most commonly seen source of soft tissue calcification. HAD does not occur in the joint cartilage except in extremely rare cases; therefore all chondrocalcinosis can be considered CPPD. This, for some reason, is confounding to many people. Many established academicians have a hard time accepting the fact that if chondrocalcinosis is present, CPPD crystals are the only possible culprit. Monosodium urate crystals in gout are not radiographically visible. CHA does not occur in cartilage. In fact, no other radiographically visible crystal in cartilage has been described. It couldn't be simpler: chondrocalcinosis equals CPPD. So what's the fuss all about? Beats me.

The joint destruction or arthropathy of CPPD is virtually indistinguishable from that of DJD. In fact, it is DJD. It's caused by CPPD crystals eroding the cartilage. There are a few features of DJD caused by CPPD that will help to distinguish it from DJD caused by trauma or overuse. The main difference is one of location. CPPD has a proclivity for the upper extremity: the shoulder, the elbow (Fig. 6.28), the radiocarpal joint in the wrist (Fig. 6.29), and the metacarpophalangeal (MCP) joints of the hand; also it tends to involve the patellofemoral joint of the knee in an isolated manner, i.e., with no DJD seen in the medial or lateral compartments. These areas are not normally involved by DJD from wear and tear. When DJD is seen in the joints that CPPD tends to involve, a search for chondrocalcinosis should be made. If necessary, a joint aspiration for CPPD crystals may be necessary to confirm the diagnosis.

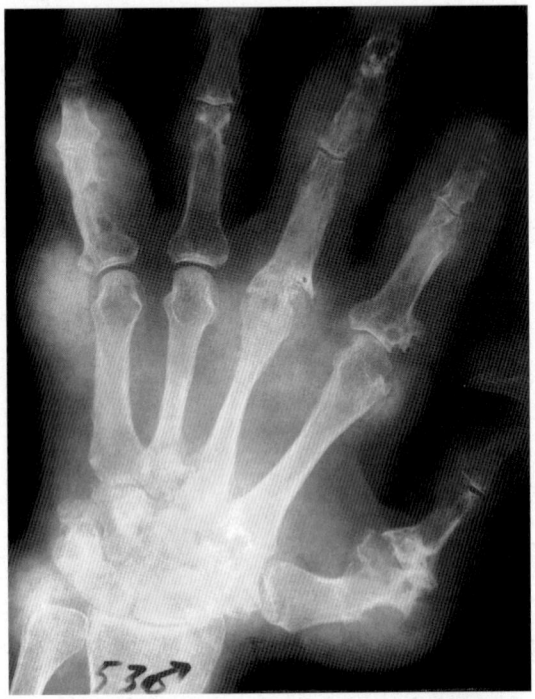

FIG. 6.25 **Advanced Gout.** Marked diffuse and focal soft tissue swelling is present throughout the hand and wrist in this patient with long-standing gout. Destructive, large, well-marginated erosions, some with overhanging edges, are noted near multiple joints. The focal areas of soft tissue swelling are called tophi, some of which are calcified. These calcify only with coexistent renal disease.

Occasionally the arthropathy of CPPD accelerates, and severe destruction occurs to such an extent that a neuropathic or Charcot joint is mimicked on the radiograph (Fig. 6.30). This has been termed a pseudo-Charcot joint. It is not a true Charcot joint because of the presence of sensation.

Three diseases have a high degree of association with CPPD. These are primary hyperparathyroidism, gout, and hemochromatosis. This is not a differential diagnosis for chondrocalcinosis. These diseases tend to occur at the same time that CPPD occurs. If the patient has one of these three disorders, he is more likely to have CPPD than is a normal person. There is probably no good reason to work up every patient with chondrocalcinosis for one of the three associated diseases, since they are so uncommon and CPPD is extremely common. Several texts list many other disorders that are supposedly associated with CPPD, such as acromegaly, diabetes, Wilson disease, and hypophosphatasia, but the recent work in this field does not support this.

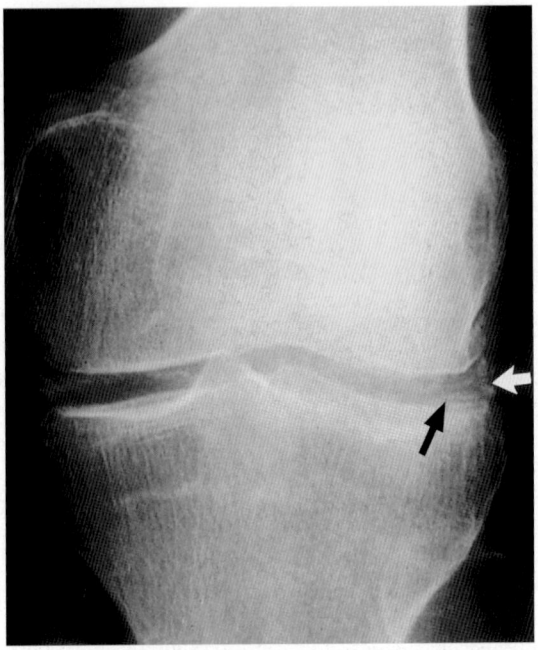

FIG. 6.26 **Chondrocalcinosis in the Knee.** Cartilage calcification, known as chondrocalcinosis, is seen in the fibrocartilage *(arrows)* and in the hyaline articular cartilage in this patient with calcium pyrophosphate dihydrate crystal deposition disease (CPPD).

COLLAGEN–VASCULAR DISEASES

Scleroderma, systemic lupus erythematosus (SLE), dermatomyositis, and mixed connective tissue disease are all grouped together as collagen–vascular diseases. The striking abnormalities in the hands in each of these disorders are osteoporosis and soft tissue wasting. SLE characteristically has severe ulnar deviation of the phalanges (Fig. 6.31). Erosions are generally not present in these diseases. Soft tissue calcifications are typically present in scleroderma (Fig. 6.32) and dermatomyositis. Mixed connective tissue disease is an overlap of scleroderma, SLE, polymyositis, and rheumatoid arthritis. Obviously it has a myriad of radiographic findings.

SARCOID

Sarcoidosis causes deposition of granulation tissue in the body, primarily in the lungs but also in the bones. In the skeletal system, it has a predilection for the hands, where it causes lytic destructive lesions in the cortex. These often have a lacelike appearance (Fig. 6.33). Sarcoid can also affect the joints in the hand, causing DJD-like changes.

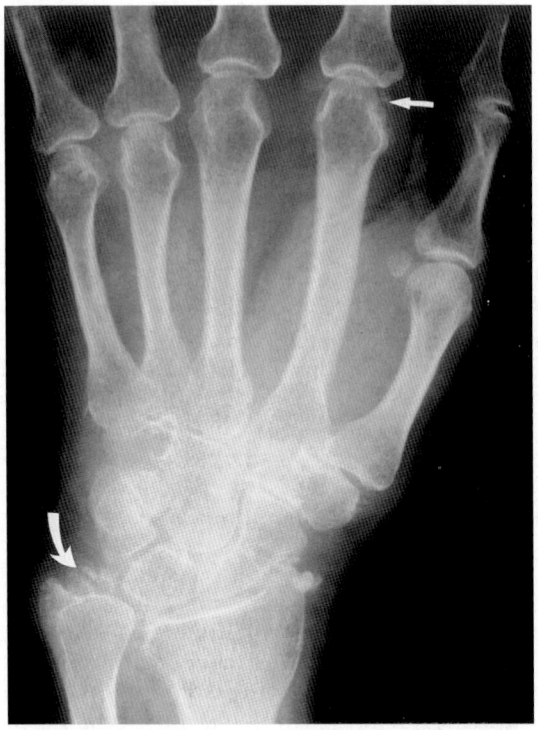

FIG. 6.27 **Chondrocalcinosis in the Wrist.** This patient with calcium pyrophosphate dihydrate crystal deposition disease (CPPD) exhibits chondrocalcinosis in the triangular fibrocartilage of the wrist *(curved arrow)*. Triangular fibrocartilage calcification is one of the more common locations for chondrocalcinosis to occur. Faint chondrocalcinosis is also present in the second MCP *(small arrow)*.

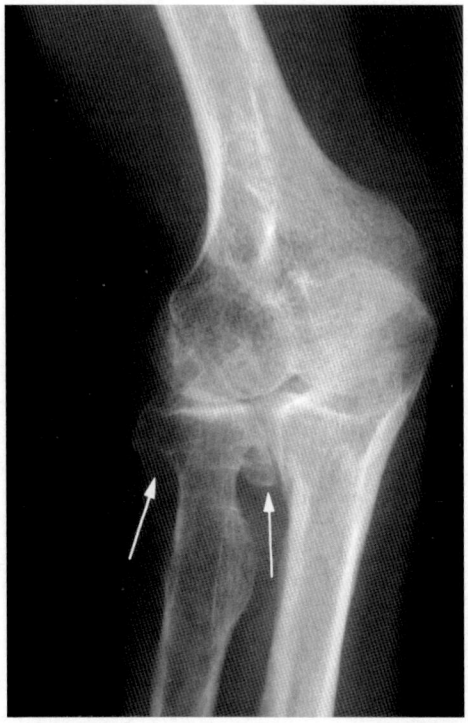

FIG. 6.28 **Calcium Pyrophosphate Dihydrate Crystal Deposition Disease (CPPD) Arthropathy.** Degenerative joint disease (DJD) of the elbow is seen in this patient with CPPD. Note the joint space narrowing with minimal sclerosis and the large osteophytes *(arrows)*. Osteophytes of this nature are termed "drooping" osteophytes and are often seen in CPPD. The elbow is an unusual place for DJD to occur except in the setting of CPPD or trauma.

HEMOCHROMATOSIS

Twenty to fifty percent of patients with hemochromatosis have a characteristic arthropathy in the hands that should suggest the diagnosis. Hemochromatosis is a disease of excess iron that gets deposited in tissues throughout the body, leading to fibrosis and eventual organ failure. The characteristic arthropathy classically involves the second through fourth metacarpophalangeal joints. The radiographic changes are essentially those of DJD (joint space narrowing, sclerosis, and osteophytes) (Fig. 6.34). Up to 50% of the patients with hemochromatosis also have CPPD; therefore when looking at the hands, a search should be made for triangular fibrocartilage chondrocalcinosis. Another finding that is often seen in hemochromatosis is called "squaring" of the metacarpal heads. They appear enlarged and blocklike as a result of the large osteophytes commonly seen in this disorder. In fact, the osteophytes are often called "drooping" because of the unusual way they hang off the joint margin.

NEUROPATHIC OR CHARCOT JOINT

The radiographic findings for a Charcot joint are characteristic and almost pathognomonic. A classic triad has been described that consists of joint destruction, dislocation, and heterotopic new bone (Fig. 6.35). Multiple other findings have been described that do not seem to be as useful as the classic triad.

Joint destruction is seen in every arthritis encountered and therefore seems very nonspecific; however, nothing causes as severe destruction in a joint as a Charcot joint. Early in the development of a Charcot joint, the joint destruction may merely appear to be joint space narrowing. It is extremely difficult to make the diagnosis this early. In the spine, instead of joint space destruction, there is disc space destruction (Fig. 6.36).

Dislocation, like joint destruction, can be present in varying degrees. Early on, the joint may have subluxation instead of dislocation.

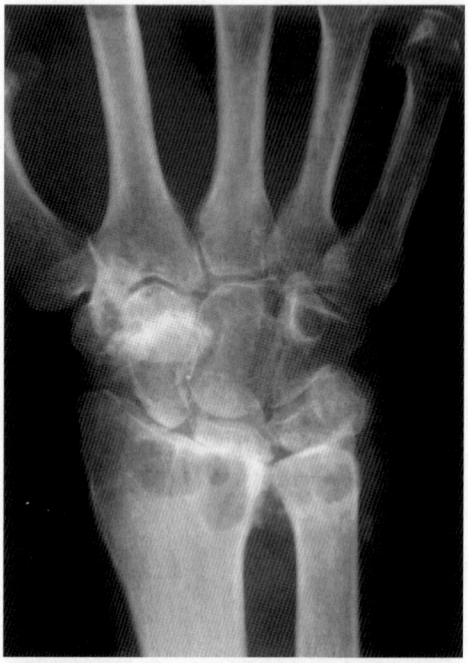

FIG. 6.29 **Calcium Pyrophosphate Dihydrate Crystal Deposition Disease (CPPD) Arthropathy.** Marked degenerative joint disease (DJD) at the radiocarpal joint is seen in this patient with CPPD. Severe joint space narrowing and sclerosis with large subchondral cysts or geodes are hallmarks of DJD. This is an unusual location for DJD except in the setting of CPPD.

Heterotopic new bone has also been termed "debris" and consists of soft tissue calcification or clumps of ossification adjacent to the joint. It, too, can be present in varying amounts.

The most commonly seen Charcot joint is in the foot of a diabetic. It typically affects the first and second tarsometatarsal joints in a fashion termed a Lisfranc fracture (Fig. 6.37). Lisfranc was Napoleon's surgeon, and he gained fame for saving the lives of soldiers with gangrenous toes from frostbite by doing a forefoot amputation at the tarsometatarsal junction.

Tabes dorsalis from syphilis is seldom seen today. I have only encountered two cases of a Charcot joint in syphilis in the past 35 years, and I've been around some pretty raunchy residents. More commonly seen is a Charcot joint in a patient with paralysis who continues to use the affected limb for support.

The shoulder can become a Charcot joint in patients with syringomyelia, which has a so-called "atrophic Charcot" appearance. This refers to its tendency to have no debris or heterotopic new bone, and the proximal humerus has a tapered appearance likened to a licked candy stick.

A pseudo-Charcot joint from CPPD (Fig. 6.30) is encountered almost as commonly as a true Charcot joint from any other cause with the exception of the Lisfranc type seen in diabetics.

HEMOPHILIA, JUVENILE RHEUMATOID ARTHRITIS, AND PARALYSIS

Why would three clinically disparate entities like juvenile rheumatoid arthritis (JRA), hemophilia, and paralysis be covered in the same section? Because this is a radiology book, and they are radiographically indistinguishable. As with several other processes covered in this book, you might as well store these three on a single neuron and save the other neuron for something important.

The classic findings for JRA and hemophilia are overgrowth of the ends of the bones (epiphyseal enlargement) associated with gracile diaphyses (Fig. 6.38). Joint destruction may or may not be present (Figs. 6.39 and 6.40). A finding that is purported to be classic for JRA and hemophilia is widening of the intercondylar notch of the knee. I find this sign variable and difficult to use. I have never seen it present when the other classic signs were not also present and obvious.

Another process that can mimic the findings in JRA and hemophilia is a joint that has undergone disuse from paralysis (Fig. 6.41). It has always been said that the reason the epiphyses are overgrown in JRA and hemophilia is because of the hyperemia; however, a lot of other things cause hyperemia without affecting the size of the epiphyses. The thing that JRA, hemophilia, and paralysis have in common is disuse. I believe that this is what causes the overgrowth of the ends of the bones seen in all three disorders.

SYNOVIAL OSTEOCHONDROMATOSIS

Synovial osteochondromatosis, a relatively common disorder, is caused by a metaplasia of the synovium, resulting in the deposition of foci of cartilage in the joint. It is most commonly seen in the knee, hip, and elbow. Most of the time these cartilaginous deposits calcify and are readily seen on a radiograph (Figs. 6.42 and 6.43). Up to 20% of the time, the cartilaginous deposits do not calcify. In these cases, all that is seen on the radiograph is a joint effusion unless erosions or joint destruction occur (Fig. 6.44).

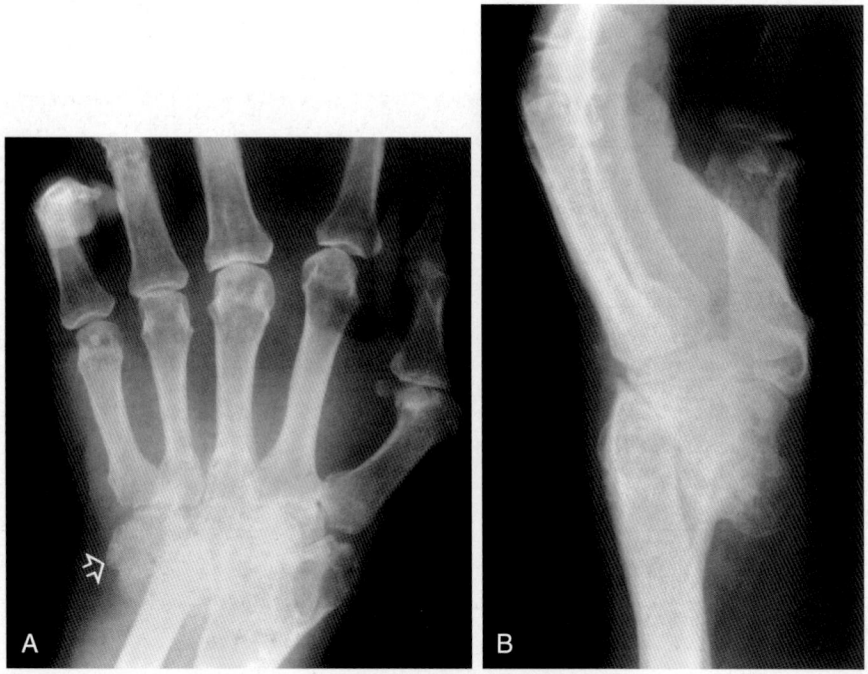

FIG. 6.30 **Pseudo-Charcot Joint in Calcium Pyrophosphate Dihydrate Crystal Deposition Disease (CPPD).** This patient with CPPD shows severe joint destruction in the carpus primarily at the radiocarpal joint. Large subchondral cysts or geodes are noted (A). Heterotopic new bone or joint debris is also seen *(arrow)*. (B) Dislocation of the radiocarpal joint is seen, with the entire carpus lying volarly in relation to the radius. The findings of severe joint destruction, heterotopic new bone, and dislocation are classic for a Charcot joint. This patient, however, had sensation in this joint; therefore it is not a true Charcot or neuropathic joint but a pseudo-Charcot joint, which is occasionally seen in CPPD.

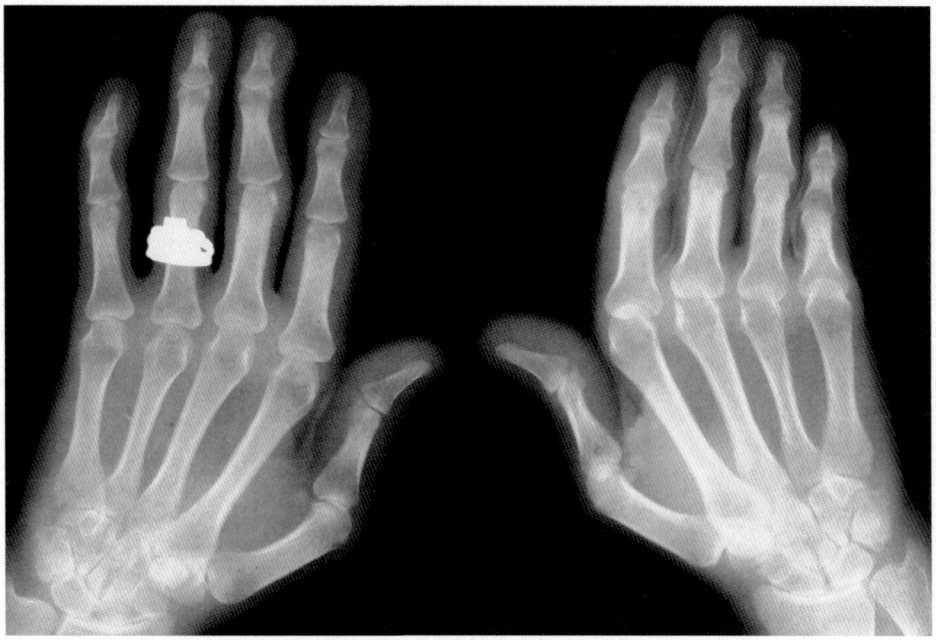

FIG. 6.31 **Systemic Lupus Erythematosus.** Marked soft tissue wasting, as noted by the concavity in the hypothenar eminence, and ulnar deviation of the phalanges, as is seen primarily in the right hand in this patient, are hallmarks of systemic lupus erythematosus (SLE).

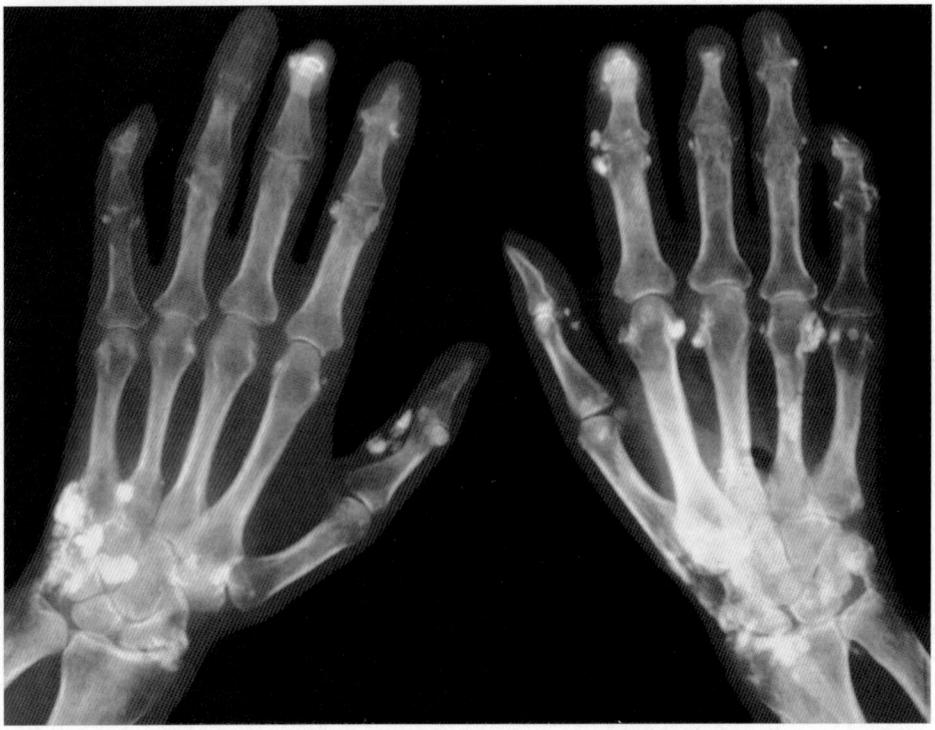

FIG. 6.32 **Scleroderma.** Diffuse subcutaneous soft tissue calcification is seen throughout the hands and wrist in this patient with scleroderma. Soft tissue wasting and osteoporosis are also present as well as bone loss in multiple distal phalanges (acro-osteolysis) secondary to the vascular abnormalities are often present in this disease.

The calcifications begin in the synovium and then tend to shed into the joint, where they can cause symptoms of free fragments or "joint mice." They then embed into the synovium and tend not to be free in the joint after a while. If the loose bodies are all of the same size, it is termed "primary" synovial osteochondromatosis. It is usually necessary to perform a complete synovectomy to relieve the symptoms. If the loose bodies are of different sizes, it is termed "secondary" synovial osteochondromatosis. This indicates it is secondary to underlying DJD in which small bits of cartilage are shed into the joint and grow as they are nourished by the synovial fluid. Since the shedding of the joint fragments occurs at varying times, the loose bodies are of different sizes. The differentiation of primary versus secondary synovial osteochondromatosis is important, as the primary type requires a synovectomy, while the secondary type requires removal of the loose bodies and treatment of the DJD, but no synovectomy.

An uncommon presentation of synovial osteochondromatosis is tumefactive synovial osteochondromatosis. This occurs when the loose bodies are so tightly packed in a joint that it appears on magnetic resonance imaging (MRI) to be a solid tumor (see discussion and figures in Chapter 3).

PIGMENTED VILLONODULAR SYNOVITIS

Pigmented villonodular synovitis (PVNS) is a chronic, inflammatory process of the synovium that causes synovial proliferation. A swollen joint with lobular masses of synovium occurs, which causes pain and joint destruction (Fig. 6.45). It virtually never calcifies. It has been termed giant cell tumor of tendon sheath and tendon sheath xanthoma when it occurs in a tendon sheath, which is not unusual. PVNS looks radiographically identical to noncalcified synovial osteochondromatosis, yet it is much less common. Therefore whenever PVNS is a consideration, mention synovial osteochondromatosis (noncalcified). MRI of a joint with PVNS shows a pathognomonic appearance of low-signal hemosiderin deposits lining the synovium (Fig. 6.46).

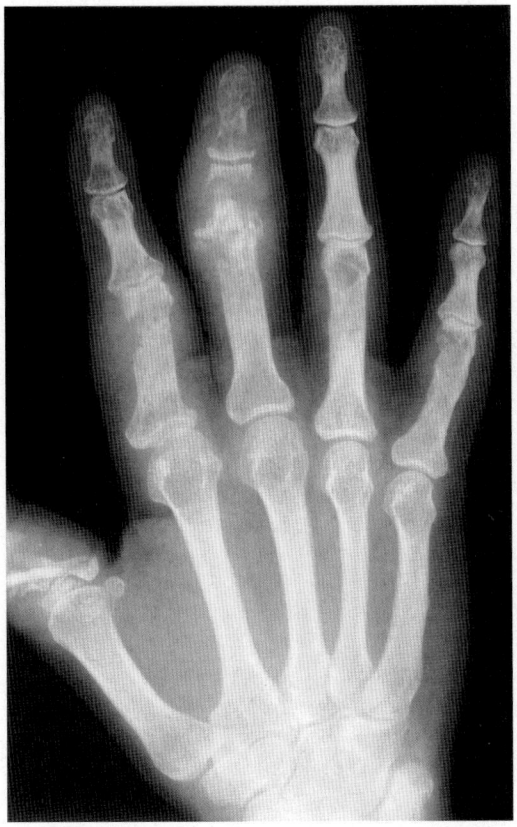

FIG. 6.33 **Sarcoid.** An anteroposterior (AP) view of the hand in this patient with sarcoid demonstrates classic changes of bony involvement with this granulomatous process. Note the lacelike pattern of destruction seen most prominently in the proximal phalanges and the distal third phalanx. Soft tissue swelling and some areas of severe bony dissolution are also noted, which occur in more advanced patterns of sarcoid. These changes are typically limited to the hands but can rarely occur in other parts of the skeleton.

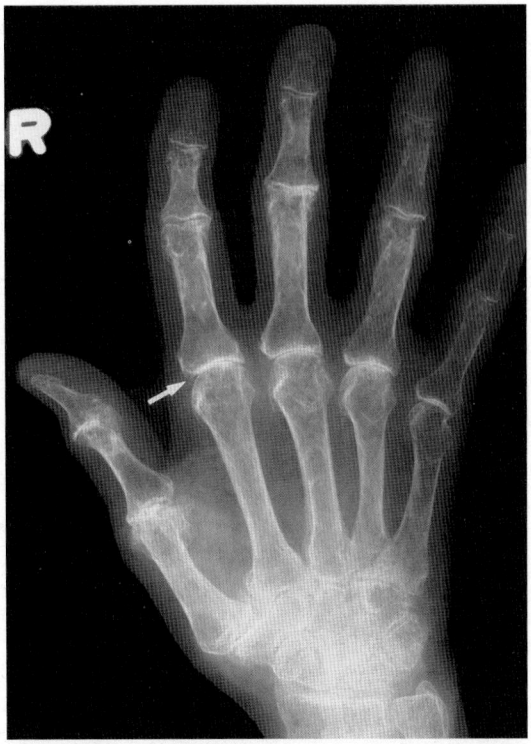

FIG. 6.34 **Hemochromatosis.** An anteroposterior (AP) view of the hand in this patient with hemochromatosis shows severe joint space narrowing throughout the hand, which is most marked at the metacarpophalangeal joints. Associated sclerosis at the metacarpophalangeal joints with large osteophytes seen off the metacarpal heads suggests degenerative joint disease (DJD). These are unusual joints for DJD to occur in, yet this is the classic appearance of hemochromatosis. No chondrocalcinosis is seen in the triangular cartilage in this patient; however, a small amount of chondrocalcinosis can be seen at the second metacarpophalangeal joint *(arrow)*. Fifty percent of patients with hemochromatosis also have pyrophosphate dihydrate crystal deposition disease (CPPD).

SUDECK ATROPHY

Also known as shoulder-hand syndrome, reflex sympathetic dystrophy, and chronic regional pain syndrome, Sudeck atrophy is a poorly understood affliction that typically occurs after minor trauma to an extremity, resulting in pain, swelling, and dysfunction. Severe osteoporosis and swelling are seen radiographically (Fig. 6.47). The disorder typically affects the distal part of an extremity, such as a hand or foot, yet intermediate joints, such as the knee and hip, are thought by some to occasionally be involved. The pain usually subsides, but the osteoporosis may persist. The swelling, with time, will subside, and the skin may become atrophic. It is important for the radiologist to recognize the aggressive osteoporosis in this disorder so the treating physician can begin aggressive physical therapy.

JOINT EFFUSIONS

Radiology residents often go to great extremes to determine whether or not a joint—be it a knee, hip, shoulder, elbow, or whatever—has an effusion. There are some good signs of joint effusions (which I will review), and there are some that are used that are invalid. The thing that amazes me is all the attention it gets because when

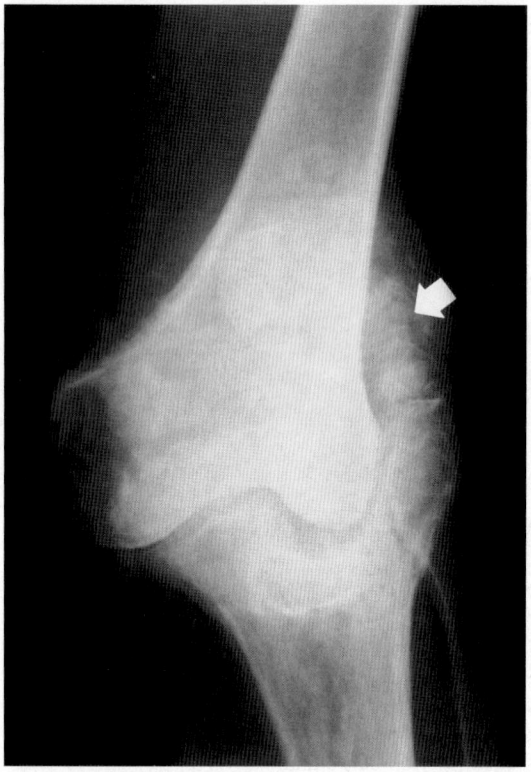

FIG. 6.35 **Charcot Joint.** An anteroposterior (AP) view of the knee in this patient with tabes dorsalis shows the classic changes of a neuropathic or Charcot joint. Note the severe joint destruction, the subluxation, and the heterotopic new bone *(arrow)*.

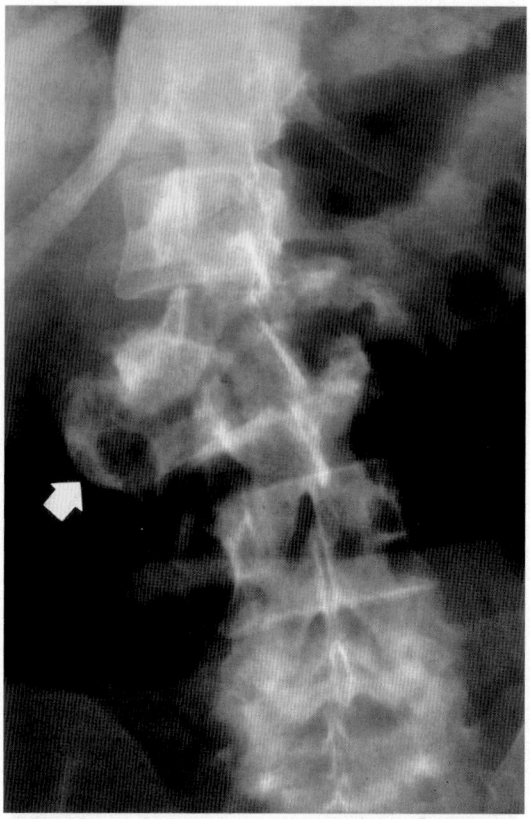

FIG. 6.36 **Charcot Spine.** An anteroposterior (AP) view of the spine in this paraplegic shows severe destruction of the L-2 and L-3 vertebral bodies and the intervening disc space, heterotopic new bone *(arrow)*, and malalignment or dislocation.

all is said and done, in most cases, it doesn't make any difference whatsoever. With the exception of the elbow (see Chapter 5) and possibly the hip, treatment is never predicated on the radiographic finding of a joint effusion.

Most joint effusions are clinically obvious and do not require radiographic validation. As mentioned earlier, the elbow is an exception. In the setting of trauma to the elbow, an effusion indicates a fracture. The radiographic signs of an elbow effusion are generally clearly seen and have proved to be valid. Clinical determination of an elbow effusion can be difficult; therefore the radiologist can be very helpful in this area (see Chapter 5 and Figs. 5.36, 5.37, and 5.38).

Clinical determination of a hip effusion is also difficult. The presence of a hip effusion can be valuable in certain clinical settings. For instance, in a patient with pain in the hip and an effusion, the joint should be aspirated to rule out an infection. If only pain were present, an aspiration would probably not be performed. The radiology literature mentions displacement of the fat stripes about the hip as being an indicator for an effusion, but this has been proved to be fallacious. The only fat pad around the hip that gets displaced with an effusion is the obturator internus, and it is seldom seen. The remainder of the fat pads are far removed from the joint capsule and are not directly influenced by the joint.

A radiographic sign in the hip that does work for indicating an effusion is called the teardrop sign. Leonard Swischuk first brought this sign to my attention by its application in pediatric patients. I have used it in adults as well with good results.[4] The teardrop is an anatomic landmark at the medial aspect of the hip joint (Fig. 6.48) that is made up of several bony structures bounding the acetabulum medially. The teardrop measurement is the distance from the medialmost part of the femoral head to the medialmost

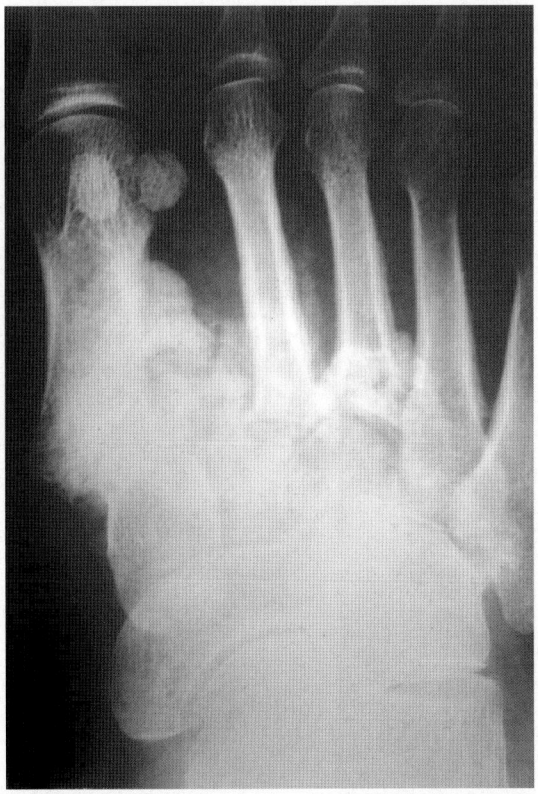

FIG. 6.37 **Lisfranc Charcot Joint.** Dislocation of the second and third metatarsals along with joint destruction and large amounts of heterotopic new bone are present in the foot of this diabetic. These findings are classic for a Charcot joint that has been termed a Lisfranc fracture–dislocation. It is most commonly seen secondary to trauma rather than as a Charcot joint, but is the most common neuropathic joint seen today.

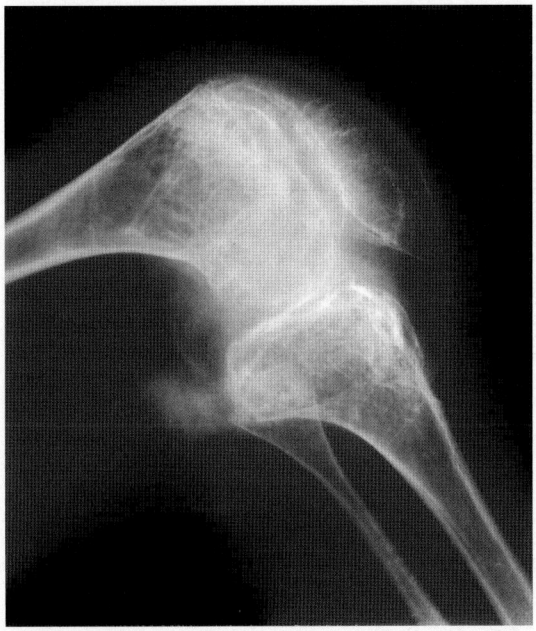

FIG. 6.38 **Juvenile Rheumatoid Arthritis (JRA).** A lateral view of the knee in this patient with JRA shows the classic findings of overgrowth of the ends of the bones and associated gracile diaphyses. These changes can also be seen in hemophilia or paralysis patients.

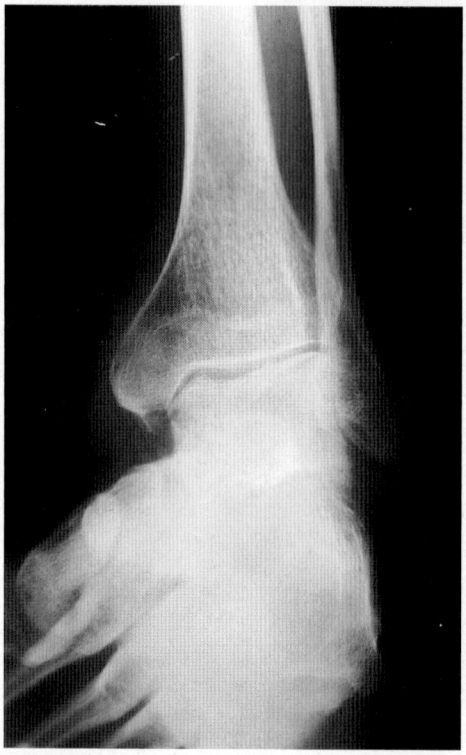

FIG. 6.39 **Hemophilia.** An anteroposterior (AP) view of the ankle in this patient with hemophilia shows subtle changes of overgrowth of the distal tibia and fibula as compared with the diameter of the diaphyses. Some joint destruction of the tibiotalar joint is also noted.

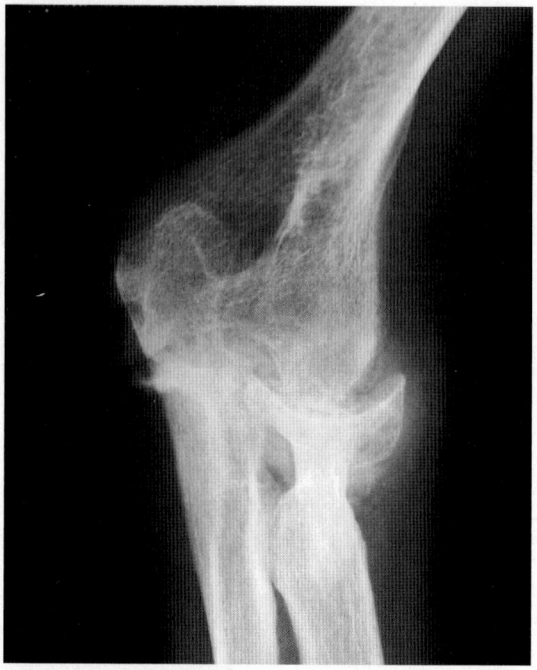

FIG. 6.40 **Hemophilia.** An anteroposterior (AP) view of the elbow in this patient with hemophilia shows overgrowth of the ends of the bones, in particular the head of the radius, and marked joint destruction. Juvenile rheumatoid arthritis (JRA) could certainly cause an appearance such as this.

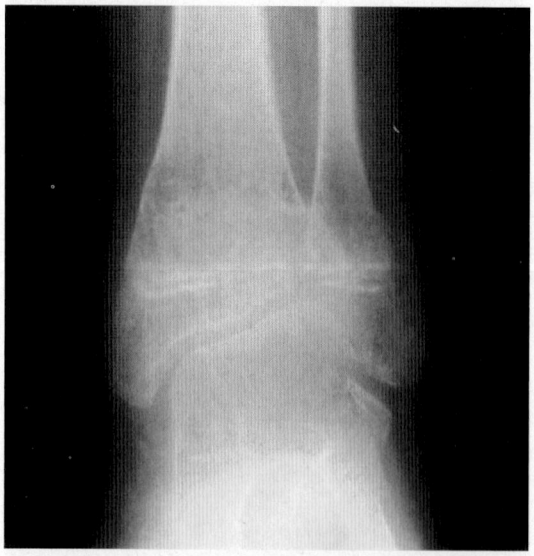

FIG. 6.41 **Muscular Dystrophy.** This patient with muscular dystrophy has changes similar to those of JRA and hemophilia, which consist of overgrowth of the ends of the bones and a tibio–talar slant. This appearance is frequently found in patients with paralysis.

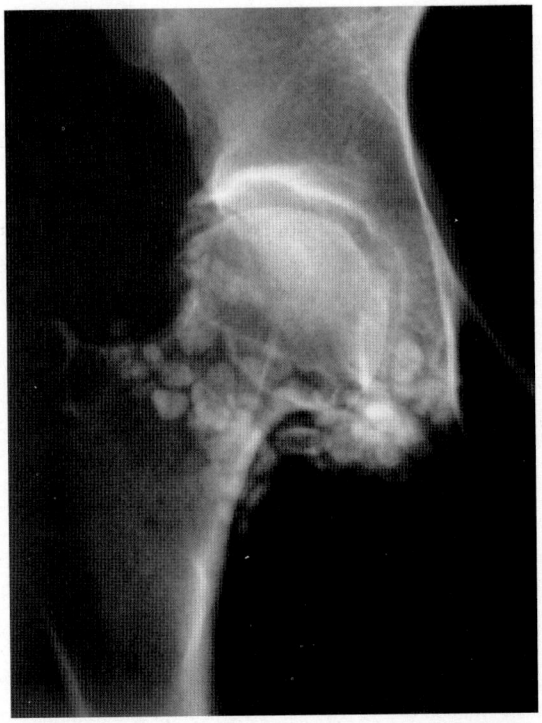

FIG. 6.42 **Synovial Osteochondromatosis.** An anteroposterior (AP) view of the hip in this patient with left hip pain shows multiple calcified loose bodies in the hip joint. The loose bodies are all of a similar size; therefore this is diagnostic of primary synovial osteochondromatosis.

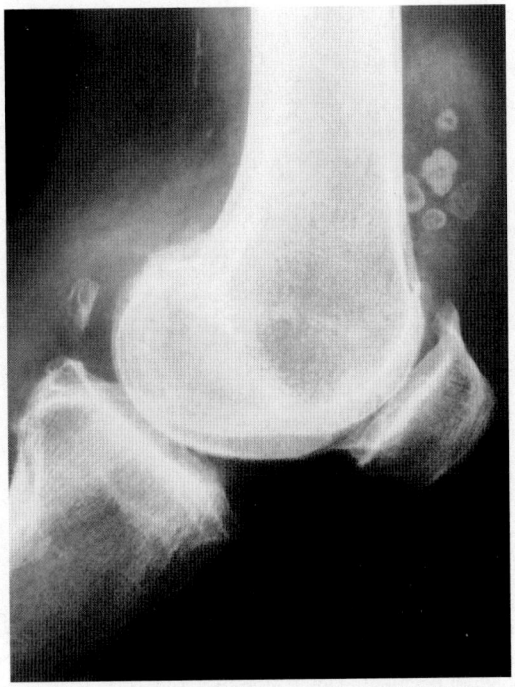

FIG. 6.43 **Synovial Osteochondromatosis.** Multiple calcified loose bodies are seen in the suprapatellar space of the knee in this patient. The loose bodies are of different sizes; therefore this is diagnostic of secondary synovial osteochondromatosis.

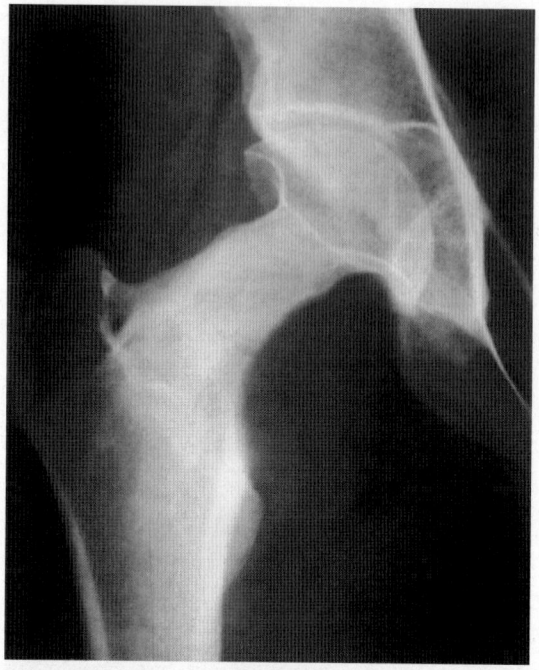

FIG. 6.44 **Synovial Osteochondromatosis without Calcification.** An anteroposterior (AP) view of the hip in this patient shows the femoral neck to be virtually whittled down, with the femoral head undercut, giving an apple core appearance. This has occurred from the pressure erosion of multiple nonossified loose bodies in the joint. This is nonossified synovial osteochondromatosis, which is probably more properly termed synovial chondromatosis. It usually does not cause this degree of bony erosion and is indistinguishable from pigmented villonodular synovitis.

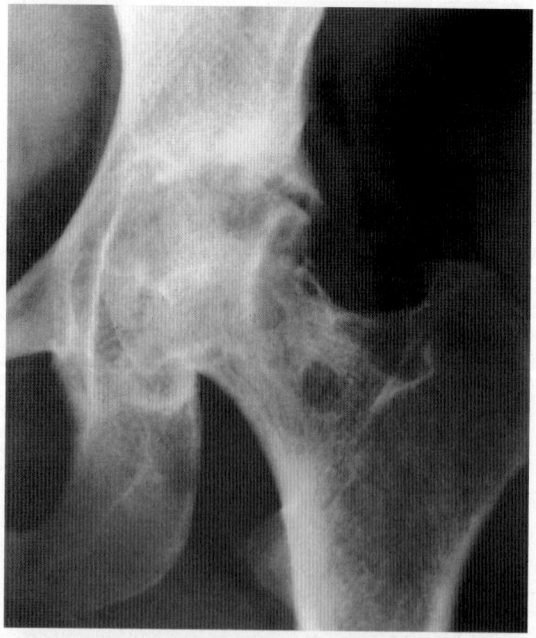

FIG. 6.45 **Pigmented Villonodular Synovitis.** An anteroposterior (AP) view of the hip in this patient shows joint space destruction and bony erosions throughout the femoral head and neck. Pigmented villonodular synovitis (PVNS) or synovial chondromatosis (nonossified) could have this appearance.

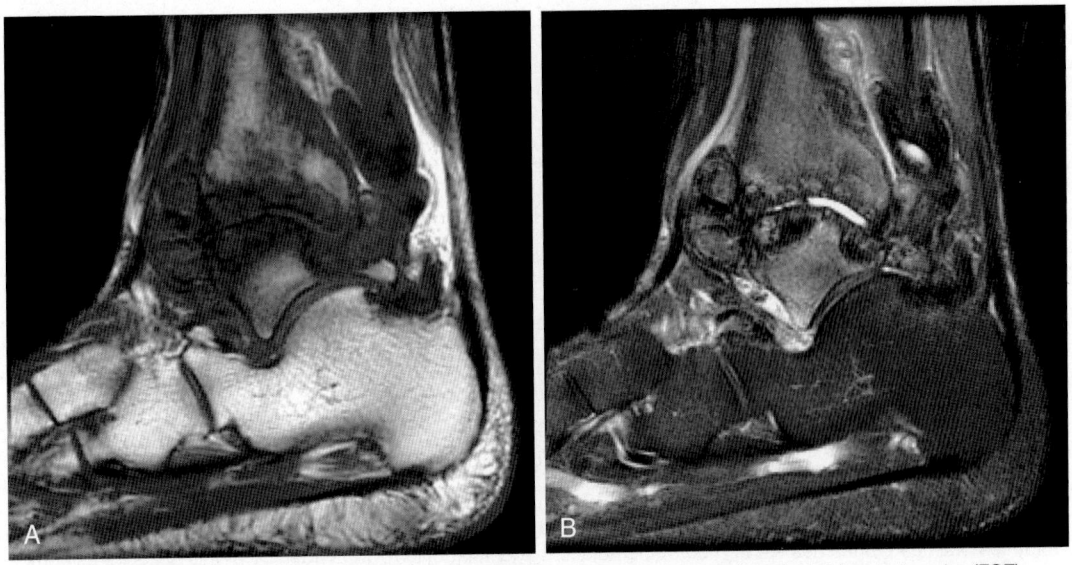

FIG. 6.46 **Pigmented Villonodular Synovitis (PVNS).** Sagittal T1-weighted (A) and fast spin-echo (FSE) T2-weighted (B) images of an ankle with PVNS show a soft tissue mass emanating from the ankle joint, which is low signal on both sequences and has very low signal hemosiderin lining parts of the synovium, which is characteristic for PVNS.

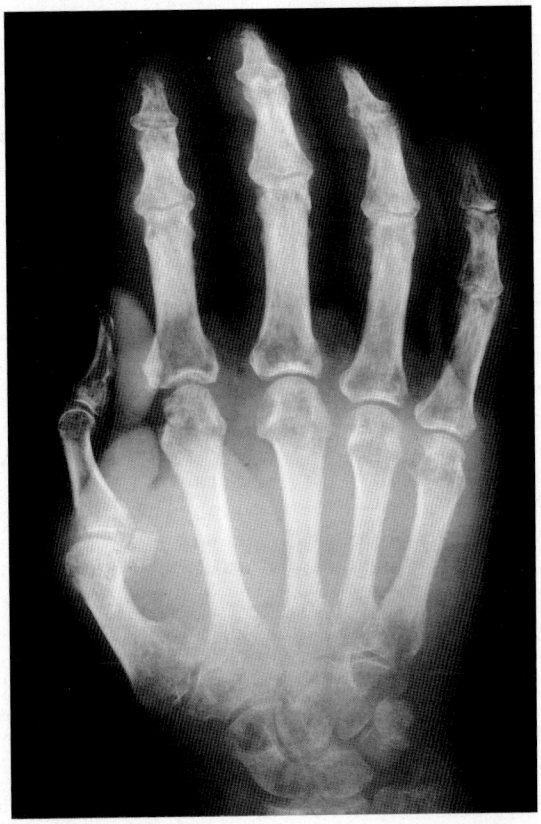

FIG. 6.47 **Sudeck Atrophy.** Diffuse soft tissue swelling and marked osteoporosis that is so aggressive it has a spotty or permeative appearance around the joints is noted in this patient with severe hand pain and dysfunction after minor trauma. This is characteristic of Sudeck atrophy.

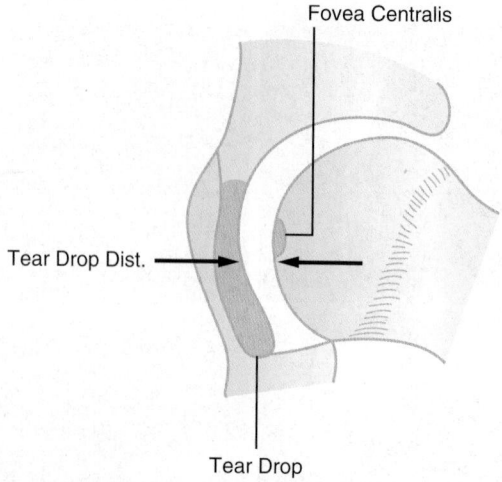

FIG. 6.48 **Drawing of the Teardrop Measurement.** The teardrop measurement is the distance from the medialmost aspect of the femoral head to the nearest portion of the adjacent acetabulum *(arrows)*. Widening of this distance as compared with the opposite hip is indicative of a joint effusion.

extent of the acetabulum (which is the teardrop). This measurement—inappropriately called the teardrop measurement—should be equal in both hips. An effusion will push the femoral head laterally and give the affected side a wider teardrop distance (Fig. 6.49). The teardrop distance is a valid indicator of an effusion in children. It is valid in adults only when no long-standing joint abnormality, such as DJD or an old fracture, is present. A difference in the teardrop distance from one hip to the other of as little as 1 mm is significant in the appropriate clinical setting. It would be better to aspirate a few normal hips rather than risk missing a hip infection that might destroy the hip if diagnosed late.

The radiographic sign for a knee effusion that seems to be the most reliable is the measurement of the distance between the suprapatellar fat pad and the anterior femoral fat pad (Fig. 6.50). A distance between these two fat pads of more than 10 mm is definite evidence for an effusion. A distance of less than 5 mm is normal. A distance of 5 to 10 mm is no-man's-land. I usually call an effusion if the distance is greater than 5 mm, realizing that I'm probably overcalling a few. I am also aware that it doesn't make any difference if there is an effusion in the knee or not—the patient gets treated the same regardless. If it were vital to the patient, you could aspirate the joint or perform an MRI study to find out. I should emphasize that we never do an MR exam just to see if there is fluid in a joint, because it is completely nonspecific.

Shoulder effusions are difficult to detect unless they are massive enough to displace the humeral head inferiorly, as with a fracture and hemarthrosis (see Chapter 5). Fortunately, as with most other joints, treatment is not based on the presence or absence of an effusion, so it hardly matters. The same is true in the ankle, wrist, and smaller joints. Ultrasound is widely available and is becoming popular for identifying joint effusions, but, again, I question why bother—it is unlikely to change the treatment.

AVASCULAR NECROSIS

Avascular necrosis (AVN), or aseptic necrosis, can occur around almost any joint for a host of reasons, including steroids, trauma, various underlying disease states, and even idiopathically. It is often seen in renal transplant patients.

The hallmark of AVN is increased bone density at an otherwise normal joint. Increased density at a joint usually indicates DJD; however, if osteophytes and joint space narrowing are not present, another disorder should be considered.

The earliest sign of AVN is a joint effusion. This often is not radiographically visible or is so nonspecific as to not help with the diagnosis unless the clinical setting had already raised suspicion for AVN. The next sign for AVN is a patchy or mottled density (Fig. 6.51). In the knee, this density increase can occur throughout an entire condyle, while in the

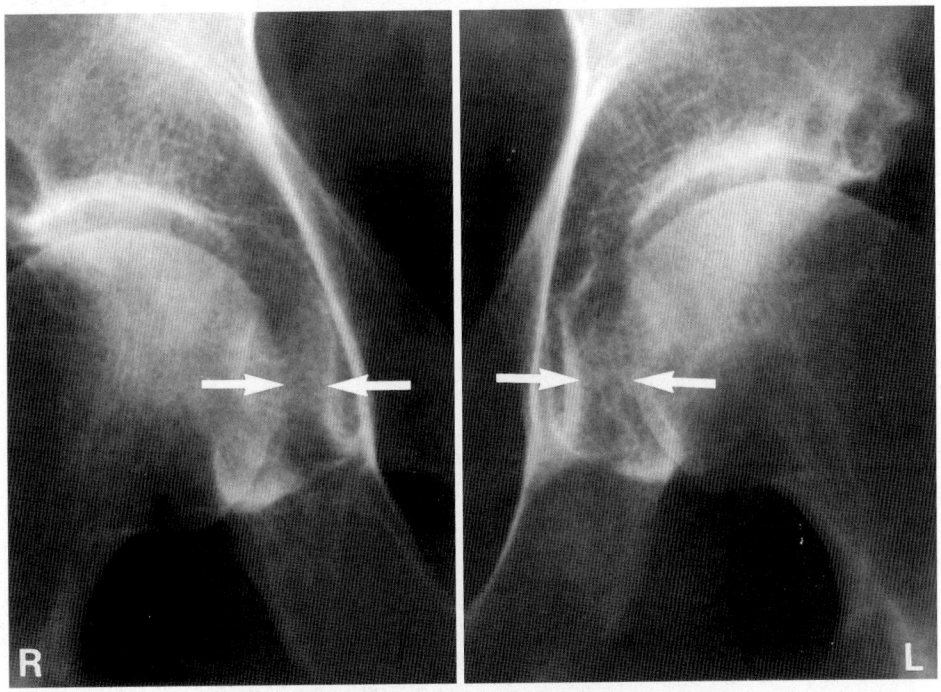

FIG. 6.49 **Widened Teardrop.** The teardrop distance in this patient on the left side *(arrows)* is slightly wider than that on the right side *(arrows)*, which is indicative of a hip joint effusion. This patient had a hip joint infection on the left side.

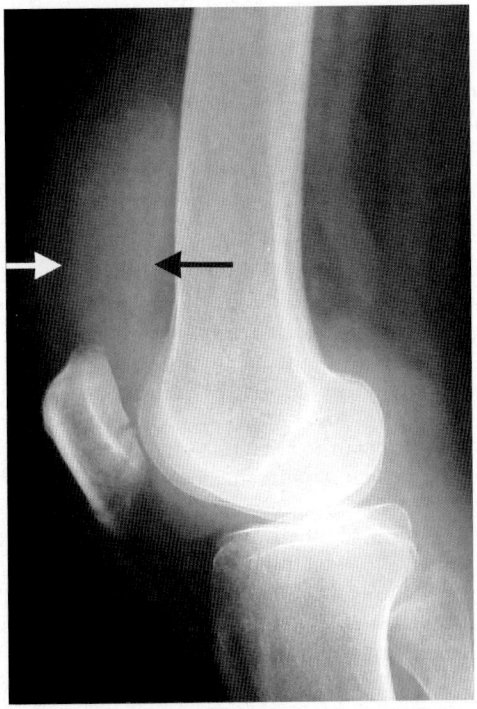

FIG. 6.50 **Knee Joint Effusion.** This patient has a fractured patella with a large joint effusion. The suprapatellar pouch is grossly distended, with the distance between the suprapatellar fat pad and the anterior femoral fat pad measuring more than 1.0 cm *(arrows)*.

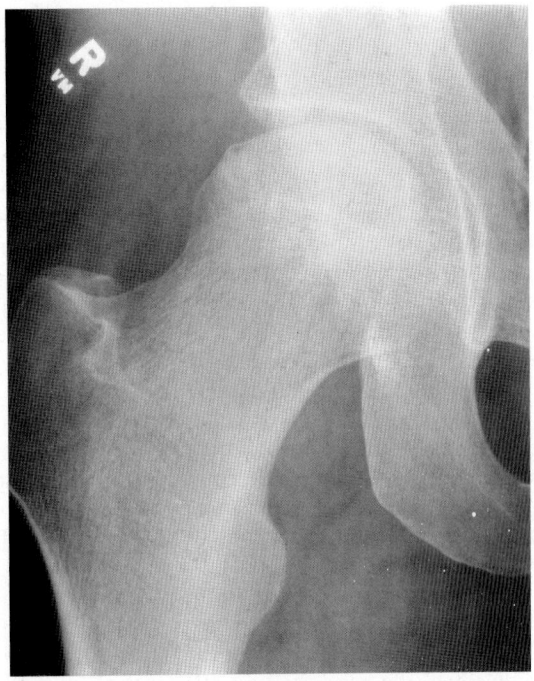

FIG. 6.51 **Early Avascular Necrosis of the Hip.** Patchy sclerosis is present throughout the femoral head in this patient with a renal transplant and avascular necrosis of the right hip. No subchondral lucency or articular surface irregularity in the weight-bearing region is yet present with the exception of a small cortical irregularity seen laterally.

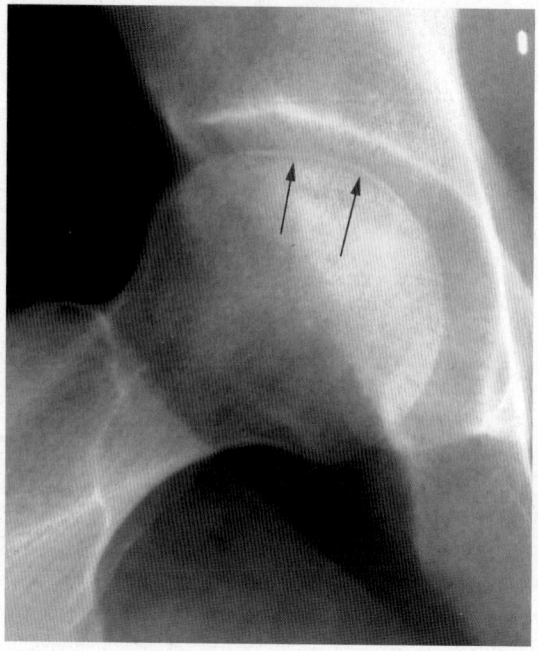

FIG. 6.52 **Avascular Necrosis of the Hip.** A definite subchondral lucency *(arrows)* is seen in the weight-bearing portion of this hip with avascular necrosis. Patchy sclerosis throughout the femoral head is also noted.

hip, it often involves the entire femoral head. Next, a subchondral lucency develops that forms a thin line along the articular surface (Fig. 6.52). This lucent line has been described as being an early indicator for AVN when, in fact, it is a late finding. Also, the lucent line stage is often not present in the evolution of AVN. Therefore using the lucent line as one of the main criteria for AVN can lead to missing early findings or missing the diagnosis completely. I would estimate that I see a lucent line in only 20% or fewer of the cases of AVN in our hospital.

The final sign in AVN is collapse of the articular surface and joint fragmentation (Fig. 6.53). I must stress that these changes all occur on only one side of a joint, which makes for an easy diagnosis, since almost everything else around joints involves both sides.

MRI plays a valuable role in the early diagnosis of AVN throughout the skeletal system but especially in the hip, where it is more sensitive than even radionuclide scans. The use of MRI in AVN of the hip is discussed more fully in Chapter 13: Magnetic Resonance Imaging: Miscellaneous Uses.

A form of AVN that is smaller and more focal than that just described is osteochondritis dissecans (OCD). For whatever reasons, the term OCD has been replaced by the term osteochondral lesion (OCL). Perhaps the absence of true dessication forced true academicians to choose a more acceptable term—I wish they'd just stick to one term, whether or not it's technically right or wrong! It is thought to be due to trauma, although many believe that it is primarily idiopathic. It is most commonly found in the knee at the medial femoral condyle (Fig. 6.54), but also is seen frequently in the dome of the talus (Fig. 6.55) and occasionally in the capitellum (Fig. 6.56). OCD, oops, I mean an OCL, often leads to a small fragment of bone being sloughed off and becoming a free fragment in the joint—a "joint mouse" (Fig. 6.54).

AVN is one of the disorders around joints in which subchondral cysts or "geodes" can occur. It is the only one of the four disorders (rheumatoid arthritis, DJD, and CPPD being the others) that can have an essentially normal joint and have a geode (Fig. 6.57). The other abnormalities will have joint space narrowing and/or osteophytes, osteoporosis, chondrocalcinosis, or other findings.

A host of names have been ascribed to epiphyseal AVN, usually with the eponym being the first person

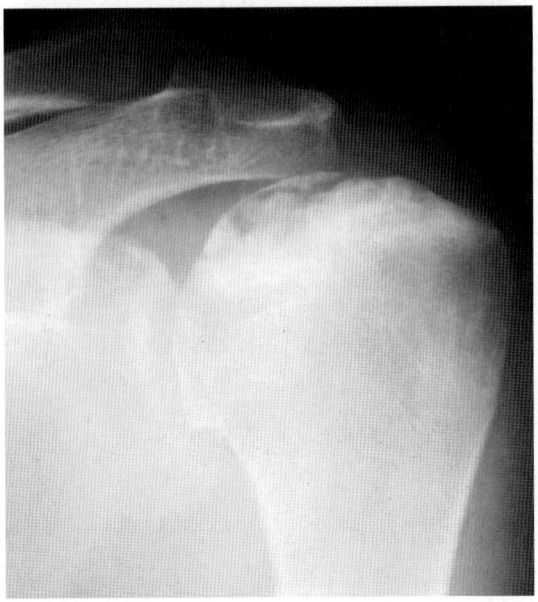

FIG. 6.53 **Avascular Necrosis of the Shoulder.** Articular surface collapse is present in this shoulder with long-standing avascular necrosis. Dense bony sclerosis is also present.

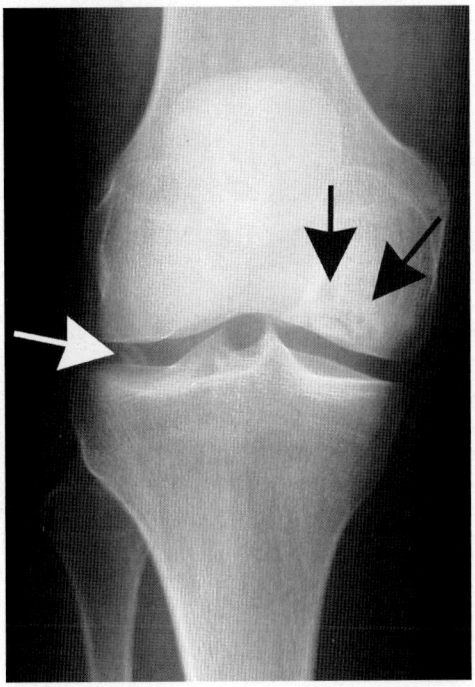

FIG. 6.54 **Osteochondral Lesion (OCL).** A small focal area of avascular necrosis in the medial condyle of the femur *(black arrows)* is present, which is an OCL. Part of the area of avascular necrosis has shed a bony fragment *(white arrow)* that is loose in the joint and known as a joint mouse.

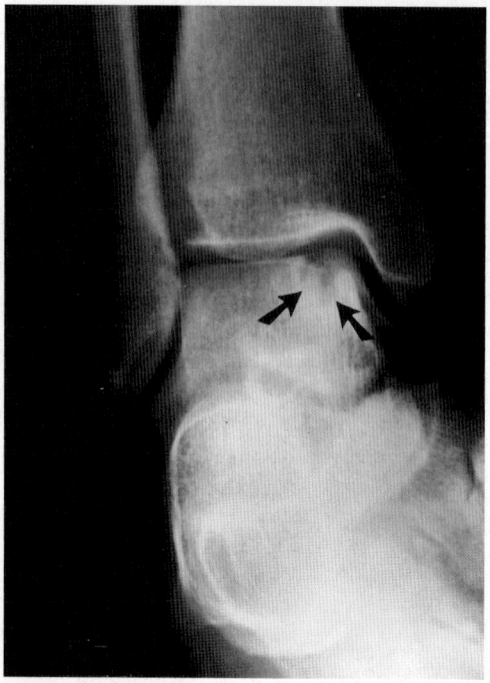

FIG. 6.55 **Osteochondral Lesion (OCL) of the Talus.** A focal area of avascular necrosis in the talus as seen here *(arrows)* is called an OCL. The talus is the second most common site after the knee and, as in the knee, can cause a joint mouse or loose body in the joint.

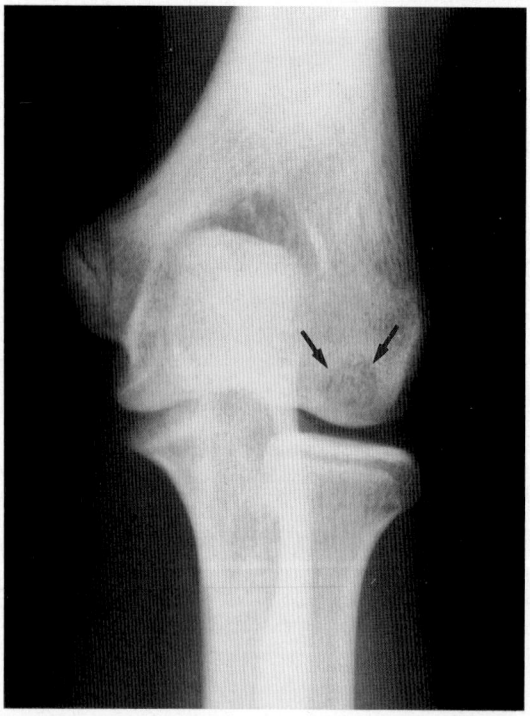

FIG. 6.56 **Osteochondral Lesion (OCL) of the Elbow.** The third most common site for an OCL is in the capitellum of the elbow. The faint lucency seen in this capitellum *(arrows)* was at first felt to be a chondroblastoma or an area of infection.

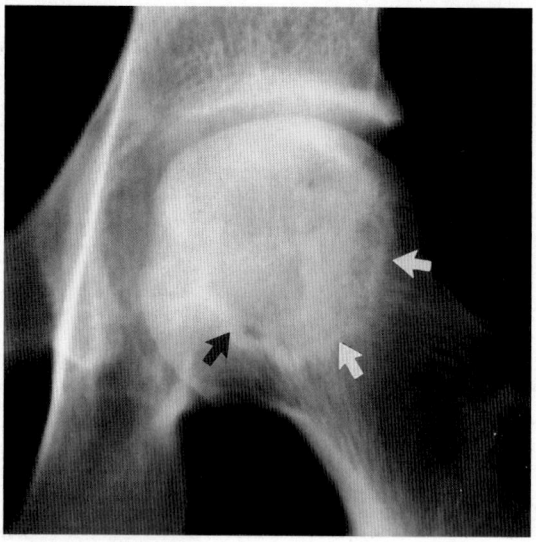

FIG. 6.57 **Geode in the Hip.** A large cystic lesion *(arrows)* is seen in this patient with avascular necrosis of the hip. Note the adjacent patchy sclerosis indicative of avascular necrosis. A subchondral cyst or geode should be considered any time a lytic lesion is found around a joint.

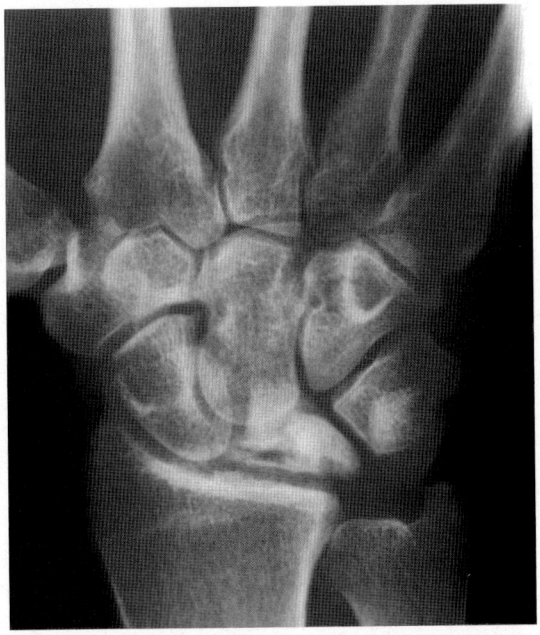

FIG. 6.58 **Kienböck Malacia.** Avascular necrosis of the lunate, or Kienböck malacia, is demonstrated in this patient. Note the increased density and partial fragmentation of the lunate.

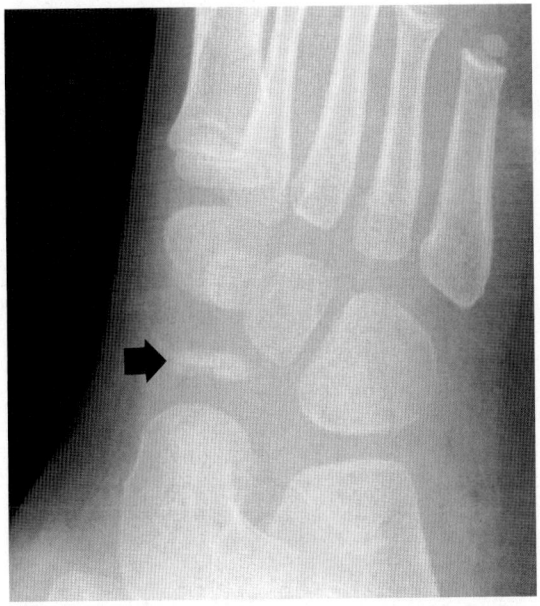

FIG. 6.59 **Köhler Disease.** Flattening and sclerosis of the tarsal navicular *(arrow)* in children is thought by many to be avascular necrosis and is called Köhler disease. Others have found this to be an asymptomatic normal variant and believe that it is an incidental finding.

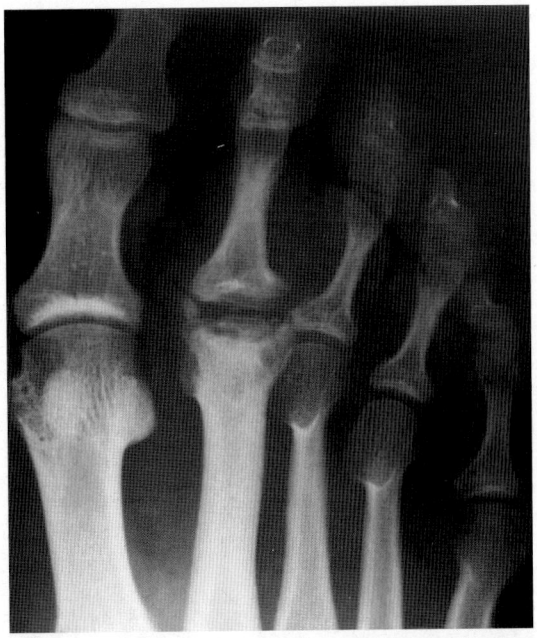

FIG. 6.60 **Freiberg's Infraction.** Flattening, collapse, and sclerosis of the second metatarsal head, as seen in this patient, is typical of avascular necrosis or Freiberg infraction. It can also involve the third or fourth metatarsal heads. Note the compensatory hypertrophy of the cortex of the second metatarsal, which is invariably found with this disorder.

to describe the disorder. These are thought to be idiopathic for the most part but can also occur secondary to trauma. A few of the more common bones involved are the following: the carpal lunate, Kienböck malacia (Fig. 6.58); the tarsal navicular, Köhler disease (Fig. 6.59); the metatarsal heads, Freiberg infraction (Fig. 6.60); the femoral head, Legg–Perthes; the ring apophyses of the spine, Scheuermann disease (Fig. 6.61); and the tibial tubercle, Osgood–Schlatter disease, also called surfer's knees.

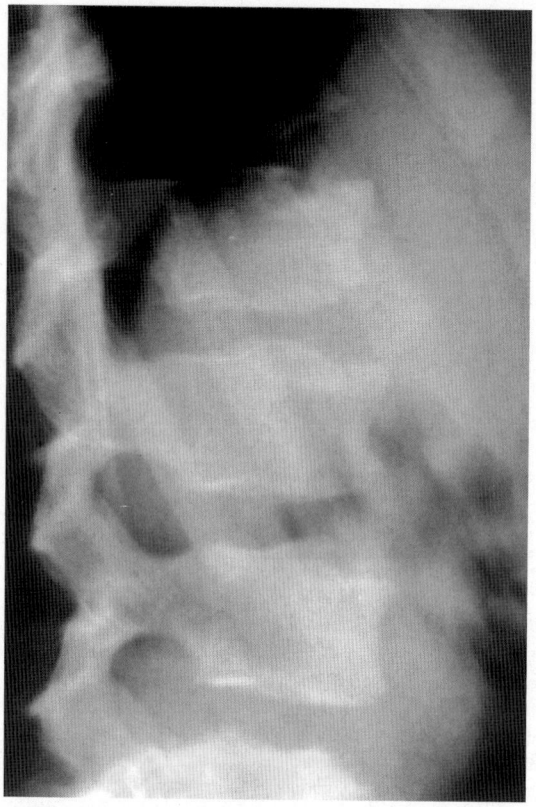

FIG. 6.61 **Scheuermann Disease.** Avascular necrosis of the apophyseal rings of the vertebral bodies is called Scheuermann disease. He originally described a painful kyphosis with multiple vertebral bodies involved. It is most commonly seen without kyphosis or pain and with only a few vertebral bodies involved.

REFERENCES

1. Forrester DM, Brown JC. *The Radiology of Joint Disease*. 3rd ed. Philadelphia: WB Saunders Co.; 1987.
2. Brower AC. *Arthritis in Black and White*. 2nd ed. Philadelphia: WB Saunders Co.; 1997.
3. Resnick D. *Diagnosis of Bone and Joint Disorders*. 4th ed. Philadelphia: WB Saunders Co.; 2002.
4. Sweeney JP, Helms CA, Minagi H, Louie KW. The widened teardrop distance: a plain film indicator of hip joint effusion in adults. *AJR*. 1987:117–119.

CHAPTER 7

Metabolic Bone Disease

Most of the literature on metabolic bone disease is steeped in biochemistry, physiology, histology, internal medicine, and other arcane pursuits that can be quite confusing for a poor radiology resident who just wants a few pearls and illustrations. Frankly, it's a tough topic. I will, by necessity, keep it simple, but this is an important topic about which every radiologist should have at least a superficial fund of knowledge. I have excluded disorders such as pseudo- and pseudo-pseudo hypoparathyroidism that are unlikely to be seen and have tried to cover the more commonly seen disorders.

OSTEOPOROSIS

Osteoporosis is diminished bone quantity in which the bone is otherwise normal. This contrasts with osteomalacia, in which the bone quantity is normal, but the bone itself is abnormal in that it is not normally mineralized. Osteomalacia results in excess nonmineralized osteoid. It is not possible in the vast majority of cases to distinguish between osteoporosis and osteomalacia on plain films.

The causes of osteoporosis are myriad, the most common of which was once called senile osteoporosis (a term that is not considered politically correct and is no longer used), or osteoporosis of aging. The preferred term for this type of osteoporosis is *primary* osteoporosis. This is seen most commonly in postmenopausal females and is a major public health concern because of the increase of spinal and hip fractures in this patient population.

Secondary osteoporosis implies that an underlying disorder, such as thyrotoxicosis or renal disease, has caused the osteoporosis. Only about 5% of osteoporosis has an underlying cause. The differential diagnosis for secondary osteoporosis is quite long and probably should not be memorized, as one cannot even be sure if it is osteoporosis or osteomalacia based on the plain films. Therefore the differential for presumed osteoporosis would have to include the causes of osteomalacia. The list gets too long to be of any real help to anyone.

The main radiographic finding in osteoporosis is thinning of the cortex. This is best demonstrated in the second metacarpal at the middiaphysis (Figs. 7.1 and 7.2). The normal metacarpal cortical thickening should be approximately one-fourth to one-third the thickness of the metacarpal (Fig. 7.3). In osteoporosis, this cortical thickness is decreased. The metacarpal cortex (and all bony cortices, for that matter) decreases normally with age and is less for women than for men of the same age. Several tables have been published that give the normal metacarpal cortical measurement, with age and sex adjustments to allow determination of normal. Unfortunately, these tables only determine the mineralization of the peripheral skeleton and do not seem to correlate to whether or not spinal or hip fractures will occur.

Measurement of the axial bone mineral content can be done by one of several methods that use computed tomography (CT) to assess the bone quantity in the spine. There is some debate over which method is superior and even whether or not knowing the bone mineral content is clinically helpful, since just knowing the age and sex of the patient is fairly accurate for predicting the bone mass quantity. Nevertheless, it is generally agreed that if a quantitative CT measurement shows bone mass to be 2 standard deviations below normal, that person has a high risk of spinal and hip fractures. Bone densitometry is widely used to identify patients, especially postmenopausal women, who are osteoporotic, so treatment can be instituted. Bisphosphonates have been widely used for treating osteoporosis, with excellent results, for the most part. A complication of long-term bisphosphonate therapy is fracture of the proximal femur.[1] These fractures occur on the lateral aspect of the proximal femoral diaphysis and are often bilateral (Fig. 7.4). If not treated, they can go on to complete fractures.

Exercise and proper diet (whatever that is) seem to help delay the onset of primary osteoporosis as much as anything. Calcium additives alone have not been shown to reverse the process of primary osteoporosis.

Because we cannot accurately give the causes of osteoporosis by looking at a radiograph and cannot even differentiate it from osteomalacia, it is a topic that is frustrating for many radiologists to deal with. Most of us would rather comment on something we can give a diagnosis on or at least a short differential. In general, when decreased bone mass is present on a radiograph, the odds are that osteoporosis is present.

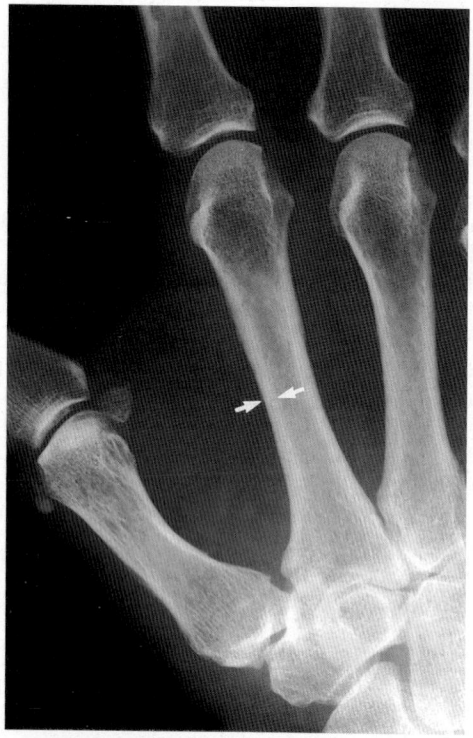

FIG. 7.1 **Mild Osteoporosis.** Mild cortical narrowing *(arrows)* at the mid second metacarpal is noted in this patient with renal osteodystrophy. Compare this cortical width with that of the normal width in Fig. 7.3.

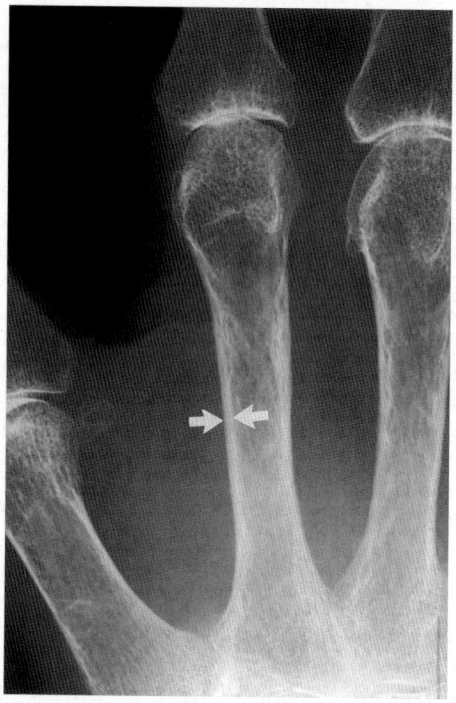

FIG. 7.2 **Marked Osteoporosis.** Marked cortical narrowing *(arrows)* of the mid second metacarpal cortex is present in this patient with severe osteoporosis. Also note the intracortical tunneling, which occurs with more rapid forms of osteoporosis.

However, because the disease process could just as easily be osteomalacia, it is recommended that the term "osteopenia" be used. This is a generic term that includes both osteoporosis and osteomalacia. When used, it also implies that the observer knows he cannot separate the two entities and is an educated person.

A type of osteoporosis that can be seen in a patient of any age is disuse osteoporosis. It results from immobilization from any cause, most commonly after treatment of a fracture. The radiographic appearance of disuse osteoporosis is different from primary osteoporosis in that it occurs somewhat more rapidly and gives the bone a patchy or even a permeative appearance (Fig. 7.5). This is from the osteocytic resorption in the cortex, causing intracortical holes. If allowed to continue with disuse, the bone would resemble any bone with marked osteoporosis (i.e., severe cortical thinning).

Occasionally, aggressive osteoporosis from disuse can mimic a permeative lesion, such as a Ewing sarcoma or multiple myeloma, because of the severe cortical patchy or permeative pattern that projects over the medullary space and resembles a medullary permeative process (Fig. 7.6). The way to differentiate a true intramedullary permeative process from an intracortical process such as osteoporosis is to observe the cortex and see if it is solid or riddled with holes (Fig. 7.7). If it is solid, you can assume the permeative process is emanating from the medullary space (Fig. 7.8); if it has multiple small holes, you have to assume the permeative pattern is from the cortical process. I call a permeative appearance that is secondary to cortical holes a pseudopermeative process to distinguish it from a true permeative process.

Another cause for a pseudopermeative process is a hemangioma. It can cause cortical holes in two ways: from focal increased blood flow or hyperemia, causing focal osteoporosis, or by the blood vessels themselves tunneling through the cortex (Fig. 7.9). I have seen more than one hemangioma operated on inadvertently because the lesion was thought to be a Ewing sarcoma—they bleed a lot.

Radiotherapy can cause cortical holes in bone and mimic a permeative pattern (Fig. 7.10). These holes

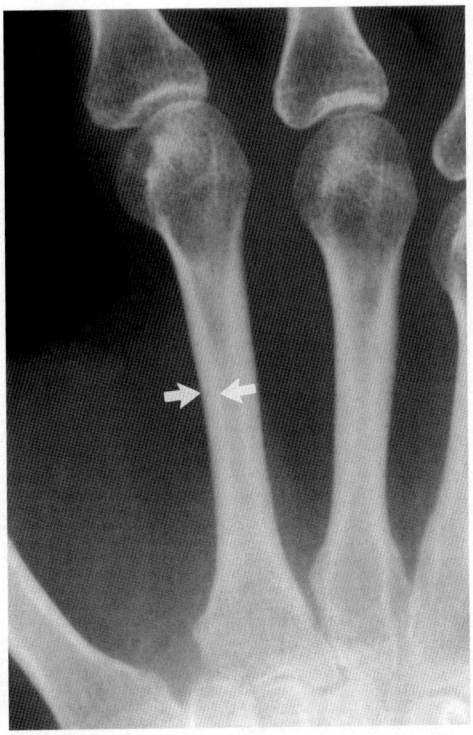

FIG. 7.3 **Normal Mineralization.** Note the cortical width *(arrows)* of the mid second metacarpal in this patient with normal mineralization. The width of the cortex is easily greater than one-third of the total width of the metacarpal.

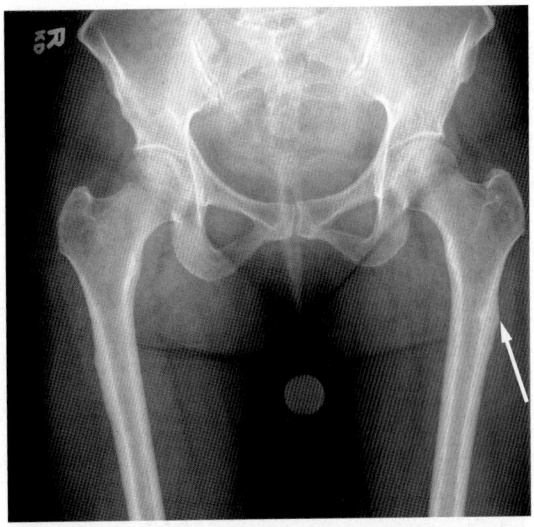

FIG. 7.4 **Femoral Fracture 2-degree Bisphosphonate Therapy.** This postmenopausal woman had been on bisphosphonates for many years and presented with left thigh pain. Focal cortical thickening *(arrow)* is characteristic for the appearance of femur fractures in bisphosphonate therapy. These can go on to a complete fracture if not protected or treated.

are often large and would not be confused with a true permeative process, but they can be small and cause confusion.

If a permeative pattern is seen in bone, the differential is usually an aggressive process such as Ewing sarcoma, infection, or eosinophilic granuloma in a young person or multiple myeloma, metastatic carcinomatosis, or primary lymphoma of bone in an older patient. If, however, the permeative pattern is seen to be a result of cortical holes (i.e., a pseudopermeative pattern), the differential is considerably kinder: aggressive osteoporosis, hemangioma, or radiation changes. This differential does not arise often, but is very useful when it does come up.[2,3]

OSTEOMALACIA

As mentioned earlier, osteomalacia is the result of too much nonmineralized osteoid. There are many causes for osteomalacia, with the most common today being renal osteodystrophy. The radiographic findings are almost identical to those of osteoporosis, and for the most part, the two disorders are indistinguishable. The only findings that are distinctive for osteomalacia are Looser fractures, which are fractures through large osteoid seams (Fig. 7.11). They are extremely uncommon but tend to occur in the pelvis and scapula.

In children, osteomalacia is called rickets. It causes the epiphyses to become flared and irregular, and the long bones undergo bending from the bone softening (Fig. 7.12). As in adults, the most common cause is renal disease, although other causes, such as biliary disease and dietary insufficiencies, are seen.

HYPERPARATHYROIDISM

Hyperparathyroidism (HPT) occurs from excess parathyroid hormone (PTH). PTH causes osteoclastic resorption in bone, which leads to osteoporosis and osteomalacia. The most common cause is renal disease, which leads to secondary HPT. Secondary HPT is due to the response of the parathyroids to hypocalcemia. Parathyroid adenomas and hyperplasia can cause primary HPT. Up to 40% of patients with primary HPT will demonstrate skeletal abnormalities radiographically.

The radiographic sign that is pathognomonic for HPT is subperiosteal bone resorption. It is seen most commonly on the radial aspect of the middle phalanges

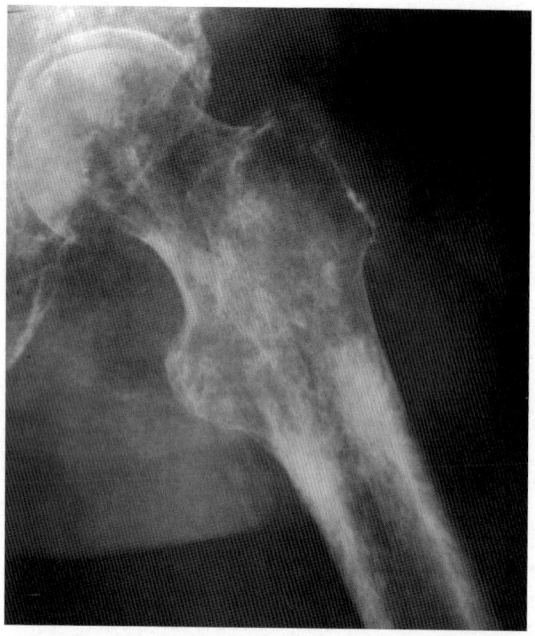

FIG. 7.5 **Aggressive Osteoporosis.** A diffuse permeative pattern throughout the proximal femur is noted in this patient, who has recently had an amputation. Note that the cortices are riddled with holes, which would indicate that this is not a true intramedullary process but an intracortical process. This is distinctive for aggressive osteoporosis and causes a pseudopermeative pattern that can be mistaken for a more sinister process.

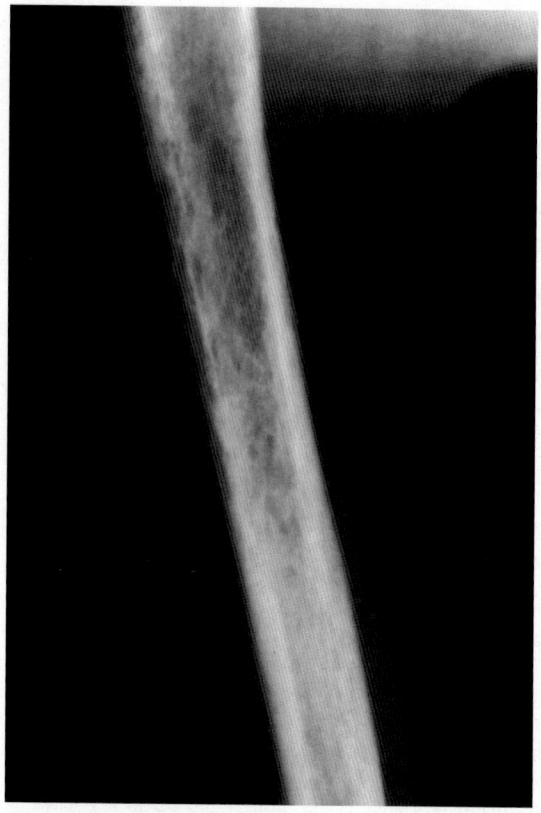

FIG. 7.6 **Cortical Holes in Osteoporosis.** This patient suffered a stroke and has aggressive osteoporosis secondary to disuse. What appears to be a diffuse permeative pattern throughout the humerus is noted, on closer inspection, to be cortical holes, which in this case are due to the aggressive osteoporosis. This type of pattern, unfortunately, often leads to a biopsy to rule out multiple myeloma or other round cell tumors.

of the hand (Fig. 7.13) but can be seen in any long bone in the body. It is occasionally seen on the medial aspect of the proximal tibia (Fig. 7.14), in the distal clavicles, and in the sacroiliac joints where it resembles bilateral sacroiliitis (Fig. 7.15). This seems to be seen more frequently in children than in adults.

Other radiographic findings include osteosclerosis, usually diffuse, but often involving the spine in a manner resembling the stripes on rugby jerseys, hence the name "rugger jersey spine" (Fig. 7.16). Brown tumors are cystic lesions that are often expansile and aggressive in appearance (Fig. 7.17). They were once said to be more common in primary HPT but are seen most commonly associated with secondary HPT today because of the overwhelming preponderance of patients with secondary disease as compared with primary. They are only rarely seen without other evidence of HPT, such as subperiosteal resorption; therefore I will not include a brown tumor in my differential diagnosis of a cystic lesion if the remainder of the bones are normal. A brown tumor can have a variety of appearances, so the only thing characteristic about it is that it is associated with subperiosteal bone resorption.

Brown tumors are uncommonly seen today, although they were frequently encountered 40 years ago. This is likely due to the widespread use of dialysis, thereby preventing hyperparathyroidism.

PTH can have an accelerating effect on bone that is undergoing slow change. In degenerative joint disease (DJD), especially in the spine, PTH can cause the affected joint or disc space to mimic infection (Fig. 7.18). PTH makes the usually sclerotic end plates fuzzy and eroded, and the narrowed disc space, which is a part of the degenerative disc disease, makes infection seem more likely. Therefore patients with renal disease who have a presumed radiographic diagnosis of joint or disc space

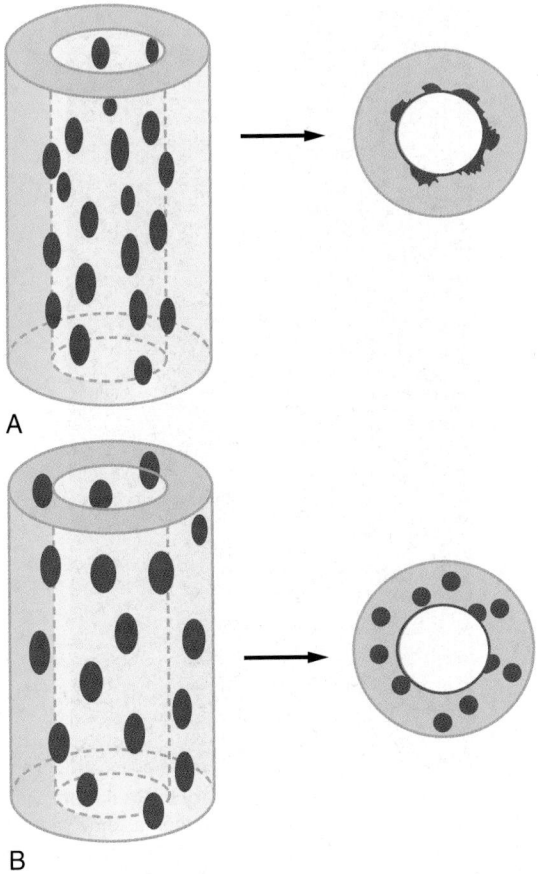

FIG. 7.7 **Schematic of Cortical Holes.** This schematic of a permeative lesion (A) shows how only the endosteum is affected with the bulk of the cortex spared. A pseudopermeative lesion (B) has the entire cortex affected. Both processes will look permeative on a plain film; however, the true permeative process will have an uninvolved cortex.

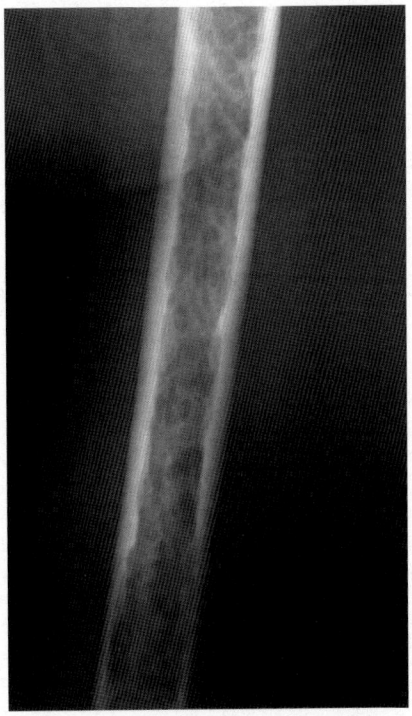

FIG. 7.8 **Permeative Appearance in Myeloma.** This patient has multiple myeloma, which has caused a diffuse permeative pattern throughout his femur. Note the solid appearance of the cortex, although there is endosteral scalloping. This is a true permeative process.

infection should not have an aspiration or biopsy unless strong clinical suspicion for infection is present.

Although subperiosteal resorption is pathognomonic for HPT, it does not seem to be found as frequently as in the past. This is likely due to better treatment of the underlying renal disease in modern medicine.

What causes the osteosclerosis in HPT? No one really knows. Several theories have evolved to explain it, but none are totally satisfactory and are best left to others to worry about.

OSTEOSCLEROSIS

The radiographic finding of diffuse increased bone density, osteosclerosis, is somewhat uncommon, yet every radiologist must have a differential diagnosis for this process. Fortunately, it is a rather short differential, and there are criteria to narrow down the list of possibilities.

Dealing with the differential diagnosis for osteosclerosis is a three-step process. First, one must recognize that the bones are truly increased in density. This sounds straightforward enough but is, in fact, often difficult to do. Technical factors can easily alter the apparent bone density and be misleading. Second, once it is determined that diffuse osteosclerosis is present, one merely has to list the disease entities that could be responsible. This is the easiest step because it merely requires memorization. I will supply a mnemonic to help your memory. Lastly, one must look for radiographic findings that are specific for each disorder to rule them out or in so as to narrow down the list of possibilities. The list of diseases that cause diffuse osteosclerosis is different with each textbook that you read. There are many disorders that have been reported to cause osteosclerosis, but you only need a list that is correct 95% to 98% of the time. Nobody expects you to include the one reported case

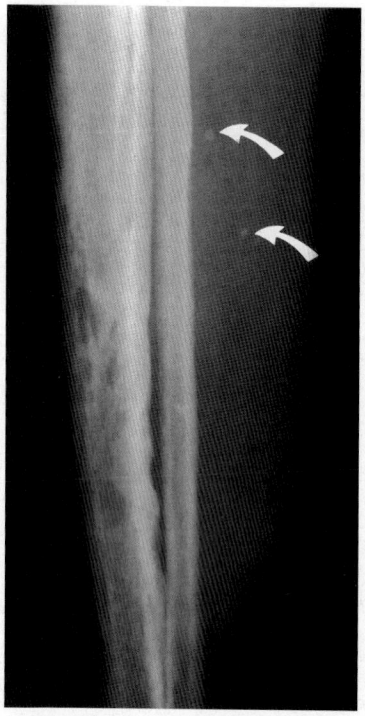

FIG. 7.9 **Hemangioma.** Cortical holes of varying sizes are seen throughout the tibia in this patient with a large hemangioma of the tibia. Also note the phleboliths present in the soft tissues *(arrows)*. It would be unlikely for osteoporosis to cause cortical holes of this size.

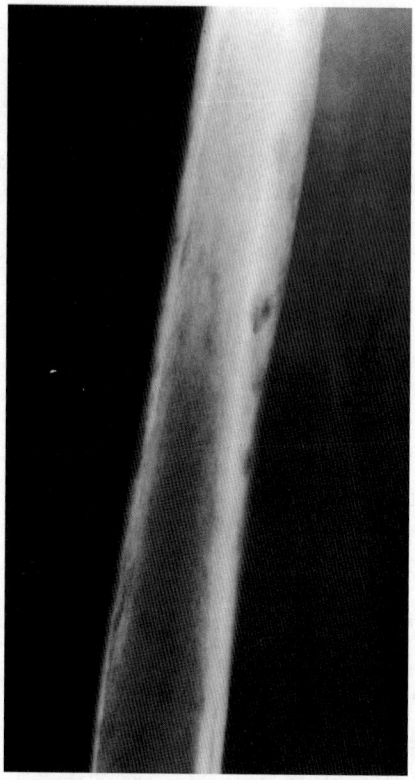

FIG. 7.10 **Osteonecrosis Secondary to Radiation.** Radiation to the femur for a soft tissue sarcoma some years before this plain film has caused large cortical holes throughout the femur. It is not likely that cortical holes of this size would be caused by osteoporosis, but they could be caused by a hemangioma.

of hunchback midget whale syndrome in your list. If you absolutely cannot bear the thought of leaving out a possibility in your differential diagnosis, you might as well just give your clinician the index from Resnick's book—it will be all-inclusive but not really useful to the clinician (not to imply that Resnick's book is not useful—it is the bible for bone radiologists).

The entities I include in the differential for diffuse osteosclerosis are the following:

- renal osteodystrophy
- sickle cell disease
- myelofibrosis
- osteopetrosis
- pyknodysostosis
- metastatic carcinoma
- mastocytosis
- Paget's disease
- athletes
- fluorosis

The mnemonic I use to remember them is "Regular sex makes occasional perversions much more pleasurable and fantastic." Hey, it's not a great mnemonic, but in the 21st century, it's not politically correct to be ribald, vulgar, off-color, coarse, crude, erotic, lewd, or even, sometimes, funny. If you want a filthy mnemonic, make up your own, you insensitive pervert.

I will cover each of these topics in generalities, trying to point out the features of each that you should look for to allow including or excluding them from the differential. A nice feature of this mnemonic is it lists the entities in their order of frequency. Not that osteopetrosis is more common than Paget's or mets, but it's more common to see osteopetrosis than either Paget's or mets presenting as diffuse bony sclerosis.

Renal Osteodystrophy

Anything that causes HPT can cause osteosclerosis, but renal disease is far and away the biggest offender. As mentioned previously, the *sine qua non* of renal osteodystrophy is subperiosteal bone resorption, seen earliest and most reliably at the radial aspect of the middle

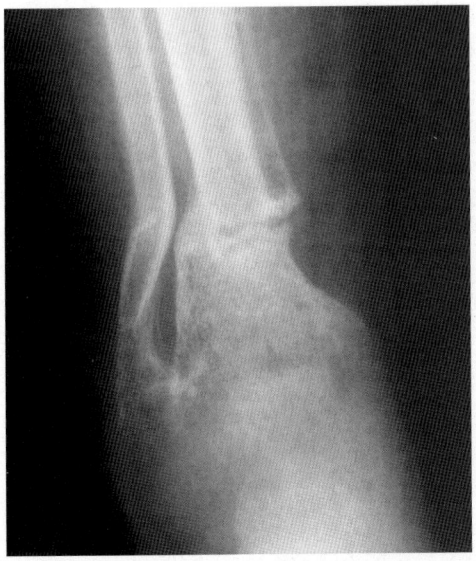

FIG. 7.11 **Looser Fractures in Osteomalacia.** A horizontal fracture of the tibia and the fibula is present in this child with osteomalacia (rickets). Fractures of this type are called Looser fractures and are virtually pathognomonic for osteomalacia; however, they are rarely seen.

phalanges of the hands. Although most patients with renal osteodystrophy will be osteopenic, about 10% to 20% will exhibit osteosclerosis, and the reasons for it are unknown.

Sickle Cell Disease

Like renal osteodystrophy, the reason for dense bones to occur in sickle cell disease is unknown. It occurs in only a small percentage of patients. Additional signs to look for are bone infarcts and H-shaped or step-off deformities of the vertebral body end plates (Fig. 7.19). These are also called "fish vertebrae" after their similarity to the vertebrae found in fish.

Myelofibrosis

Also called agnogenic myeloid metaplasia, myelofibrosis is a disease caused by progressive fibrosis of the marrow in patients over 50 years of age. It leads to anemia with splenomegaly and extramedullary hematopoiesis. Whenever osteosclerosis is seen in a patient over the age of 50, a search for a large spleen and extramedullary hematopoiesis should be made (Fig. 7.20).

Osteopetrosis

Also called marble bone disease, this uncommon hereditary abnormality results in extremely dense bones throughout the skeleton (Fig. 7.21). There is a congenita and a tarda form with different degrees of

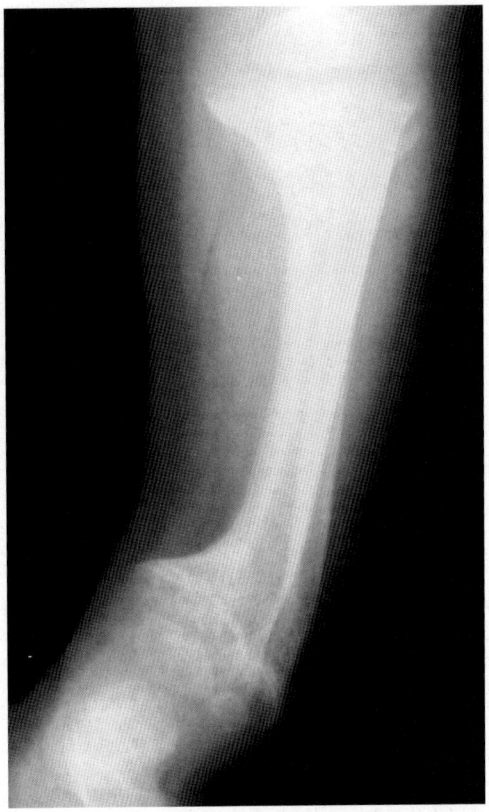

FIG. 7.12 **Rickets.** Osteomalacia in children causes fraying and splaying of the epiphyses as well as bending of the bone secondary to bone softening. This condition has been termed rickets and is most commonly seen in renal disease.

severity in each. It is not so rare that you will never see a case; therefore I include it in this differential list. A characteristic finding is the "bone-in-bone" appearance often seen in the vertebral bodies, in which the vertebrae have a small replica of the vertebral body inside the normal one (Fig. 7.22). Also characteristic is the "sandwich vertebrae" in which the end plates are densely sclerotic, giving the appearance of a sandwich (Fig. 7.23). These findings do not have to be present to make the diagnosis, but their absence makes the diagnosis less likely.

Pyknodysostosis

This is the other congenital abnormality with dense bones that should be considered in the differential diagnosis for osteosclerosis. Like osteopetrosis, it is rare but is seen from time to time in busy radiology practices. These patients are typically short and have hypoplastic mandibles. The distinguishing

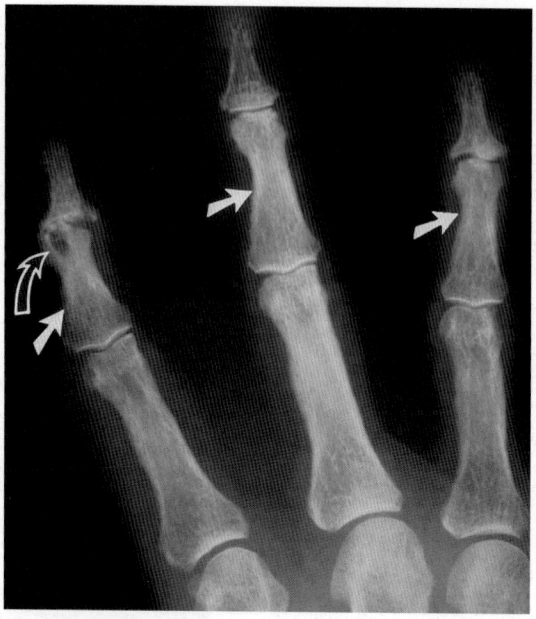

FIG. 7.13 **Hyperparathyroidism.** Subperiosteal bone resorption is noted along the radial aspect of the middle phalanges *(arrows)*, which is pathognomonic for hyperparathyroidism. The lytic lesion seen in the distal part of the middle phalanx *(curved arrow)* is either a brown tumor or a geode.

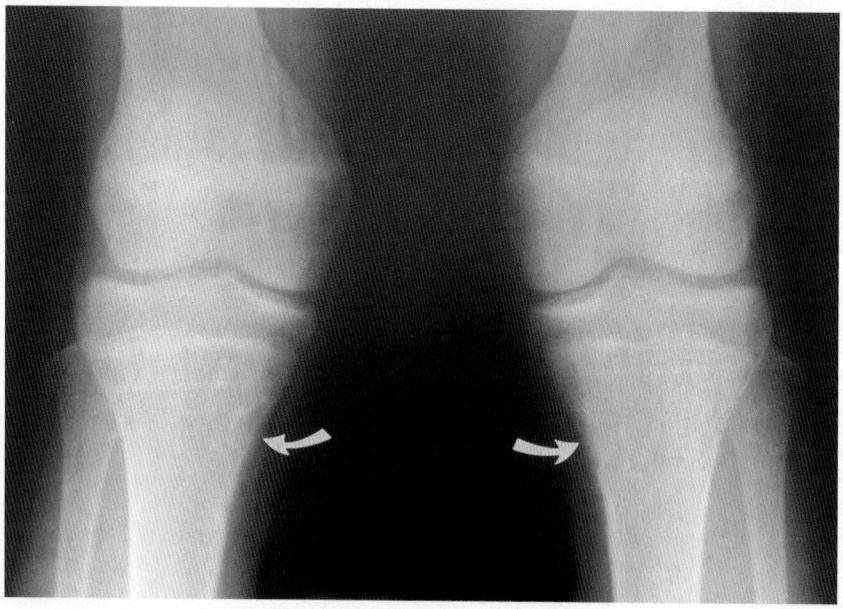

FIG. 7.14 **Hyperparathyroidism.** Subperiosteal bone resorption is noted along the medial aspect of the proximal tibias *(arrows)*. This is pathognomonic for hyperparathyroidism.

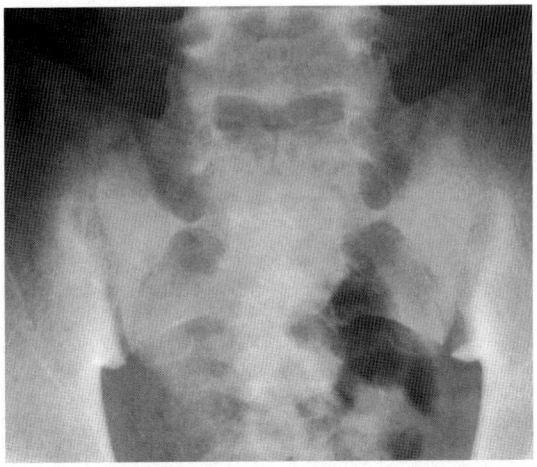

FIG. 7.15 **Hyperparathyroidism with Sacroiliac (SI) Joint Subperiosteal Erosion.** Bilateral SI joint widening and erosions can be seen in this patient with renal disease. This is due to subperiosteal resorption and is a frequent finding in children with hyperparathyroidism.

radiographic finding that is essentially pathognomonic is that the distal phalanges often have the appearance of chalk that has been put into a pencil sharpener—they are pointed and dense (Fig. 7.24). Nothing else does this, but unfortunately pyknodysostosis does not do this in every case. Another name for this disorder is Toulouse–Lautrec syndrome; this famous artist was apparently afflicted with pyknodysostosis.

Metastatic Carcinoma. Only rarely will diffuse metastatic carcinoma cause a problem in diagnosis. I have seen only a handful of cases in which diffuse metastatic disease mimicked diffuse osteosclerosis, and in every case, the primary tumor was prostate or breast carcinoma. If cortical destruction or a lytic component is present, the differential diagnosis is simplified, so these should be searched for.

Mastocytosis

This is another uncommon disorder that can cause uniform increased bone density. Unfortunately, there are no other plain-film findings that might help with the diagnosis. These patients have thickened small-bowel folds with nodules, but, of course, to see them, an upper gastrointestinal contrast study must be performed (Fig. 7.25). Mastocytosis is rare enough that you might be justified in leaving it out of your differential—you won't miss many, but it messes up the mnemonic.

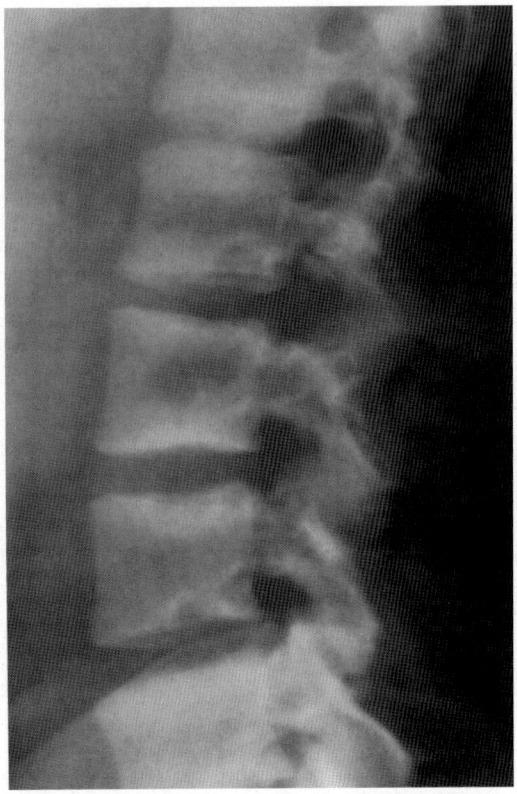

FIG. 7.16 **Hyperparathyroidism.** Sclerotic bands are seen along the vertebral body end plates. This has been termed a "rugger jersey spine" and is characteristic for hyperparathyroidism. Note how the sclerotic bands in the rugger jersey spine such as this are much less distinct and more fuzzy than the sclerotic bands seen in osteopetrosis in Fig. 7.23.

Paget's Disease

Although Paget's disease in bone is common, diffuse Paget's disease that could be confused with one of the other diseases in the differential diagnosis of generalized osteosclerosis is very rare—I have seen only one or two cases ever. Paget's classically causes bony enlargement (Fig. 7.26), but this is not always present. It occurs most commonly in the pelvis (Fig. 7.27), where it has been said the iliopectineal line on the pelvic brim must be thickened if Paget's is present. In fact, the iliopectineal line is usually, but not always, thickened. Paget's can occur in any bone in the body, including the smaller bones of the hands and feet (Fig. 7.28). It has been spread through the teaching files of many institutions (I have seen many statements in teaching files that have never made the literature that have served me well and others

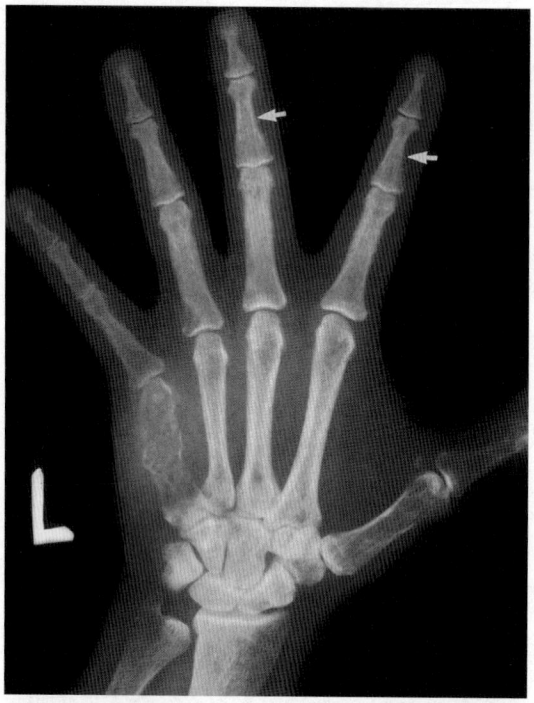

FIG. 7.17 **Hyperparathyroidism.** Lytic lesions are seen in the fifth metacarpal and at the base of the fourth proximal phalanx in this patient with hyperparathyroidism. Note the subperiosteal bone resorption seen along the radial aspect of the middle phalanges *(arrows)*. Any cystic lesion in a patient with hyperparathyroidism should be considered a brown tumor until proved otherwise.

that have misled me) that the fibula is the only bone that Paget's never affects. I must agree that the fibula is usually spared—even with profound disease all around it—but I have certainly seen exceptions to this rule.

Three distinct phases are radiographically visible in Paget's: a lytic phase, a sclerotic phase, and a mixed lytic–sclerotic phase (Fig. 7.29). The lytic phase often has a sharp leading edge, called a "flame-shaped" or "blade of grass" leading edge. In a long bone, with the sole exception being the tibia, Paget's always starts at the end of the bone; therefore if a lesion is present in the middle of a long bone and does not extend to either end, you can safely exclude Paget's disease.

So why is Paget's in this differential if it so rarely fits? Good question. You can probably safely leave it out without missing too many cases, but it's good to at least think about, since it is so readily diagnosed once you do think of it. Also, it does occasionally involve a large area, such as the entire pelvis, and makes the observer think that the entire skeleton might be involved.

When Paget's involves the skull, it often causes thickening of the base of the skull (Fig. 7.30), whereas entities that cause osteosclerosis due to marrow disease (sickle cell and myelofibrosis) will spare the base of the skull since it contains no marrow. This point is best illustrated by thalassemia in which the calvarium is thickened by marrow hyperplasia, while the base of the skull is spared (Fig. 7.31).

Athletes

I see radiographs on professional athletes quite often and continue to be impressed by the degree of increased cortical thickness these people possess. No question about it: increased stress causes hypertrophy of bone as well as of muscle. I see radiologists routinely question the presence of diffuse increased bone density in this set of patients, enough so that I have added normal athletes to my differential diagnosis for osteosclerosis.

Fluorosis

This is another uncommon disorder that could probably be left off the list without danger of missing too many cases. Fluorosis is usually a result of chronic intake in certain areas that have large amounts of fluoride present in the drinking water. It can also be a result of long-term therapy with sodium fluoride for osteoporosis. A radiographic finding that patients with fluorosis often have is ligamentous calcification. If I have a patient with dense bones and no ligamentous calcifications, I will put fluorosis lower on the list but not eliminate it. If ligamentous calcifications are present, it will go to the top of the list. Calcification of the sacrotuberous ligament is said to be characteristic for fluorosis.

CONCLUSION

There are other categories of disease that could be covered in a chapter on metabolic bone disease, but most of the remaining disorders are exceedingly rare and not likely to be seen by most radiologists on a routine basis. Excellent texts are available for additional details on the diseases I have mentioned as well as for learning about the less common entities.

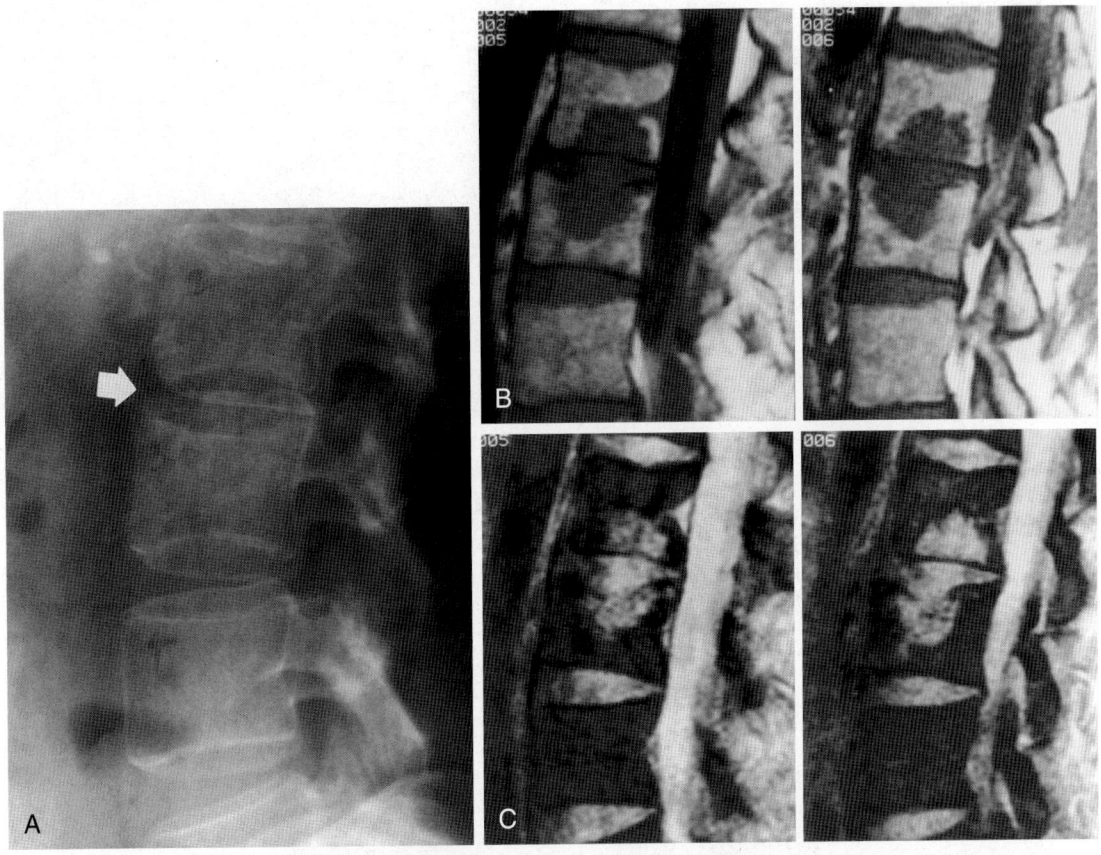

FIG. 7.18 **Parathyroid Hormone (PTH) Discitis.** (A) A lateral plain film of the lumbar spine reveals disc space narrowing with erosion of the end plates at the L2-3 level *(arrow)*. This is a typical appearance of disc infection. (B) A sagittal T1-weighted image of the lumbar spine reveals disc space narrowing and low signal extending into the end plates and vertebral bodies adjacent to the L2-3 disc. (C) A T2-weighted image shows high signal in the L2-3 disc and in the tissue extending into the vertebral bodies. This is the classic magnetic resonance imaging (MRI) appearance of disc infection with involvement of the vertebral bodies. However, this patient has renal osteodystrophy, and hyperparathyroidism can cause changes in the joints and the disc spaces identical to infection. Clinical correlation must be used to avoid an unnecessary biopsy.

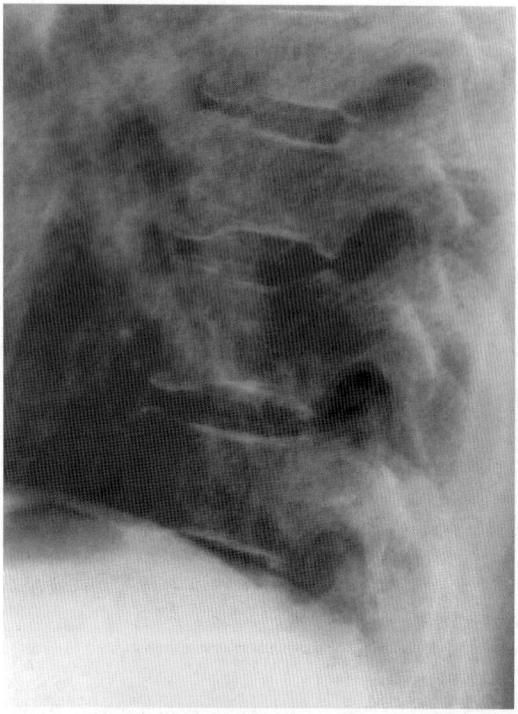

FIG. 7.19 **Sickle Cell Disease.** Step-off deformities *(arrows)* are seen in the end plates of multiple vertebral bodies in this patient with sickle cell disease. Although the bones do not show osteosclerosis, the visible trabeculae are somewhat coarsened. The step-off deformities in the spine are characteristic for sickle cell disease. These are also called "fish vertebrae."

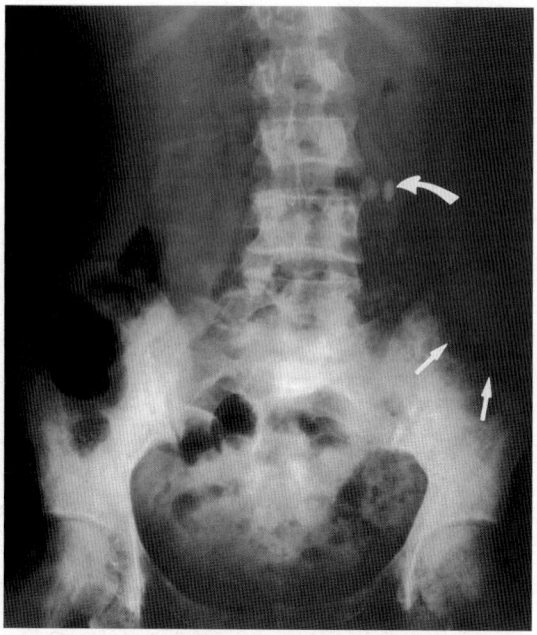

FIG. 7.20 **Myelofibrosis.** Uniform increased bone density seen most prominently throughout the pelvis is present in this patient with myelofibrosis. Note the grossly enlarged spleen *(arrows)* and the opaque iron tablets (curved arrow), which are taken for the anemia often present in this disorder.

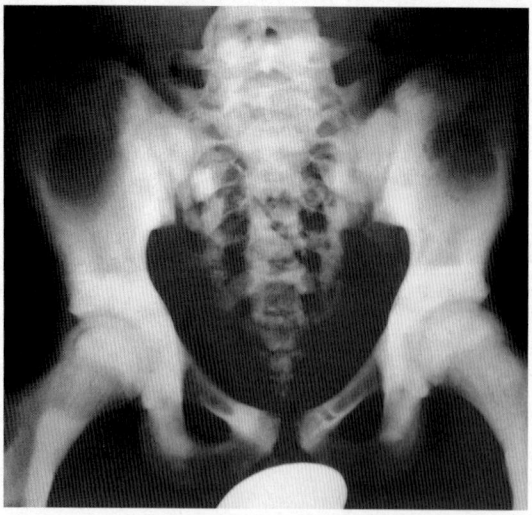

FIG. 7.21 **Osteopetrosis.** Diffuse bony sclerosis is present throughout the skeleton in this patient with osteopetrosis.

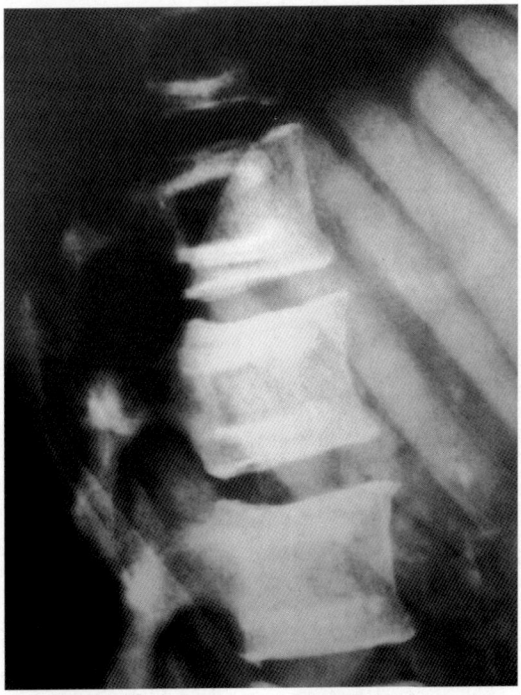

FIG. 7.22 **Osteopetrosis.** A "bone-in-bone" appearance is present in the vertebral bodies in this patient with osteopetrosis. This is often seen in osteopetrosis and is occasionally seen in other disorders.

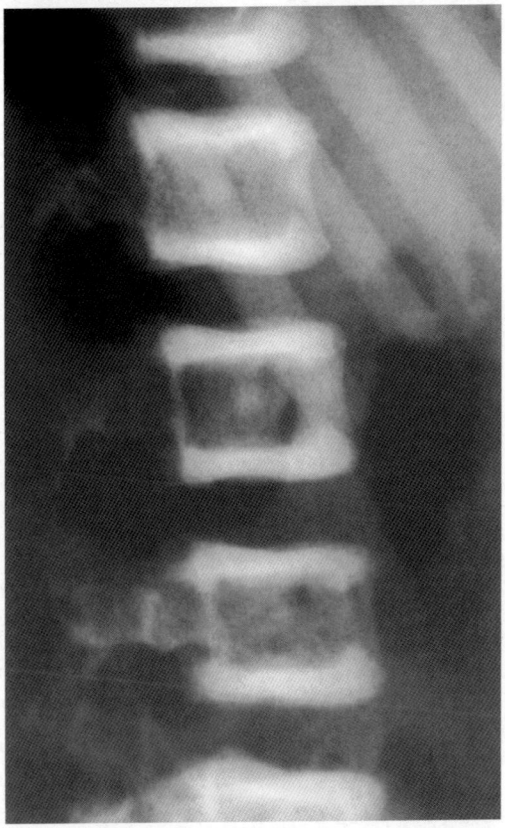

FIG. 7.23 **Osteopetrosis.** "Sandwich vertebrae" are seen in the vertebral bodies in this patient with osteopetrosis. This is virtually pathognomonic for osteopetrosis when present and should not be confused with the ill-defined bands of sclerosis seen in the rugger jersey spine of hyperparathyroidism.

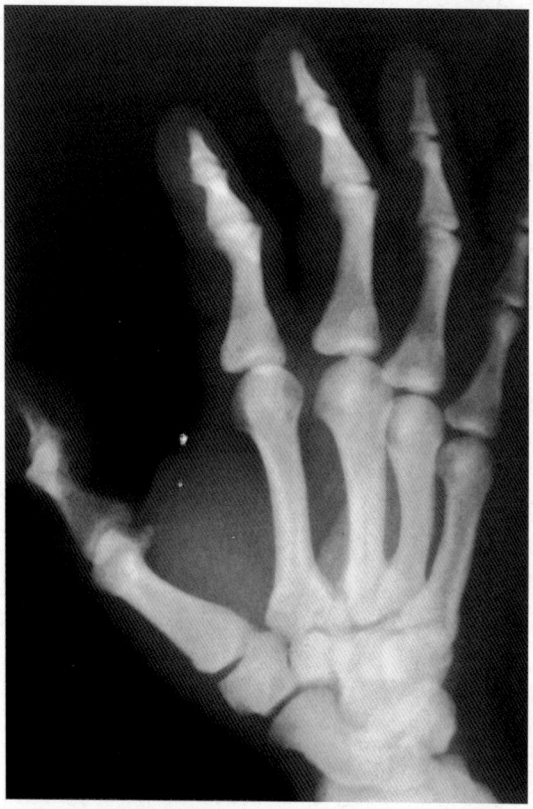

FIG. 7.24 **Pyknodysostosis.** Dense sclerosis is seen throughout the hand in this patient with pyknodysostosis. A pathognomonic finding is seen in the distal phalanges, where the tufts are absent and the phalanges are pointed and sclerotic.

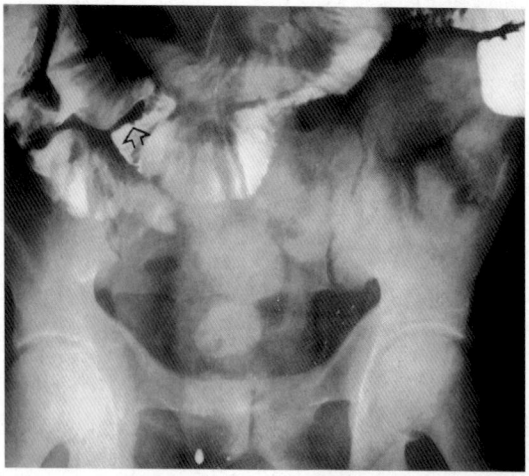

FIG. 7.25 **Mastocytosis.** Uniform dense bones are noted throughout the pelvis in this patient with mastocytosis. Note the thickened small-bowel folds with nodules *(arrow)*, which are often seen in mastocytosis.

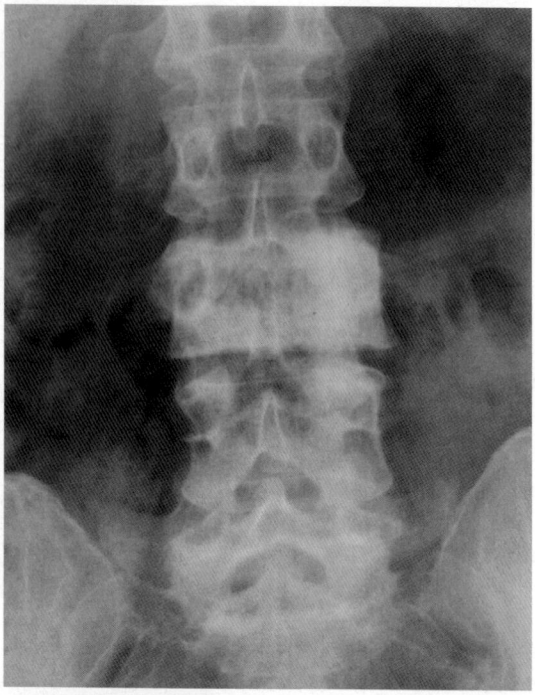

FIG. 7.26 **Paget's Disease.** Dense sclerosis with bony overgrowth is seen in the L-3 vertebral body in this patient with Paget's disease. The left L-3 pedicle is particularly dense and overgrown.

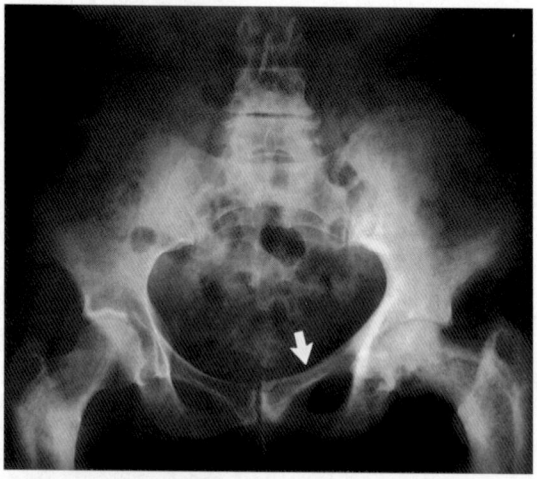

FIG. 7.27 **Paget's Disease.** Dense bony sclerosis with some bony enlargement is seen throughout the left pelvis and proximal femur. Note the thickening of the iliopectineal line on the left side *(arrow)* as compared with the right side. This is not an example of diffuse dense bones; therefore the differential diagnosis is considerably shorter.

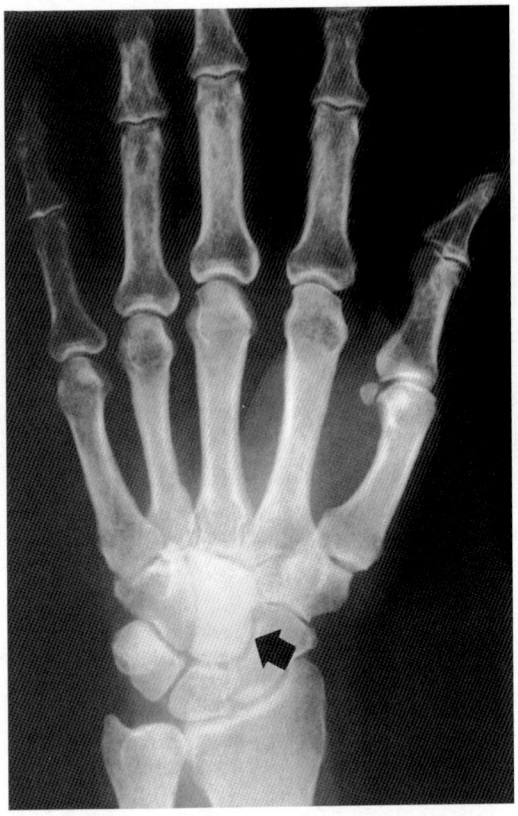

FIG. 7.28 **Paget's Disease.** Dense sclerosis of the capitate *(arrow)* is seen in this patient. Although no definite bony overgrowth is appreciated, it is not unusual for Paget's disease to affect a single bone uniformly such as this.

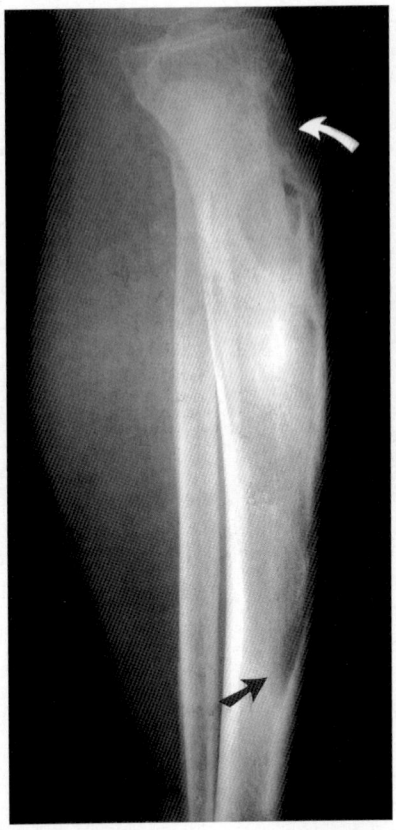

FIG. 7.29 **Paget's Disease.** A "flame-shaped" or "blade of grass" appearance is seen in the distal tibia *(arrow)* in this patient with Paget's disease of the tibia. The sclerotic phase of Paget's disease is seen in the midtibia in this patient, whereas the proximal tibia has an area of apparent cortical destruction *(curved arrow)*, which is suspicious for sarcomatous degeneration.

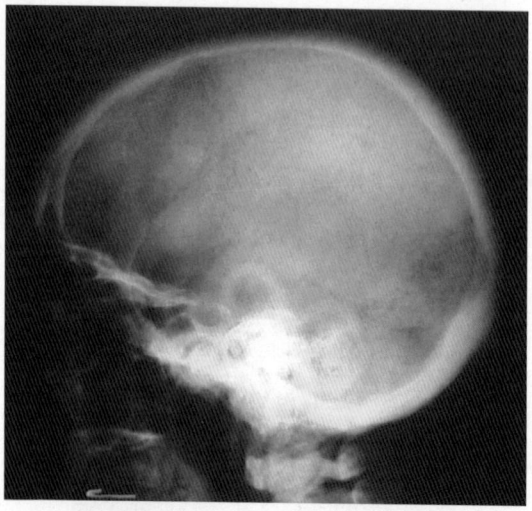

FIG. 7.30 **Paget's Disease.** This patient with Paget's disease shows marked thickening of the base of the skull on this lateral skull film.

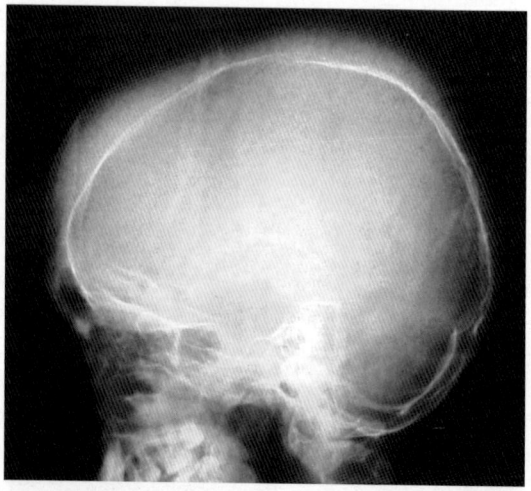

FIG. 7.31 **Thallassemia.** This patient with thallassemia has marked thickening of the calvarium with sparing of the base of the skull.

REFERENCES

1. Schilcher J, Michaelsson K, Aspenberg P. Bisphosphonate use and atypical fractures of the femoral shaft. *NEJM*. 2011;364:1728–1737.
2. Hall FM. Bone-mineral screening for osteoporosis. *Opinion. AJR*. 1987;149:120–122.
3. Helms C, Munk P. Pseudopermeative skeletal lesions. *Br J Radiol*. 1990;63:461–467.

CHAPTER 8

Miscellaneous Conditions

There are a host of bony conditions, diseases, and syndromes that do not fit conveniently into any of the preceding chapters yet should be given some mention in an attempted overview of musculoskeletal radiology. Many of these are simply "Aunt Minnies" and only require you to have seen them once or twice to recognize them. I have severely limited the things I have included in this chapter—it could easily have dozens of other entities, but none are very common. Besides, I need to have something to add in future editions. These are listed alphabetically for lack of a more scientific basis.

ACHONDROPLASIA

The most common cause of dwarfism is achondroplasia, a congenital, hereditary disease of failure of endochondral bone formation. The femurs and humeri are more profoundly affected than the other long bones, although the entire skeleton is abnormal. The spine typically has narrowing of the interpedicular distances in a caudal direction (Fig. 8.1), the opposite of normal where the interpedicular distances get progressively wider as one proceeds down the spine. I know of no other entity that has narrowing of the interpedicular distance, and I have never seen a case of achondroplasia without this narrowing. The long bones are short but have normal width, giving them a thick appearance.

AVASCULAR NECROSIS

The term avascular necrosis (AVN), also called osteonecrosis, refers to the lack of blood supply with subsequent bone death and ensuing bony collapse in an articular surface. The etiology of AVN is an extensive differential that most commonly includes trauma, steroids, aspirin, sickle cell disease, collagen vascular diseases, alcoholism, and idiopathic (Table 8.1).[1] The radiographic appearance ranges from patchy sclerosis (Fig. 8.2A) to articular surface collapse and fragmentation (Fig. 8.3). Just before collapse, a subchondral lucency is occasionally seen (Fig. 8.4); however, this is a late and inconstant sign of AVN. Magnetic resonance (MR) imaging is extremely valuable in demonstrating the presence and extent of AVN (Fig. 8.2B), even when plain films are apparently normal. MR imaging is currently considered to be the most efficacious way to evaluate a joint for AVN.[2] It is useful not only in AVN of the hips, but also of the knee, wrist, foot, and ankle.

ENGELMANN

Also known as diaphyseal dysplasia, this congenital disorder is manifested by diaphyseal cortical thickening, which primarily involves the long bones, particularly the lower extremity (Fig. 8.5). Although it can be asymptomatic and incidental, these children can have a painful, waddling gait, and it can progress dramatically, causing severe medullary encroachment with subsequent anemia.

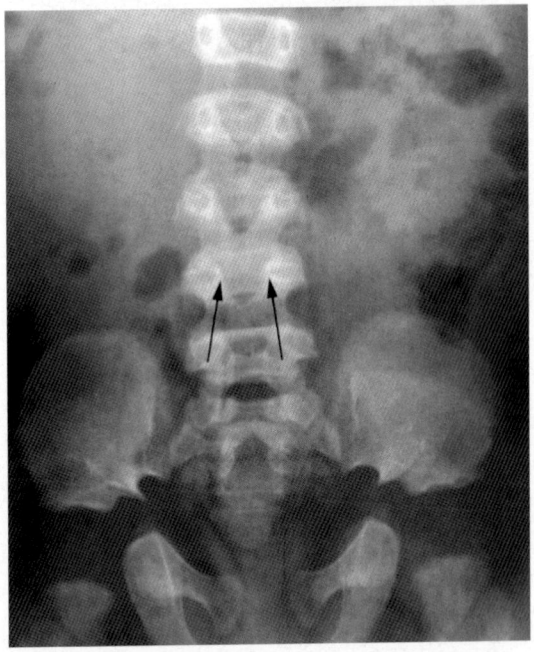

FIG. 8.1 **Achondroplasia.** An anteroposterior (AP) plain film of the spine in this patient with achondroplasia demonstrates narrowing of the interpedicular distance *(arrows)* in a caudal direction, which is characteristic of this disorder. Ordinarily, the interpedicular distance widens in each vertebra in a caudal direction.

TABLE 8.1 Common causes of avascular necrosis	
Trauma	Collagen vascular diseases
Steroids	Alcoholism
Aspirin	Idiopathic
Sickle cell disease	

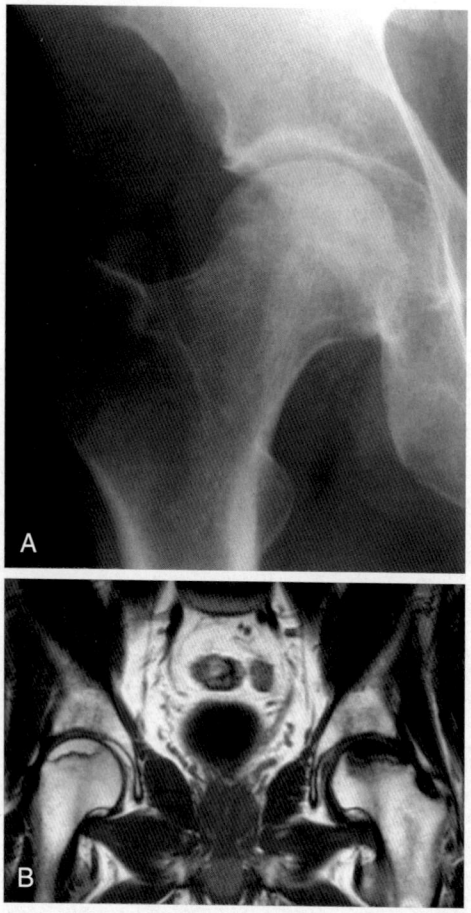

FIG. 8.2 **Avascular necrosis.** (A) A plain film of the hip in this patient with avascular necrosis (AVN) shows faint patchy sclerosis throughout the femoral head. This is a relatively early plain-film finding for AVN. Coronal (B) T1WI in another patient with bilateral AVN of the hips shows two different appearances, with low signal on the left side and high signal on the right. Each is consistent with AVN.

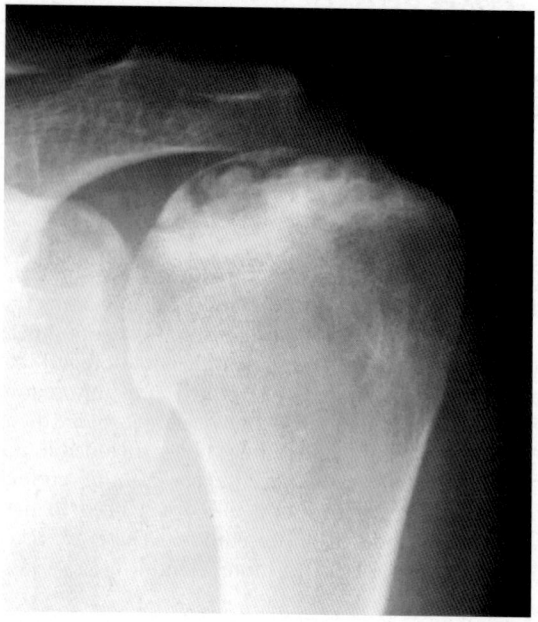

FIG. 8.3 **Avascular necrosis.** An anteroposterior (AP) plain film of the shoulder reveals articular surface collapse in this patient who was treated with steroids for systemic lupus erythematosus. This is an advanced stage of avascular necrosis (AVN).

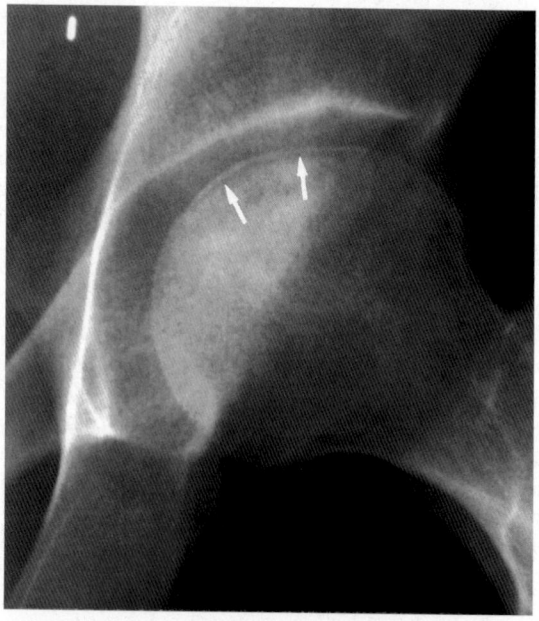

FIG. 8.4 **Avascular necrosis.** An anteroposterior (AP) frog-leg lateral view of the hip in this patient with sickle cell disease shows a subchondral lucency *(arrows)* and patchy sclerosis in the femoral head, indicative of avascular necrosis (AVN). This is a relatively advanced stage of AVN. The subchondral lucency is often better demonstrated with the frog-leg lateral view.

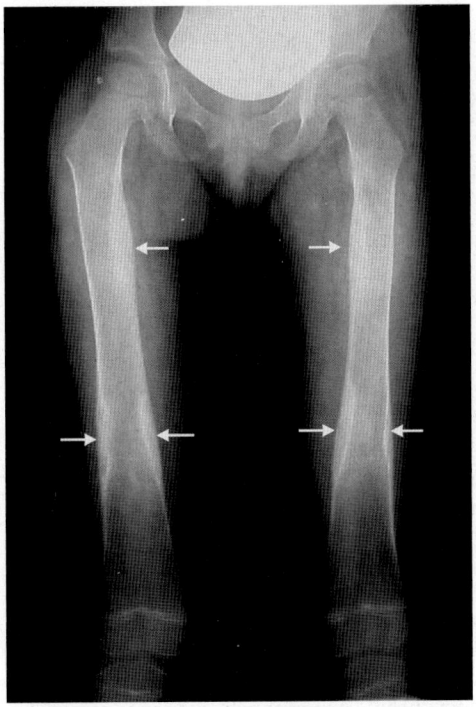

FIG. 8.5 **Engelmann.** An anteroposterior (AP) film of the femurs shows bilateral cortical thickening that is localized to the diaphyses.

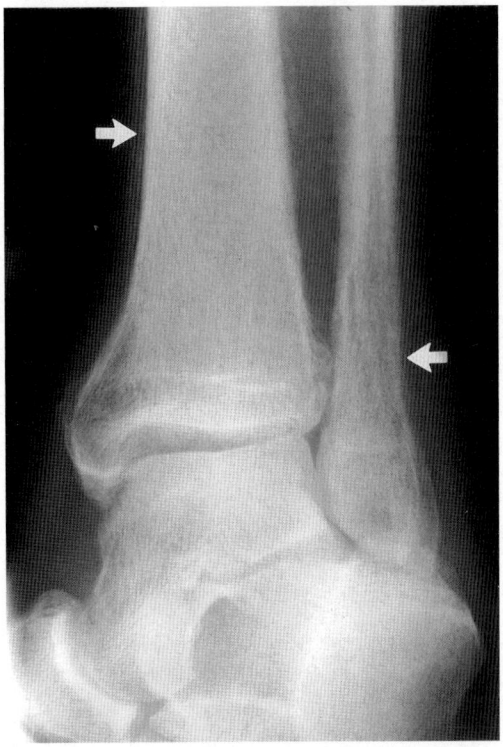

FIG. 8.6 **Hypertrophic pulmonary osteoarthropathy (HPO).** Periostitis can be seen along the shafts of the distal tibia and fibula *(arrows)* in this patient with bronchogenic carcinoma and leg pain. This is characteristic for HPO.

HYPERTROPHIC PULMONARY OSTEOARTHROPATHY

Hypertrophic pulmonary osteoarthropathy (HPO) is manifested by clubbing of the fingers and periostitis, usually in the upper and lower extremities (Fig. 8.6), which may or may not be associated with bone pain. It is most commonly seen in patients with lung cancer, but many other etiologies have been reported, including bronchiectasis, gastrointestinal disorders, and liver disease. The actual mechanism of formation of periostitis secondary to a distant malignancy or other process is unknown. The differential diagnosis for periostitis in a long bone without an underlying bony abnormality would include HPO, venous stasis, thyroid acropachy, pachydermoperiostosis, and trauma (Table 8.2).

TABLE 8.2
Periostitis without underlying bony lesion

Trauma	Venous stasis
Hypertrophic pulmonary osteoarthropathy	Thyroid acropachy
	Pachydermoperiostosis

MELORHEOSTOSIS

Melorheostosis is a rare, idiopathic disorder characterized by thickened cortical new bone that accumulates near the ends of long bones, usually only on one side of the bone, and has an appearance likened to "dripping candle wax" (Fig. 8.7). It can affect several adjacent bones and can be symptomatic. Many feel there is some relation or overlap among melorheostosis, osteopathia striata, and osteopoikilosis (mentioned later in this chapter), all of which present with varying patterns of increased cortical bone.

MUCOPOLYSACCHARIDOSES (MORQUIO, HURLER, AND HUNTER SYNDROMES)

The mucopolysaccharidoses are a group of inherited diseases characterized by abnormal storage and excretion in the urine of various mucopolysaccharides

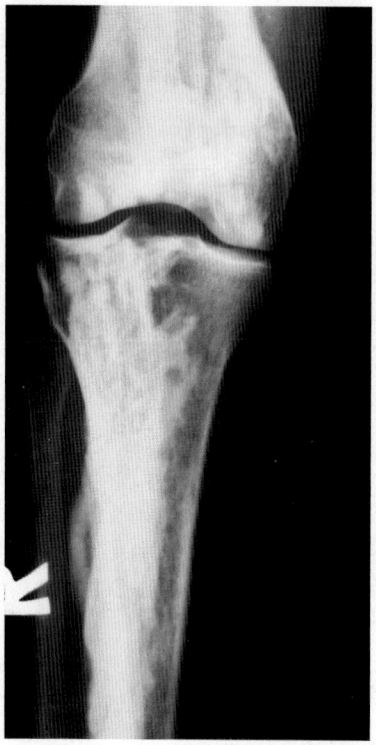

FIG. 8.7 **Melorheostosis.** Dense, wavy, new bone is seen adjacent to the lateral tibial cortex, which has a "dripping candle wax" appearance that is classic for melorheostosis. A similar pattern can be seen in the distal femur.

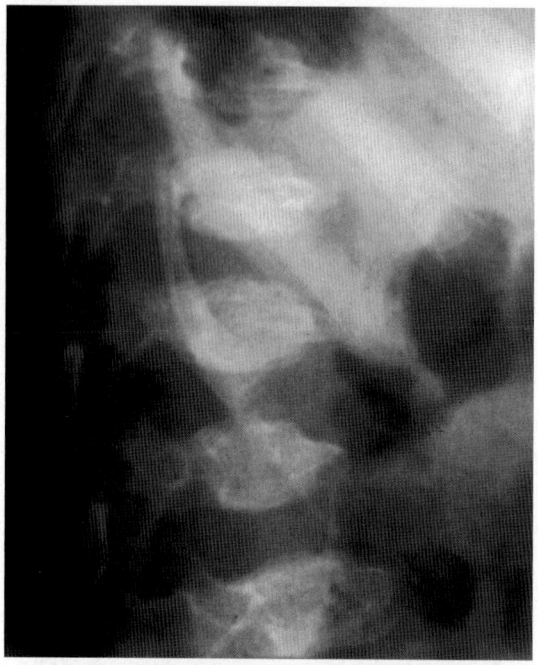

FIG. 8.8 **Morquio.** A lateral plain film of the spine reveals a central "beak" or anterior bony projection off of the vertebral bodies in this patient with Morquio syndrome.

such as keratan sulfate (Morquio) and heparan sulfate (Hurler). These patients have short stature, primarily from shortened spines, and characteristic plain-film findings. In the spine, patients with Morquio have platyspondyly (generalized flattening of the vertebral bodies) with a central anterior projection, or "beak," off of the vertebral body, as viewed on a lateral plain film (Fig. 8.8). Hurler and Hunter show platyspondyly with a "beak" that is anteroinferiorly positioned (Fig. 8.9) (remember "middle" beak for Morquio and "hind" beak for Hurler and Hunter). The pelvis in these disorders is similar in appearance to that of achondroplasts with wide, flared iliac wings and broad femoral necks. A characteristic finding in the hands is a pointed proximal fifth metacarpal base that has a notch appearance on the ulnar aspect (Fig. 8.10).

MULTIPLE HEREDITARY EXOSTOSES

Also known as diaphyseal aclasis, this is a not uncommon hereditary disorder that seems to affect multiple

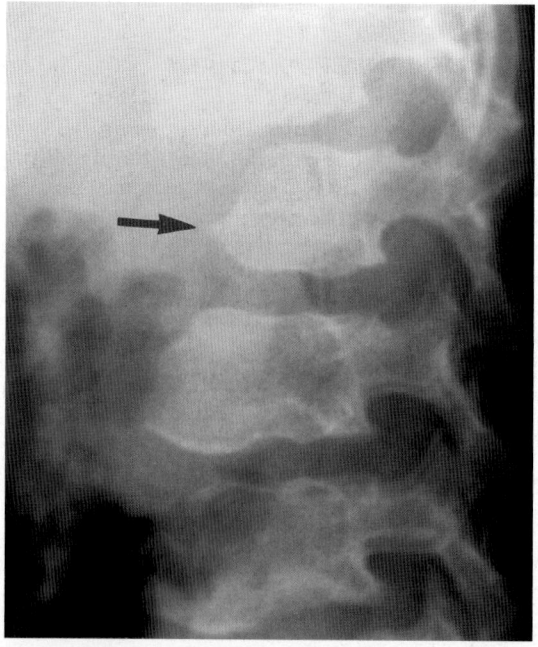

FIG. 8.9 **Hurler.** A lateral plain film of the spine in this patient with Hurler syndrome shows an inferiorly placed bony projection extending anteriorly off of the vertebral bodies *(arrow)*.

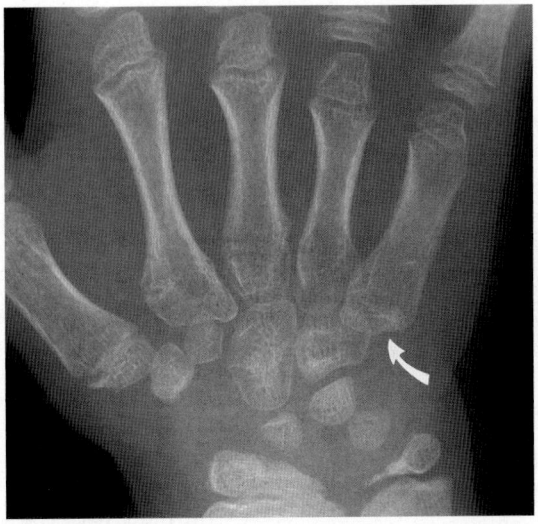

FIG. 8.10 **Hurler.** An anteroposterior (AP) plain film of the hand in this patient with Hurler syndrome shows a notch *(arrow)* at the base of the fifth metacarpal, which is a characteristic finding in all of the mucopolysaccharidoses.

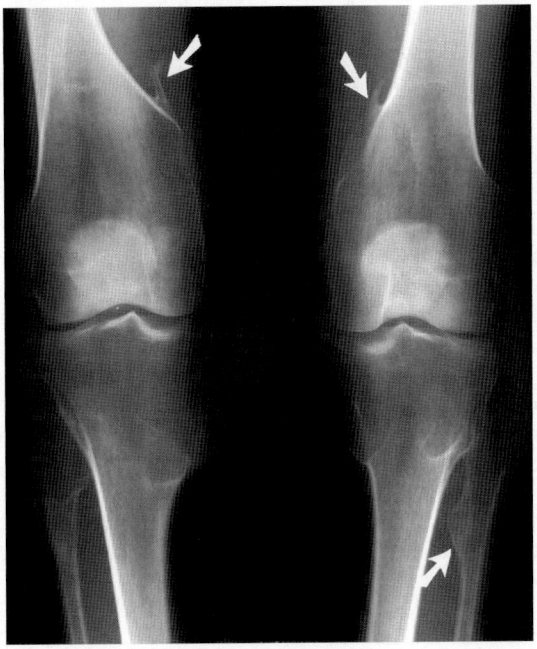

FIG. 8.11 **Multiple hereditary exostosis.** The knees are involved in virtually every case of multiple hereditary exostosis. They typically show not only multiple exostoses *(arrows)*, but also marked undertubulation (widening) in the metaphyses.

members of a family with multiple osteochondromas, or exostoses. An osteochondroma is a cartilage-capped bone outgrowth, which may be pedunculated or sessile in appearance. In the multiple hereditary form, the knees are virtually always involved (Fig. 8.11). The incidence of malignant degeneration in this population has been reported to be as high as 20%, but this is a gross overestimation, with the actual incidence

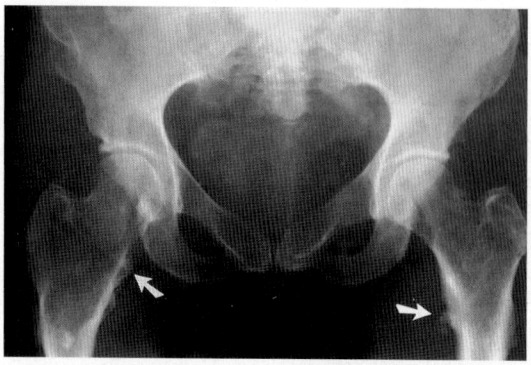

FIG. 8.12 **Multiple hereditary exostosis.** The femoral necks are often involved in multiple hereditary exostosis. They will show undertubulation, as in this example, and usually have one or more exostoses *(arrows)*. Note the involvement of the superior pubic rami and the symphysis.

probably less than 1%. As with solitary osteochondromas, the more axially situated lesions are more prone to undergo malignant degeneration, while the more peripheral lesions are less likely to do so. The proximal femurs are frequently involved and have a characteristic appearance (Fig. 8.12).

OSTEOID OSTEOMA

The etiology of osteoid osteoma is unknown. Is it an infection (bacterial or viral), a slow-growing tumor, a dessert topping? Nobody knows. It is a painful lesion that occurs almost exclusively in patients under the age of 30 that is treated successfully with surgical excision or, more commonly today, percutaneous radiofrequency ablation. Aspirin often gives dramatic relief of the pain and can be used for conservative treatment in lieu of surgery. A classic clinical picture for an osteoid osteoma is "night pain relieved by aspirin." However, many osteoid osteomas do not have this presentation, and most painful musculoskeletal lesions are worse at night and relieved by aspirin, so this can lead to confusion.

Radiographically, an osteoid osteoma is said to have a typical appearance, but in fact it has many different appearances, which can make diagnosis difficult.[3] The classically described radiographic appearance is a cortically based sclerotic lesion in a long bone that has a small lucency within it, which is called the nidus (Fig. 8.13A). It is the nidus that causes the pain and the surrounding reactive sclerosis. If the nidus is surgically removed or ablated percutaneously with radiofrequency, complete cessation of pain is the rule. Computed tomography (CT) and radionuclide bone scanning are often very helpful in demonstrating the exact location of the nidus (Figs. 8.13B and C).

If the nidus of an osteoid osteoma is located in the medullary rather than the cortical portion of a bone, or if it is located in a joint, there is much less reactive sclerosis present. This gives the lesion a different overall appearance than the more common cortical lesion in that it does not appear as sclerotic. Up to 80% of osteoid osteomas are located intracortically, with the remainder being in the intramedullary part of a bone. Rarely, an osteoid osteoma will present in the periosteum, causing tremendous periostitis.

The nidus itself is usually lucent but often develops some calcification within it. It then has the appearance of a sequestrum, as is seen in osteomyelitis. If the nidus calcifies completely, it blends in with the surrounding sclerosis and cannot be seen on most radiographs. Therefore the diagnosis of an osteoid osteoma is not dependent on seeing a nidus.

Since an osteoid osteoma resembles osteomyelitis, regardless of the appearance of the nidus, it can be difficult to differentiate the two radiographically. In fact, it cannot be done with plain films, CT scan, or MR imaging. However, because the nidus is extremely vascular, it avidly accumulates radiopharmaceutical bone-scanning agents. An osteoid osteoma will have an area of increased uptake corresponding to the area of reactive sclerosis but, in addition, will demonstrate a second area of increased uptake corresponding to the nidus (Figs. 8.13 to 8.15). This has been termed the "double density" sign.[4] In contrast, osteomyelitis has a photopenic area corresponding to the plain-film lucency, which represents an avascular focus of purulent material. The natural history of an osteoid osteoma is presumed to be spontaneous regression since they are rarely seen over the age of 30.

OSTEOPATHIA STRIATA

Also known as Voorhoeve disease, this disorder is manifested by multiple 2- to 3-mm-thick linear bands of sclerotic bone aligned parallel to the long axis of a bone (Fig. 8.16). It usually affects multiple long bones and is asymptomatic; hence it is usually an incidental finding.

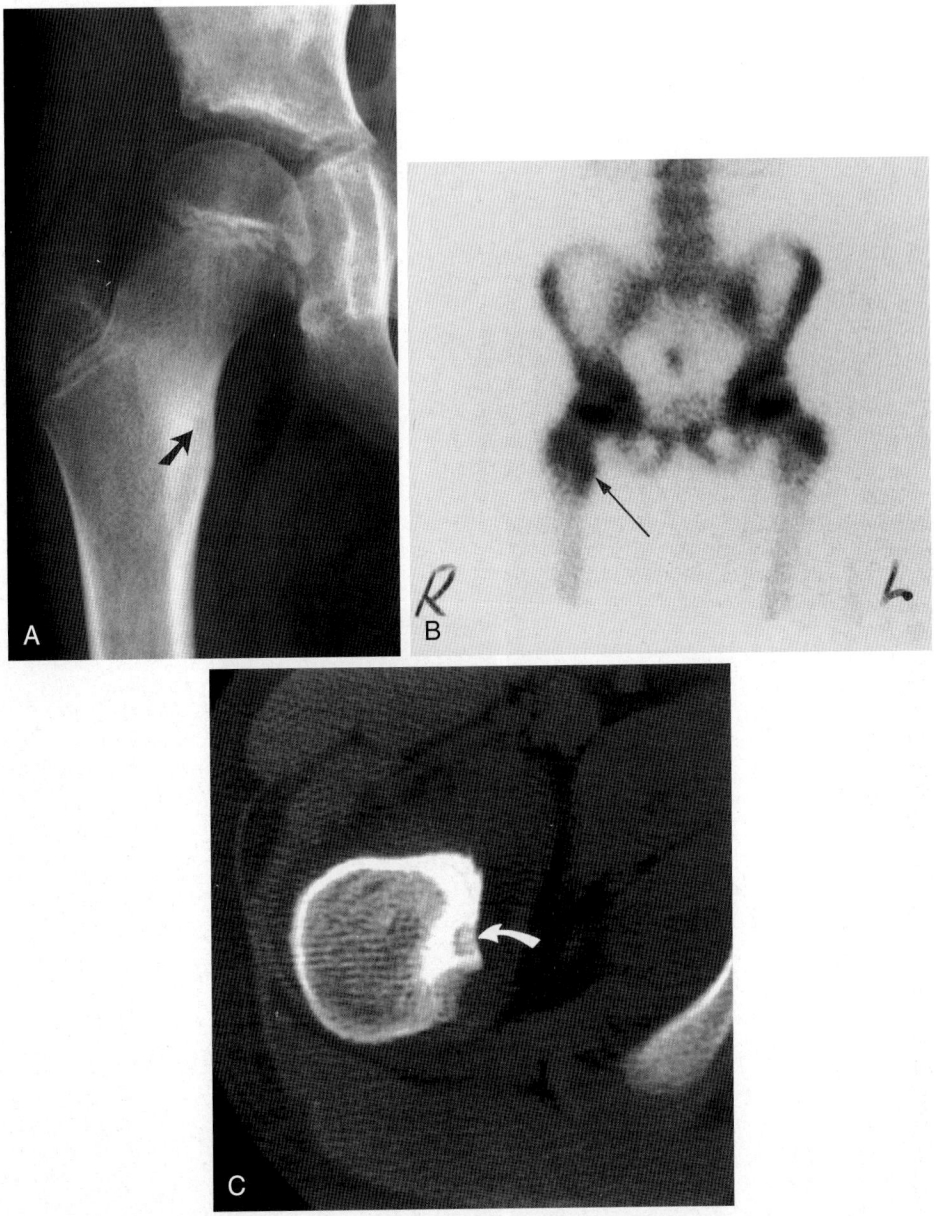

FIG. 8.13 **Osteoid osteoma.** (A) An anteroposterior (AP) plain film of the femur in a child with hip pain shows an area of sclerosis medially near the lesser trochanter with a small lucency *(arrow)*, which is the nidus of an osteoid osteoma. Osteomyelitis could have this identical appearance. (B) A radionuclide bone scan shows increased uptake in the proximal femur, which corresponds to the reactive new bone seen on the plain film. In addition, however, note the second smaller area of increased radionuclide uptake within the larger area *(arrow)*. This corresponds to the nidus itself. This pattern on a bone scan is called the double density sign. (C) A computed tomography (CT) scan of the femur shows the sclerosis medially and the lucent nidus *(arrow)* to better advantage. The CT and the bone scan give the surgeon a more precise anatomic location of the nidus than the plain film.

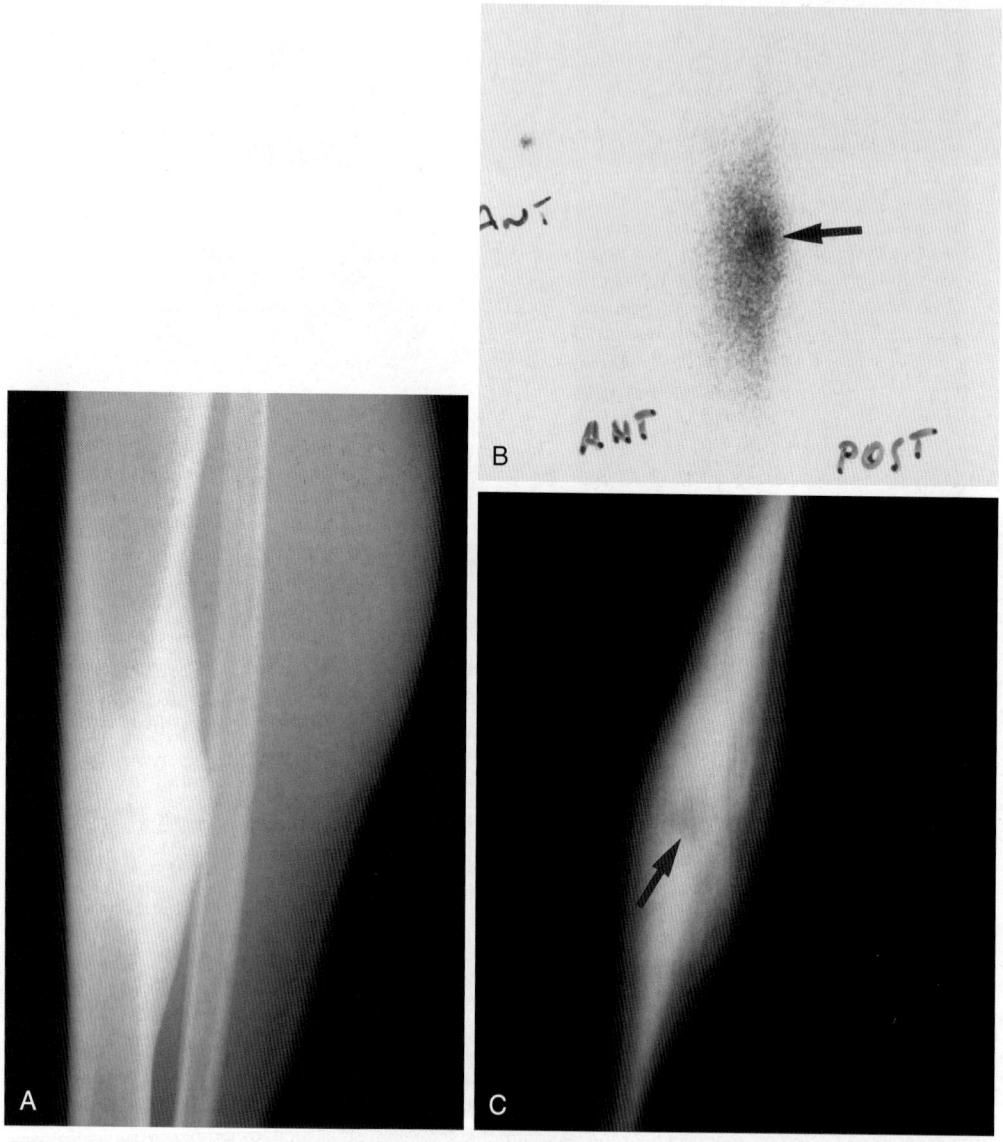

FIG. 8.14 **Osteoid osteoma.** (A) A lateral plain film of the tibia in this child with leg pain shows cortical thickening in the posterior diaphysis. No lucency in the sclerotic area could be identified. (B) A radionuclide bone scan reveals uptake corresponding to the area of sclerosis in the tibia, with a more marked area of uptake centrally *(arrow)*, which is the double density sign of an osteoid osteoma. (C) The surgical specimen shows the nidus *(arrow)* as a faint lucency within the sclerotic bone.

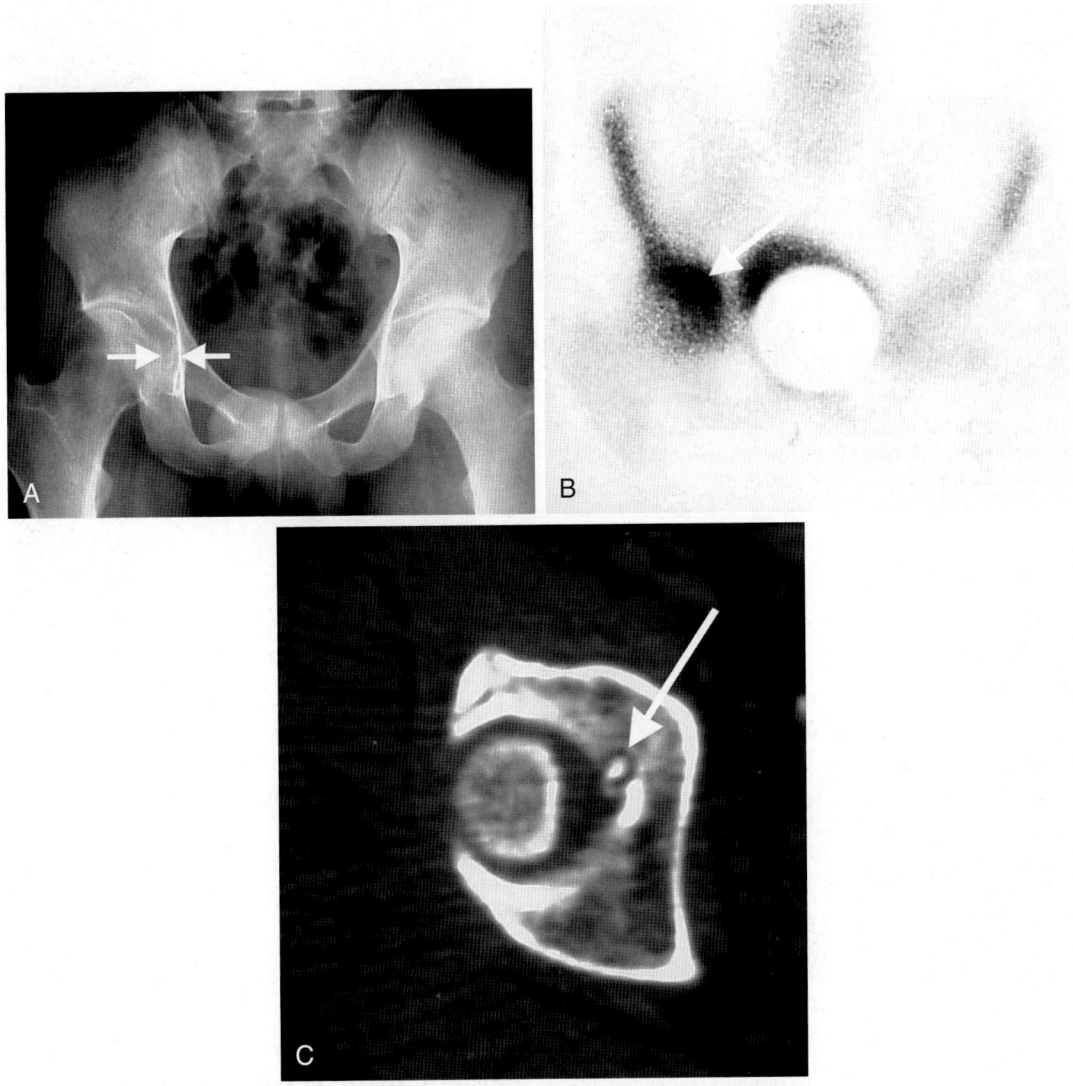

FIG. 8.15 **Osteoid osteoma.** (A) A plain film of the hips in this 24-year-old male with right hip pain shows a widened tear drop *(arrows)* measurement on the right as compared to the left. This indicates a joint effusion. No other abnormality was found, so an aspiration arthrogram was performed to exclude infection. It was normal except for a joint effusion, which was culture negative. A radionuclide bone scan (B) was done to see if avascular necrosis (AVN) or a stress fracture was the source of the pain. It revealed increased uptake throughout the acetabulum with a second area of increased uptake *(arrow)* corresponding to a double-density sign. A computed tomography (CT) scan (C) through the acetabulum shows a lucent nidus, which is partially calcified *(arrow)*. This is characteristic for an osteoid osteoma; however, osteomyelitis with a sequestrum could have an identical appearance except for the bone scan double-density sign.

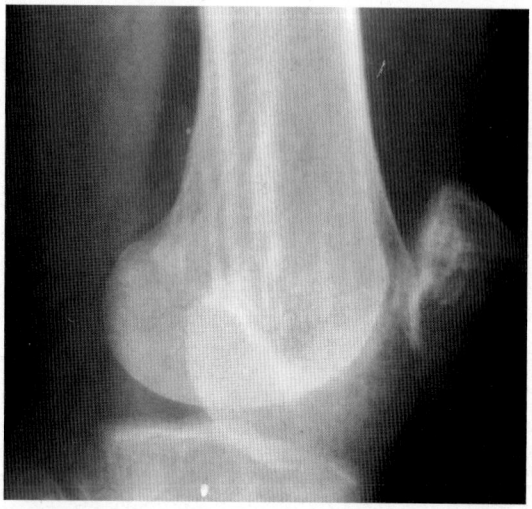

FIG. 8.16 **Osteopathia striata.** Multiple linear dense streaks are seen in the distal femur, which are characteristic of osteopathia striata.

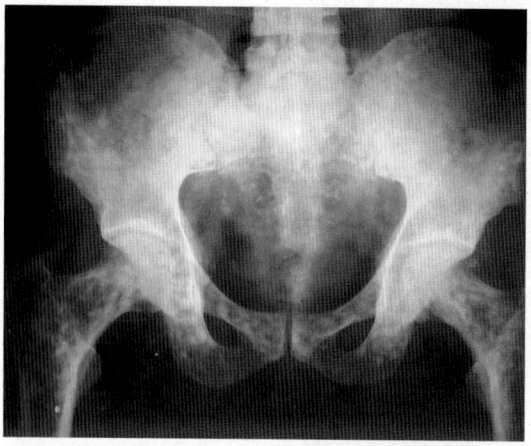

FIG. 8.17 **Osteopoikilosis.** An anteroposterior (AP) of the pelvis reveals multiple small round sclerotic foci throughout the pelvis and femurs. This is diagnostic of osteopoikilosis. This is occasionally mistaken for metastatic disease.

OSTEOPOIKILOSIS

Osteopoikilosis is a hereditary, asymptomatic disorder that is usually an incidental finding of multiple small (3–10 mm) sclerotic bony densities affecting primarily the ends of long bones and the pelvis (Fig. 8.17). It has virtually no clinical significance other than that it can be confused for diffuse osteoblastic metastases.

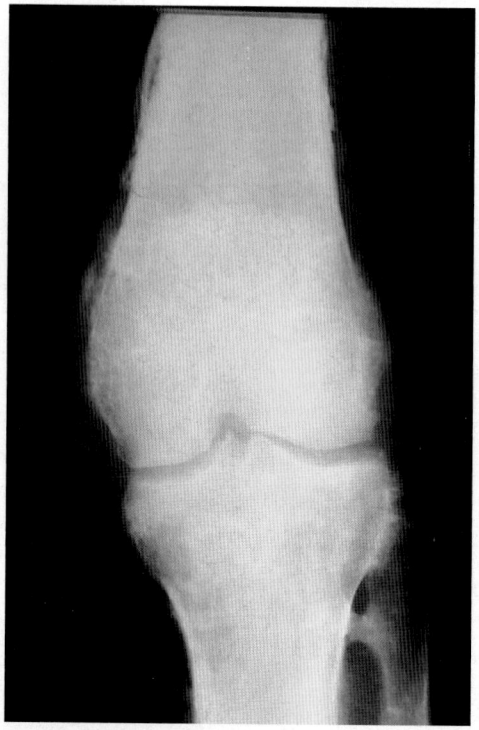

FIG. 8.18 **Pachydermoperiostosis.** An anteroposterior (AP) film of the knee in this 50-year-old black man shows extensive periostitis about the knee, which is characteristic for pachydermoperiostosis.

PACHYDERMOPERIOSTOSIS

Pachydermoperiostosis is a rare, familial disease that is manifested by periostitis in the extremities, thickening of the skin of the extremities and face, and clubbing of the fingers. It seems to be more common in the African-American population. The periosteal reaction is similar to that of HPO (Fig. 8.18), but pachydermoperiostosis is rarely painful.

PAINFUL BONE MARROW EDEMA

Painful bone marrow edema was first described in the hip and called idiopathic transient osteoporosis of the hip (ITOH). It was initially described on plain films in young (30–50 years old) males with a sudden onset of severe hip pain of unknown etiology that was self-limited (usually lasting 6 months or so) and treated with palliation. When MRI was developed, this entity was found to have a characteristic appearance of diffuse edema throughout the femoral head and neck (Figs. 8.18 and 8.19). It commonly affects the knee and is seen on MRI as extensive high T2 signal in the medial or lateral condyle

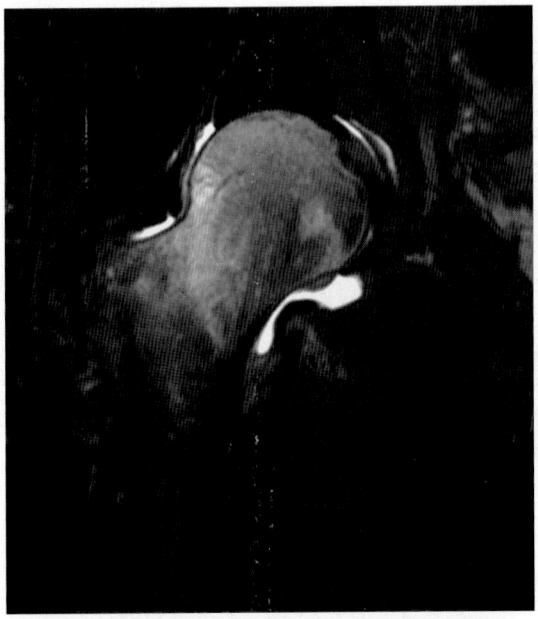

FIG. 8.19 **Idiopathic transient osteoporosis of the hip.** A coronal T2WI of the hip in a patient with sudden onset of pain and no trauma shows diffuse high signal throughout the hip, which is characteristic of idiopathic transient osteoporosis of the hip (ITOH).

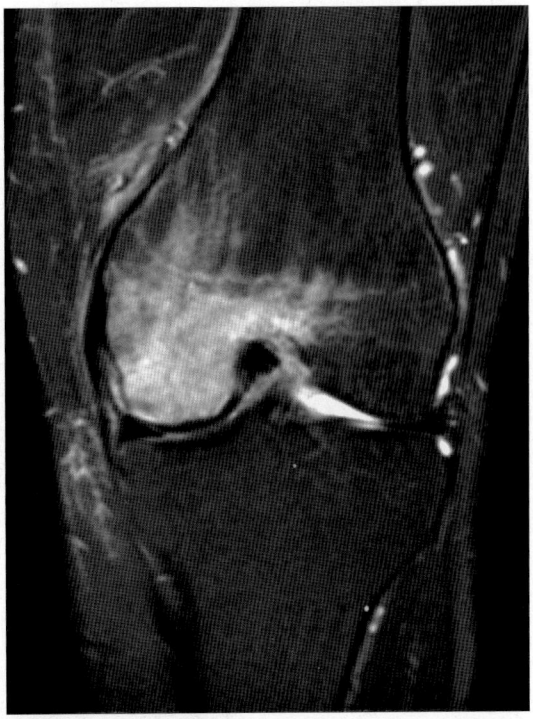

FIG. 8.20 **Painful bone marrow edema of the knee.** A coronal T2WI of the knee in a patient with sudden onset of knee pain and no trauma shows diffuse high signal in the medial femoral condyle. The adjacent cartilage was normal. This is characteristic for painful bone marrow edema.

(Figs. 8.18–8.20) and less commonly in the tibial plateau. The increased signal is out of proportion to any internal derangement or cartilage abnormality. The absence of trauma excludes a contusion, which could have this appearance. These patients need protected weight bearing so they do not develop subchondral fractures. In fact, about half have a tiny fracture visible on their initial MRI, and some show a fracture has occurred after weight bearing when a follow-up MRI is performed.

The foot and ankle are frequently affected with painful bone marrow edema. The appearance in the ankle is somewhat different from the hip and knee in that it typically has a "spotted" appearance with small foci of high T2 signal scattered throughout (Figs. 8.18–8.21). It is not unusual for a patient to have recurrent episodes of painful bone marrow edema in several joints (hip, knee, or ankle) months or years apart. This is known as regional migratory osteoporosis.[5]

SARCOID

Sarcoidosis is a noncaseating granulomatous disease that primarily affects the lungs. When the musculoskeletal system is involved, the hands are mainly affected, with the spine and long bones only infrequently involved. Sarcoid causes a characteristic "lack-like" pattern of bony destruction in the hands (Fig. 8.22). Multiple phalanges are typically affected in either one or both hands. It is so radiographically characteristic that there is almost no differential diagnosis for this pattern.

SLIPPED CAPITAL FEMORAL EPIPHYSIS

The epiphysis of the femoral head (called the capital epiphysis) has a tendency to slip medially. This is seen primarily in young teenage boys who are overweight, although it can be seen in hyperparathyroidism or idiopathically. It can be identified on an anteroposterior of the pelvis or hips by drawing a line along the lateral femoral neck and noting that in normals this line intersects about a quarter of the epiphysis (Fig. 8.23). In patients with a slipped capital epiphysis, this line intersects little or none of the slipped epiphysis. This process is often found bilaterally and is treated by internally fixing the epiphysis with pins.

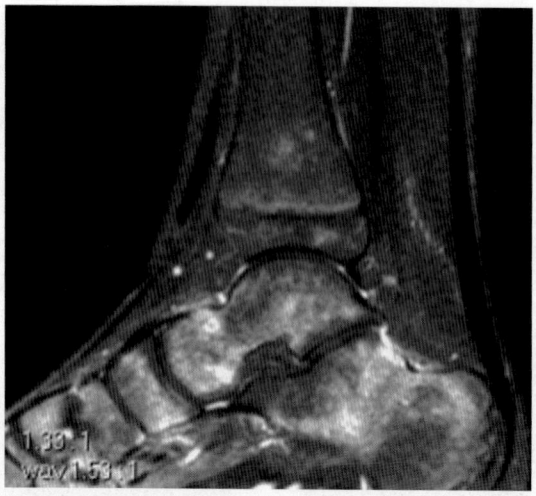

FIG. 8.21 **Painful bone marrow edema of the ankle.** A sagittal T2WI of the ankle in a patient with sudden onset of ankle pain shows a spotted appearance of high signal around the ankle, which is typical for painful bone marrow edema in the ankle.

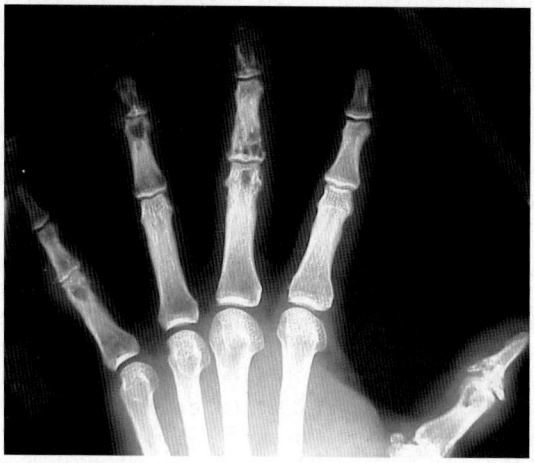

FIG. 8.22 **Sarcoid.** An anteroposterior (AP) plain film of the hands in a patient with sarcoidosis shows multiple lytic lesions, many of which demonstrate a "lacelike" pattern.

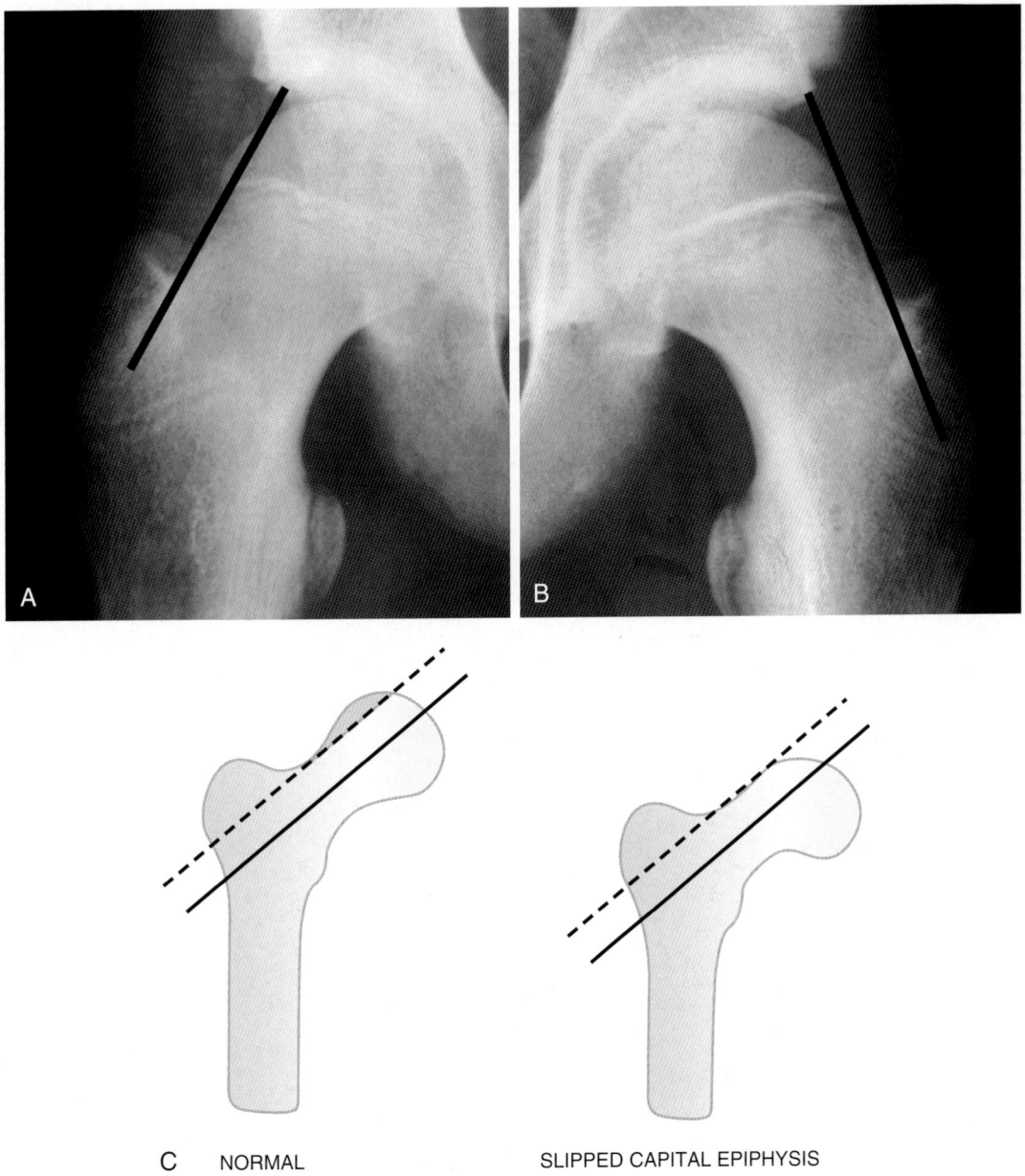

FIG. 8.23 **Slipped capital femoral epiphysis.** A plain film of the hips in this child shows medial slippage of the left femoral capital epiphysis (B) as compared to the right (A). Although the amount of slippage is slight and difficult to appreciate at first glance, note that a line drawn along the lateral femoral neck on the normal side (A) intersects a portion of the femoral epiphysis, whereas on the left side (B), a similar line misses most of the epiphysis. A schematic of the normal hip and a hip with a slipped capital epiphysis (C) shows how a line parallel to the femoral neck *(solid line)* that is then moved to the lateral aspect of the femoral neck *(dotted line)* intersects part of the epiphysis *(shaded)* in the normal and misses the epiphysis in a slipped epiphysis.

REFERENCES

1. Mankin H. Nontraumatic necrosis of bone (osteonecrosis). *N Engl J Med*. 1992;326:1473–1479.
2. Mitchell D, Kressel H, Arger P, Dalinka M, Spritzer C, Steinberg M. Avascular necrosis of the femoral head: morphologic assessment by MR imaging, with CT correlation. *Radiology*. 1986;161: 739—42.
3. Marcove R, Heelan R, Huvos A, Healey J, Lindeque B. Osteoid osteoma. Diagnosis, localization, and treatment. *Clin Orthop Relat Res*. 1991;267: 197—201.
4. Helms CA, Hattner RS, Vogler III J. Osteoid osteoma: radionuclide diagnosis. *Radiology*. 1984;151(3): 779—84.
5. Korompilias AV, Karantanas AH, Lykissas MG, Beris AE. Bone marrow edema syndrome. *Skeletal Radiology*. 2009;38:425–436.

CHAPTER 9

Magnetic Resonance Imaging of the Knee

Magnetic resonance (MR) imaging of the knee has developed into one of the most frequently requested exams in radiology. This is not just because many people injure their knees, but because of its high accuracy in depicting internal derangements. Accuracy reports of knee MR imaging vary from 85% to 95%, with many investigators feeling that MR imaging of the knee is, in fact, more accurate than arthroscopy. Very few top orthopedic surgeons will operate on a knee without an MRI to serve as a "road map." Although some surgeons feel MR imaging is too expensive for routine use in every patient, there are studies that show enormous financial savings (not to mention decreased patient morbidity) in performing an MR exam on every patient who is a candidate for knee arthroscopy. Many of these patients do not need subsequent arthroscopy, and those who do benefit from a more complete preoperative assessment (not directly reflected in financial savings but clearly beneficial for surgical planning).[1] MR imaging of the knee has a very high negative predictive value; therefore a normal MR imaging knee exam is highly accurate in excluding an internal derangement.[2,3]

Maximum diagnostic accuracy can be obtained in several ways. First, and most obvious, is to obtain high-quality images. This includes using the appropriate imaging protocol. Employing an inappropriate protocol is probably the number one error committed in knee MR imaging. Second, knowing the basic MR imaging signs for internal derangements is key in achieving a high accuracy rate. Third, knowing the imaging pitfalls, such as normal variants that can mimic pathology, will further aid in diagnostic accuracy. Proper protocols, basic imaging signs, and pitfalls will be discussed in detail in this chapter.

IMAGING PROTOCOL

The proper imaging protocol is essential for a high diagnostic accuracy rate. A sagittal T1-weighted (or proton density) sequence is essential for examining the menisci. Four- or five-millimeter-thick slices with a small (12–14 cm) field of view and at least a 192 matrix are recommended. The knee should be imaged using a dedicated knee coil and externally rotated about 5 to 10 degrees (do not exceed 10 degrees) to put the anterior cruciate ligament (ACL) in the plane of imaging. T2 spin-echo or T2* gradient-echo sagittal images are obtained primarily to examine the cruciate ligaments and cartilage. With T2 spin-echo images, meniscal tears may be difficult to see; however, they will be picked up on the proton density images. Thus the menisci and the cruciate ligaments are examined primarily on the sagittal images. Although the menisci and the cruciate ligaments can be seen on the coronal and axial images, it is uncommon for those images to show an abnormality that is not seen on the sagittal images.

Coronal images are obtained to examine the collateral ligaments and to look for meniscocapsular separations. These abnormalities can most often only be seen with T2-weighted images. T1 coronal images are therefore a waste of time, as there is nothing to be seen on these images that cannot be equally well seen on the sagittal images. T2* gradient-echo coronals or fast spin-echo (FSE) T2 sequences in the coronal plane are imperative. FSE (also called turbo spin-echo, or TSE) sequences should have fat suppression applied or fluid cannot be distinguished from fat.

A few centers continue to use T1-weighted coronal images without realizing that they give no additional information and in fact can hide significant abnormalities. Why would they do this? T1-weighted coronal images were part of everyone's protocol when we first began to use MR imaging in the knee. Articles, book chapters, and speakers (including me) would give the standard protocol, not thinking enough about what each sequence was showing us. I remember reading out a knee study in the late 1980s with one of the radiology residents, and I asked him to hedge on the diagnosis of a partial tear of the medial collateral ligament (MCL) and request a repeat exam with T2-weighted coronals to rule out a meniscocapsular separation. This was the second or third time that week that the resident had been so instructed, so he asked, "Why don't we just routinely do a T2 coronal—we don't see anything on the T1 coronal and we often have to hedge or repeat the exam with a T2 coronal?" I just said for him to worry about dictating the cases; I and others would take care of setting up the protocols. Well, 2 weeks later, he rotated to another service, and we began doing T2 coronal images as part of our standard knee protocol. Uppity residents!

Axial images were initially used by the technicians as a scout view. They were then found to be useful for viewing the patellofemoral cartilage and for identifying and characterizing fluid collections. As in the coronal images, to afford an opportunity to see any pathology, T2 images must be obtained.

We have found that fat-suppressing the sagittal T1 or proton-density meniscus-sensitive sequence increases the dynamic range of signal in the meniscus and makes meniscal pathology more conspicuous. It gets rid of all the distracting high signal in the marrow, making it easier to visualize the meniscus.

The use of FSE sequences with a short TE (FSE proton density) has been shown in several reports to be useful for meniscal tears, and yet others have reported a decreased sensitivity. What is the truth? The truth is that every published report I can find shows a sensitivity of around 80% for FSE proton density sequences, whereas conventional spin-echo sequences have a sensitivity closer to 95%. It is very controversial, but basically everyone's results are the same (80% sensitivity); only the conclusions differ.[4] If you're willing to decrease your sensitivity for meniscal tears from 95% to 80% to save 3 minutes (the only advantage of FSE), then your time is more valuable than your diagnostic accuracy. Get another job!

The protocol I currently recommend consists of a sagittal proton density–weighted spin-echo series with fat suppression and sagittal, coronal, and axial FSE T2 with fat suppression (Table 9.1). Many acceptable variations of this protocol exist. Many centers, for various reasons, prefer not to use FSE images and instead use gradient-echo.

MENISCI

The normal meniscus is a fibrocartilaginous, C-shaped structure that is uniformly low in signal on both T1- and T2-weighted sequences (Fig. 9.1). With T2* sequences, the menisci will usually demonstrate some internal signal. With T1-weighted images, any signal within the meniscus is abnormal, except in children, where some signal is

TABLE 9.1
Knee Protocol

	TR/TE	Nex	Matrix	Fat Sat	Thickness (mm)	FOV
Sagittal	2000/20	1	192	yes	4	14
Sagittal	4000/70	2	192	yes	4	14
Coronal	4000/70	2	192	yes	4	14
Axial	4000/70	2	192	yes	4	14

Fat Sat, Fat suppression; *FOV*, field of view; *Nex*, number of excitations.

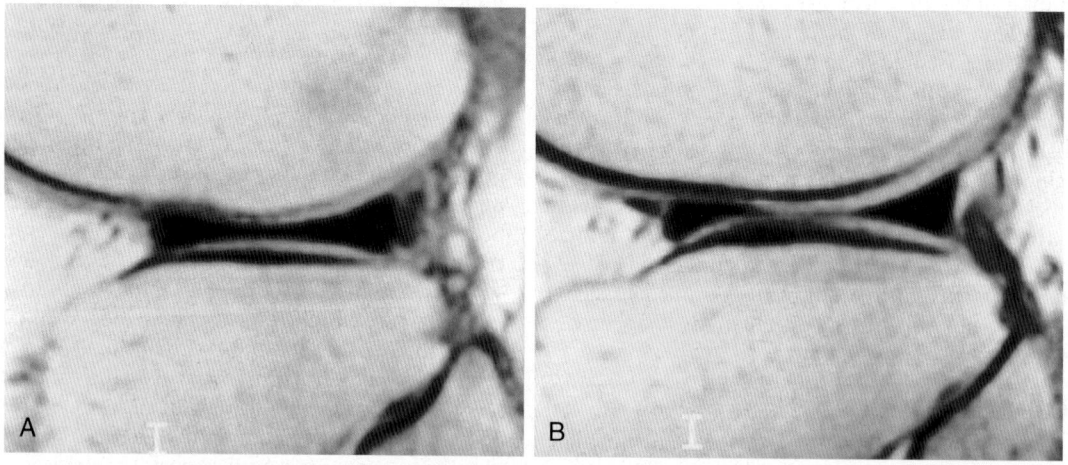

FIG. 9.1 **Normal Meniscus.** (A) A T1-weighted sagittal image through a normal lateral meniscus demonstrates uniform low signal in the meniscus. This is a section through the body of the meniscus since it has a bowtie configuration. Two sections of the body should be seen in each meniscus with 4- or 5-mm-thick slices. (B) In the same T1-weighted sequence, this sagittal image demonstrates uniform low signal in the anterior and posterior horns of this normal lateral meniscus. (Anterior is to the left.)

normal and represents normal vascularity. Meniscal signal that does not disrupt an articular surface is representative of intrasubstance degeneration (Fig. 9.2), which is myxoid degeneration of the fibrocartilage. It most likely represents aging and normal wear and tear. It is not felt to be symptomatic and cannot be diagnosed clinically or with arthroscopy. Some choose, therefore not to mention intrasubstance degeneration in the radiology interpretation.

When high signal in a meniscus disrupts the superior or inferior articular surface, a meniscal tear is diagnosed (Figs. 9.3 and 9.4). Care must be taken to be sure that the signal actually disrupts the articular surface of the meniscus before calling a tear. When high signal approaches the articular surface of the meniscus, it seems many radiologists tend to overcall it whether or not it disrupts the surface. This is evidenced not only from my experience of watching residents and fellows, but also by noting that most published series on accuracy of knee MR imaging have a lower specificity than sensitivity (i.e., there are more false positives than false negatives). One way to aid in avoiding false positive calls is to cover up the meniscus with a card, or your thumbnail, leaving only a thin margin of the articular surface of the meniscus visible. If this margin of articular surface of the meniscus is seen as a straight, uninterrupted line, no tear of the meniscus is present. If the thin margin is interrupted, a meniscal tear is present.

Meniscal tears have many different configurations and locations, with an oblique tear extending to the inferior surface of the posterior horn of the medial meniscus the most common type. In a small but significant percentage of cases (around 10%), it can be virtually impossible to be certain if meniscal high signal disrupts an articular surface. In these cases, it is recommended that the surgeon be advised that it is too close to call. The surgeon can then rely on his clinical expertise to decide if arthroscopy is warranted, and, if it is, the MR will guide him to where the questionable tear is located. DeSmet showed that signal that disrupts the surface of the meniscus on only one sagittal image should be considered a sign of an equivocal tear.[5] He found only 56% of the medial menisci and 30% of the lateral menisci were torn if only one sagittal image showed the "tear." If these equivocal cases are excluded, the remaining cases will have an extremely high accuracy rate.

Another very common meniscus tear, one that is frequently missed by radiologists, is a bucket handle tear. This is a vertical longitudinal tear that can result in the inner free edge of the meniscus becoming displaced into the intercondylar notch (Fig. 9.5). It is most easily recognized by observing on the sagittal images that only one image is present, which has the bowtie appearance

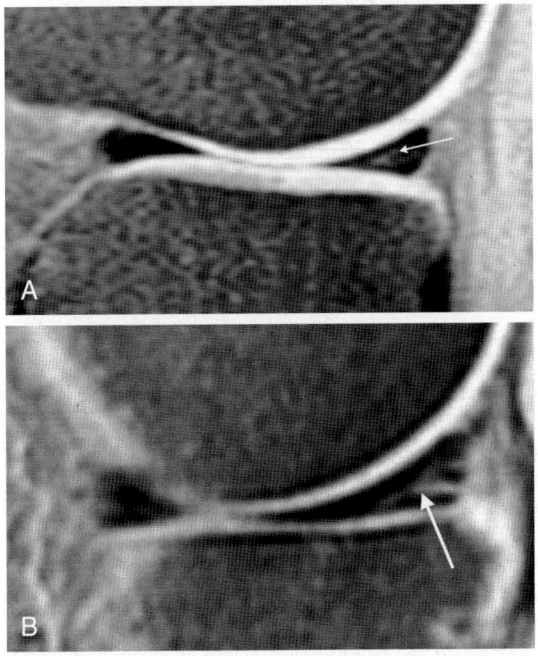

FIG. 9.2 **Intrasubstance Degeneration.** (A) Faint intermediate signal can be seen in the posterior horn of this meniscus *(arrow)*, which does not disrupt the articular surface of the meniscus. This is intrasubstance degeneration. (B) Linear high signal is present in the posterior body segment of the meniscus *(arrow)*. The signal does not disrupt the articular surface; therefore this represents intrasubstance degeneration.

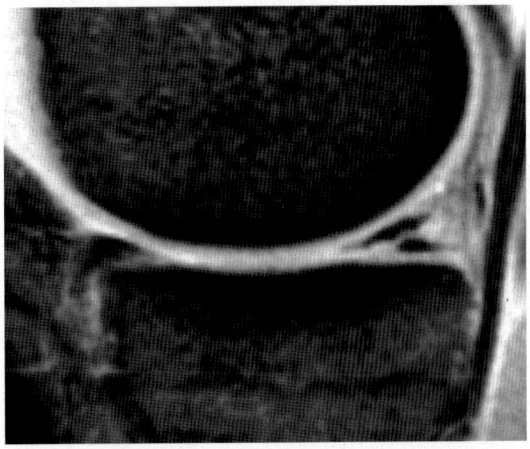

FIG. 9.3 **Meniscal Tear.** This fat-suppressed T1-weighted sagittal image shows linear high signal in the posterior horn of the meniscus, which disrupts the inferior articular surface. This is the appearance of an oblique meniscal tear.

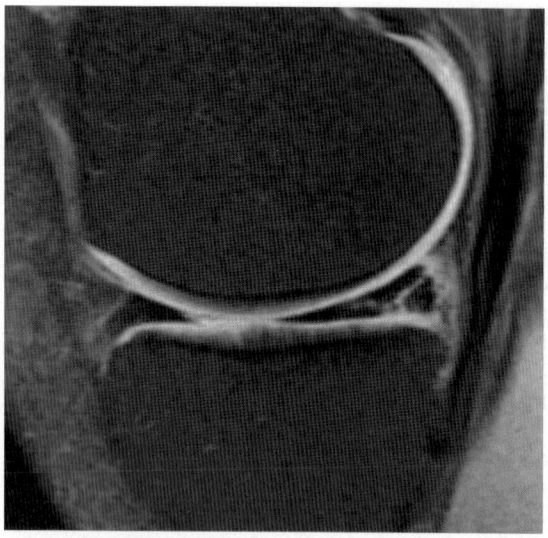

FIG. 9.4 **Meniscal Tear.** This fat-suppressed T1-weighted sagittal image shows linear high signal in the posterior horn of the meniscus, which disrupts the inferior articular surface and has a stellate appearance. This is a complex meniscal tear.

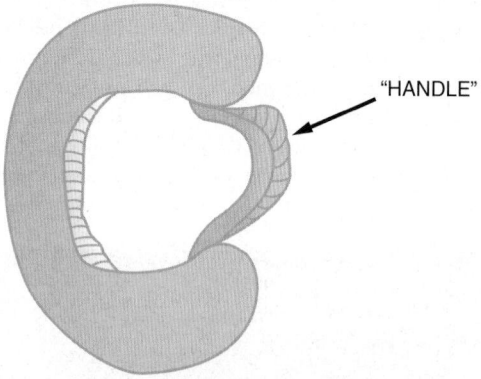

FIG. 9.5 **Bucket Handle Tear.** This drawing illustrates a bucket handle tear with the torn free edge of the meniscus displaced as the "handle" of the bucket.

of the body segment of the meniscus (Fig. 9.6). Normally, two contiguous sagittal images with a bowtie shape are seen, since the normal meniscus is 9 to 12 mm in width, and the sagittal images are 4 to 5 mm in thickness. On the coronal images, a bucket handle tear may reveal the meniscus to be shortened and truncated; however, often the torn meniscus remodels and truncation cannot be appreciated (Fig. 9.7). The displaced inner edge of the meniscus (the "handle" of the bucket) should be seen in the intercondylar notch on sagittal or coronal views (Fig. 9.8).

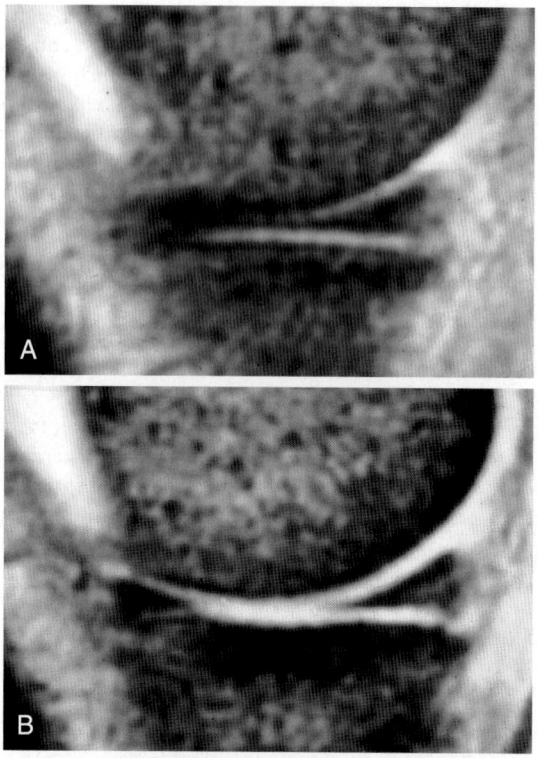

FIG. 9.6 **Bucket Handle Tear.** Sagittal gradient-echo images through the medial meniscus at its most medial aspect reveal one bowtie, indicative of the body of the meniscus (A), with the adjacent image (B) having apparent normal anterior and posterior horns. However, since there should be two consecutive sagittal images with a bowtie configuration, this indicates a bucket handle tear. (Anterior is to the left.)

Another meniscus tear that is diagnosed by having too few bowtie segments present in the sagittal plane is a radial tear or parrot beak tear. This is a tear of the free edge of the meniscus (Fig. 9.9), which is a common tear. It should be suspected when only one bowtie segment is present, and the adjacent sagittal image shows a small gap (a bucket handle tear will have a large gap) in the expected bowtie (Fig. 9.10). The apparent anterior and/or posterior horn triangles will often be rounded or truncated instead of pointed.

Use of the "bowtie sign," that is, having two consecutive sagittal images that demonstrate a bowtie configuration, is one of the most useful signs I can give beginners in evaluating a knee MR image.[6] It will allow a bucket handle tear to virtually never be overlooked and, as the next section describes, can be used to diagnose a discoid meniscus. There are four pitfalls to be aware of in applying the bowtie sign (Table 9.2). First, if the knee and the menisci are very small, as in a

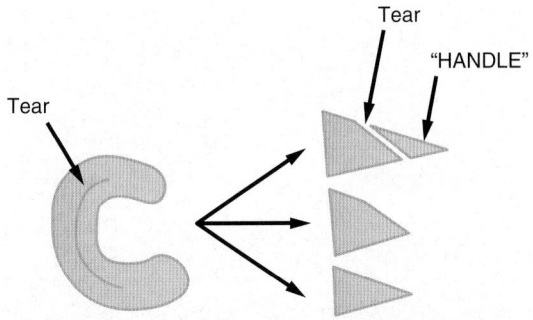

FIG. 9.7 **Schematic of Bucket Handle Tear.** This drawing shows how a vertical longitudinal tear, as shown on the axial view (left), can appear on the coronal views *(right).* Prior to the free edge being displaced, the tear may be seen *(top, right);* after the free edge (or "handle") displaces, the remaining meniscus may appear truncated *(center, right);* after weight bearing, the truncated meniscus smooths out to a sharp triangle that is simply decreased in width from the normal *(bottom, right).*

child's knee, only one bowtie may be observed without a bucket handle tear being present. However, there will be only two or three sagittal images that demonstrate the anterior and posterior horns. A normal-sized knee will have two bowties and three or four images that show the anterior and posterior horns. Also, in a small knee, both the medial and lateral menisci will have only one bowtie image, and bucket handle tears involving both the medial and lateral menisci are very rare.

The second pitfall in the bowtie sign is seen in older patients—over the age of 60. Patients older than 60 often have worn down the inner free edges of their menisci so that they will only have one sagittal image of the body seen, followed by four or five images that show the anterior and posterior horns—usually a good sign for a bucket handle tear. This, unlike the pitfall described in children or small knees, does not necessarily occur in both menisci. How do I differentiate this from a real bucket handle tear? First, degenerative joint disease is always present, and, second, no displaced meniscal fragment can be found.

A third pitfall to be aware of in using the bowtie sign is that the sign only works if the entire meniscus is covered with sagittal images. If the tech doesn't begin the sagittal images at the far medial or lateral aspects of the knee, the meniscus will not be imaged in its entirety. One will quickly learn to appreciate whether or not the entire meniscus is covered.

The fourth pitfall is seen in knees with prior surgery in which a partial meniscectomy has been performed. This can be differentiated from a bucket handle tear by the lack of a displaced fragment (no handle of the bucket). In fact, all four of the pitfalls mentioned can be recognized by the inability to see a displaced meniscal fragment.

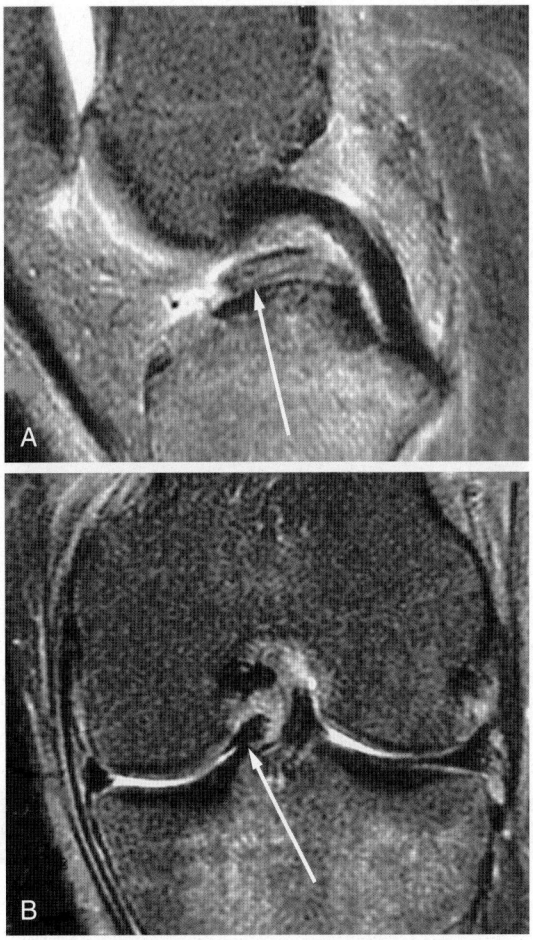

FIG. 9.8 **Displaced Fragment in Bucket Handle Tear.** (A) Sagittal and (B) coronal T2-weighted images through the intercondylar notch in a patient with a bucket handle tear reveals the displaced free fragment or "handle" *(arrows)* just anterior to the posterior cruciate ligament.

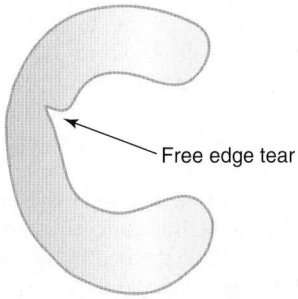

FIG. 9.9 **Parrot Beak Tear.** This drawing shows the appearance of a radial free edge meniscal tear called a parrot beak tear.

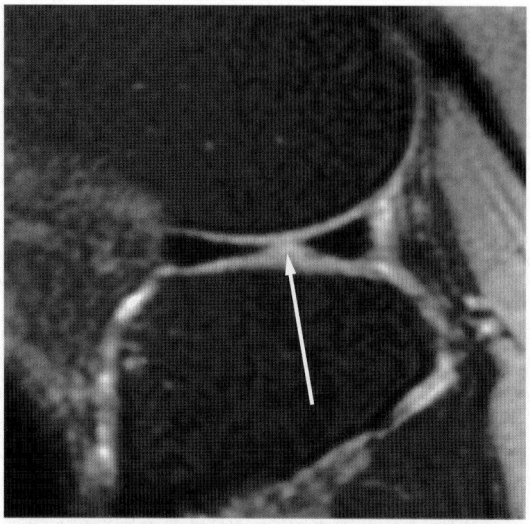

FIG. 9.10 **Radial Tear.** Sagittal images through the body of the medial meniscus in a patient with a radial tear showed a normal bowtie configuration in the most medial image, with the next adjacent image *(shown here)* having a small gap *(arrow)*, which indicates a disruption of the free edge of the meniscus. Note the rounded tip of the apparent anterior horn, which is further evidence of a torn free edge or parrot beak tear.

TABLE 9.2 Pitfalls in "Bowtie" Sign
1. Small knee with small menisci
2. Older patients (>60) who may have fraying and degeneration of free edge
3. Incomplete coverage
4. Prior surgery

A discoid meniscus is a large disc-like meniscus that can have many different shapes—lens shaped, wedged, flat, and others. It is not known if it is congenital or acquired, but most are found in children or young adults. It is seen laterally in up to 3% of the population, with a discoid medial meniscus being rare. A discoid meniscus is felt to be more prone to tear than a normal meniscus and can be symptomatic even without being torn. Although they are easily identified on coronal images by noting meniscal tissue extending into the tibial spines at the intercondylar notch (Fig. 9.11), they are most reliably diagnosed by noting more than two consecutive sagittal images that show the meniscus with a bowtie appearance (Fig. 9.12). Hence the bowtie sign can be used to diagnose a bucket handle tear (fewer than two bowties) or a discoid meniscus (more than two bowties). If thinner slices than 4 or 5 mm are used, the bowtie sign can be adjusted to whatever slice thickness is employed.

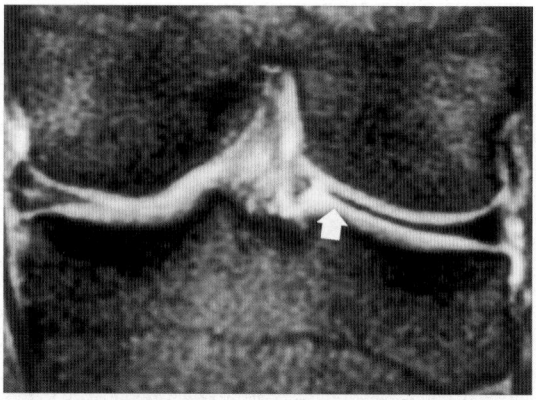

FIG. 9.11 **Discoid Lateral Meniscus.** A coronal gradient-echo image through the intercondylar notch shows a large lateral meniscus with meniscal tissue extending into the notch medially *(arrow)*.

The lateral meniscus often has what appears to be a tear on the anterior horn near its upper margin, which is a pseudotear from the insertion of the transverse ligament (Fig. 9.13). This can easily be differentiated from a real tear by following it medially across the knee in Hoffa fat pad to where it inserts onto the anterior horn of the medial meniscus. Although less common than on the lateral meniscus, a pseudotear from the insertion of the transverse ligament onto the anterior horn of the medial meniscus can be seen.

Meniscal cysts occur in about 5% of cases and can cause pain, even if the meniscus is not torn. The etiology is unknown, but they occur more frequently in discoid menisci. If the meniscus is not torn, the surgical approach used by some is percutaneous with decompression and packing performed, whereas if a meniscus tear is associated with the cyst, it is approached intraarticularly. Hence accurate diagnosis of a tear is imperative. The intrameniscal portion of the cyst typically does not get fluid-bright in signal on T2 sequences (Fig. 9.14), which has misled many radiologists into discounting the presence of a cyst. A meniscal cyst will enlarge the meniscus and give it a swollen appearance unless it decompresses into the soft tissues (called a parameniscal cyst) or into the joint via a meniscus tear. Decompression into a parameniscal cyst does not indicate a meniscus tear. A meniscus tear, by definition, has to disrupt the articular surface of the meniscus. Although a meniscus with a meniscal cyst is more likely to tear than an otherwise normal meniscus, up to 40% are not torn.[7] Many reports cite that menisci with cysts are torn up to 98% of the time—this is simply not true.

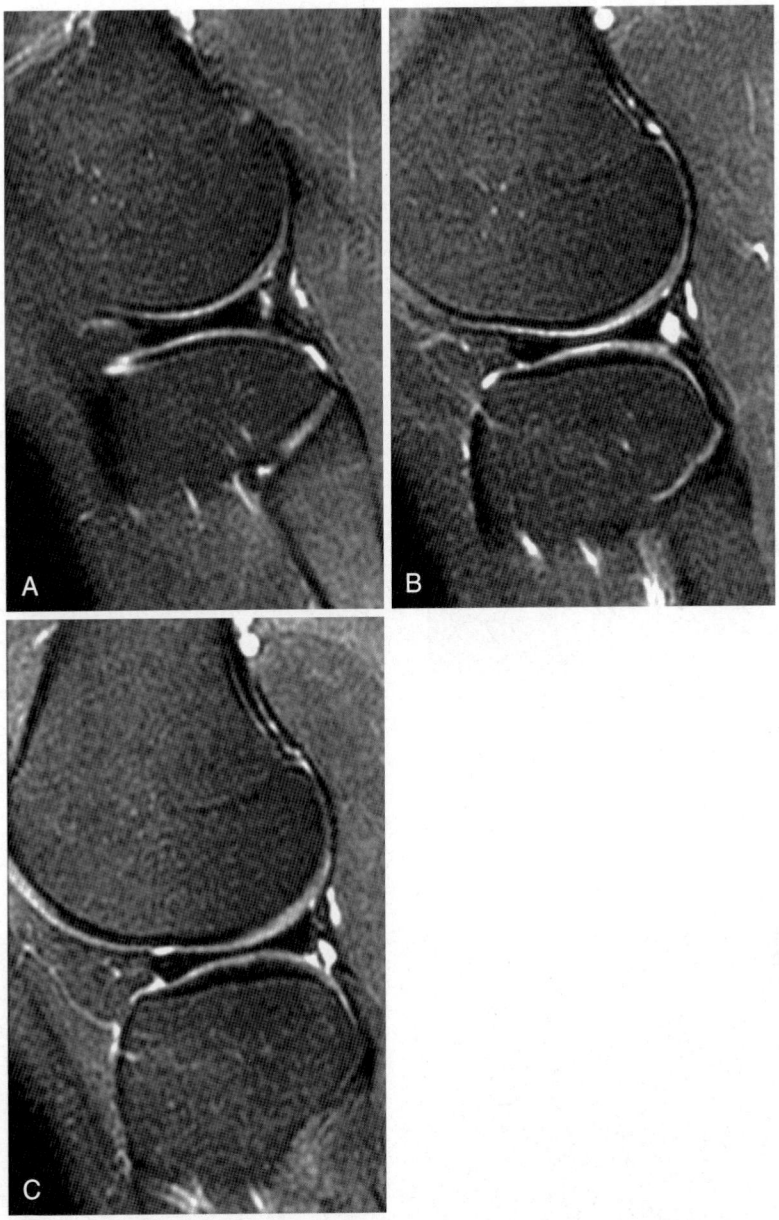

FIG. 9.12 **Discoid Lateral Meniscus.** Three consecutive 5-mm-thick T1-weighted images through the lateral meniscus, beginning with the most lateral (A) and extending medially (B and C); each show the meniscus to have a bowtie configuration. Since only two images should have a bowtie shape, indicative of the body of the meniscus, this is diagnostic of a discoid lateral meniscus (Fig. 9.11 is a coronal image of the same knee). (Anterior is to the left.)

CRUCIATE LIGAMENTS

MR imaging of the cruciate ligaments is more accurate than is MR imaging of the menisci, with accuracy reported near 100% in several published series.[8] The normal ACL is seen in the intercondylar notch as a linear, predominantly low-signal structure on T1- or proton density–weighted images that often shows some linear striations near its insertion onto the medial tibial spine when viewed on sagittal images (Fig. 9.15A). T2 images are imperative for obtaining the highest accuracy in diagnosing ACL tears, as fluid and hemorrhage will often obscure the ligament on T1-weighted images (Fig. 9.15B).

A torn ACL is most often simply not visualized (Fig. 9.16), although sometimes the actual disruption will be seen (Fig. 9.17). Partial tears or strains of the ACL are manifested by high signal and/or laxity in an otherwise intact ligament. The diagnosis of a partial tear or strain is generally not critical on MR imaging, as the treatment afforded the patient is dependent primarily on the diagnosis of a complete tear. In most instances, the arthroscopist cannot tell a partial tear from an intact ACL.

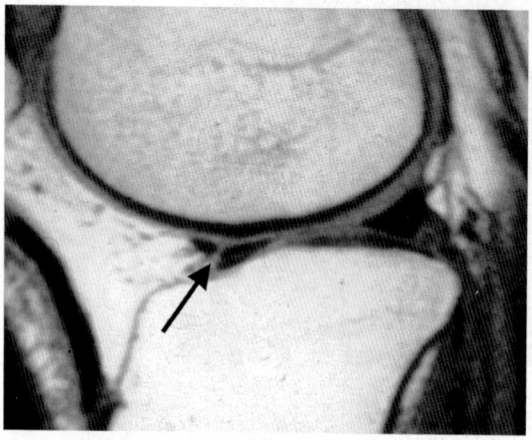

FIG. 9.13 **Pseudotear From a Transverse Ligament.** A sagittal T1-weighted image through the lateral meniscus shows linear high signal through the upper anterior horn *(arrow)*, which resembles a tear. This is the insertion of the transverse ligament onto the meniscus (see Fig. 9.1B for another example). (Anterior is to the left.)

An entity that has been mistaken for a torn ACL is an ACL cyst (Fig. 9.18). The etiology is unknown, but it basically represents fluid in and around the fibers of the ACL, giving it a swollen, "drumstick" appearance on sagittal images. It has been mistakenly diagnosed as a tumor with subsequent radical removal (oops!) in one published report. It is an incidental finding with little or no clinical significance. It is found in about 1% of all knees. Even though it often gets misdiagnosed as an ACL tear on MRI, it virtually never confuses a surgeon into operating because the knee is stable.

The normal posterior cruciate ligament (PCL) is a gently curved, uniformly low-signal structure (Fig. 9.19), which is infrequently torn and even less frequently repaired by surgeons. When torn, it typically has a thickened appearance with diffuse intermediate signal throughout (Fig. 9.20). It typically appears intact but has undergone a plastic deformation that renders it unstable, much like overstretching the elastic in your socks. In only a third of cases can an actual ligament disruption or avulsion off of the femur or tibia be seen.[9] Many orthopedic surgeons do not even inspect the PCL at arthroscopy

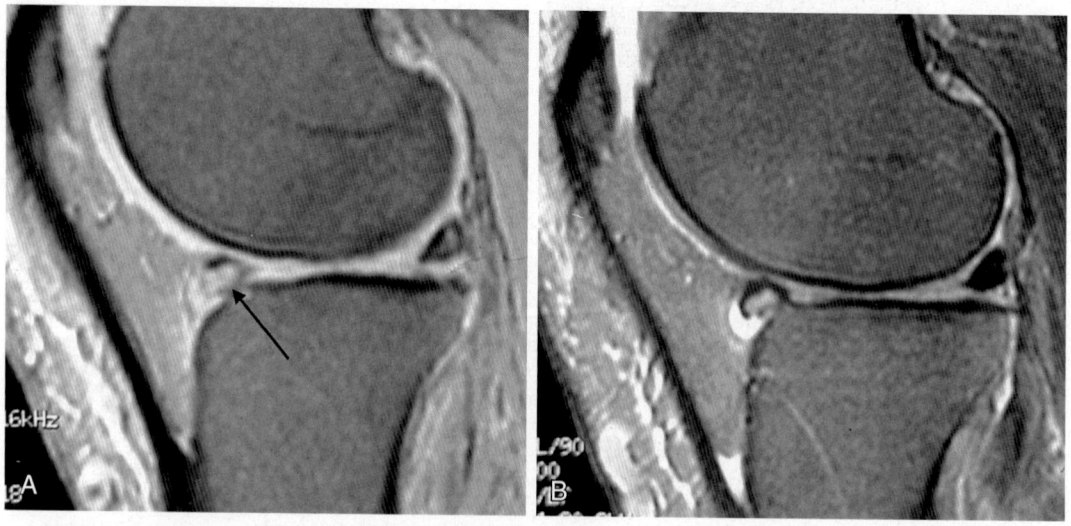

FIG. 9.14 **Meniscal Cyst.** A sagittal proton-density weighted image (A) through the medial meniscus shows a swollen anterior horn filled with increased signal *(arrow)*. A T2-weighted image (B) shows high signal similar to fluid in the parameniscal portion, whereas the intrameniscal signal is only intermediate.

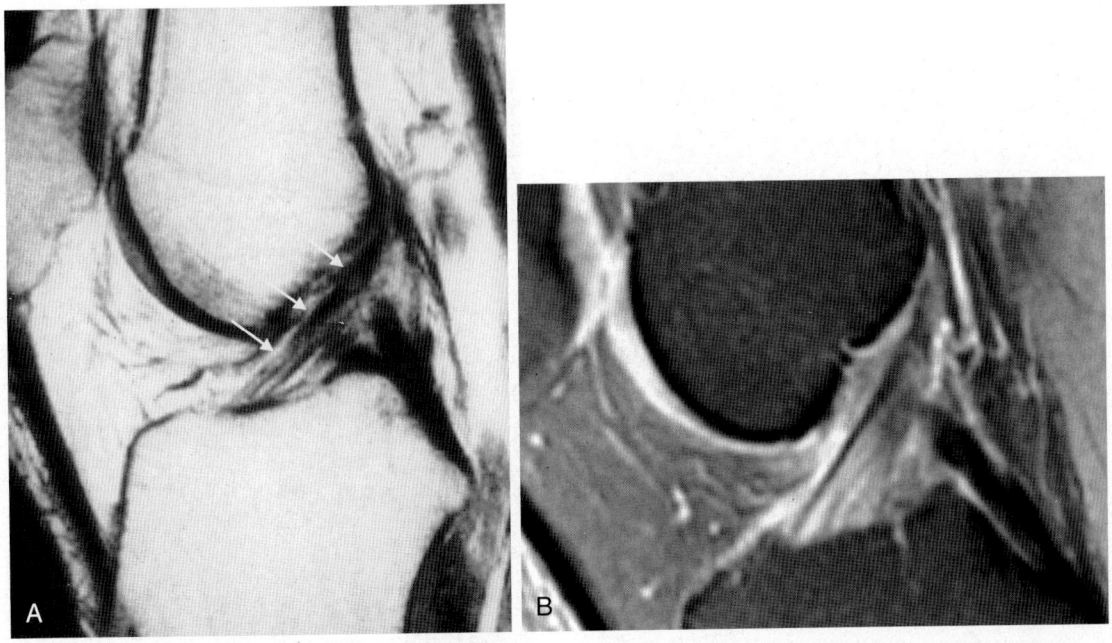

FIG. 9.15 **Normal Anterior Cruciate Ligament.** (A) A sagittal T1-weighted image through the intercondylar notch shows the normal appearance of the anterior cruciate ligament (ACL) *(arrows).* (B) A sagittal T2-weighted image with fat suppression through the intercondylar notch in another patient shows a normal ACL.

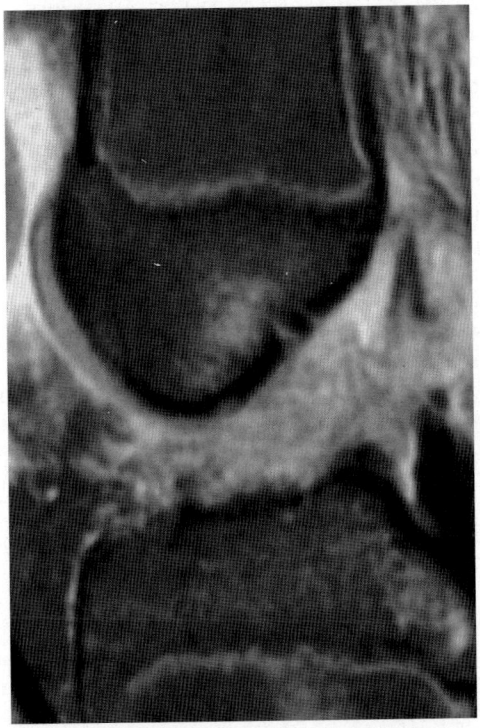

FIG. 9.16 **Torn Anterior Cruciate Ligament (ACL).** This sagittal T2-weighted image with fat suppression through the intercondylar notch fails to show the ACL. This is a fairly typical example of a completely torn ACL.

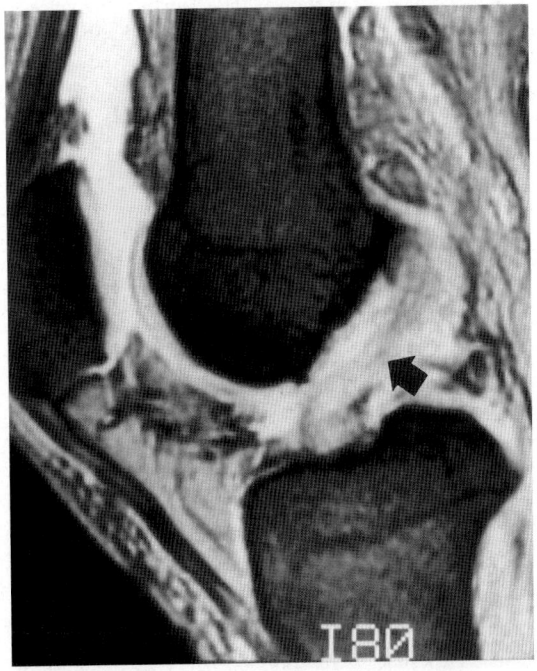

FIG. 9.17 **Torn Anterior Cruciate Ligament (ACL).** A sagittal gradient-echo image through the intercondylar notch shows fibers of a torn ACL, which are disrupted centrally *(arrow).*

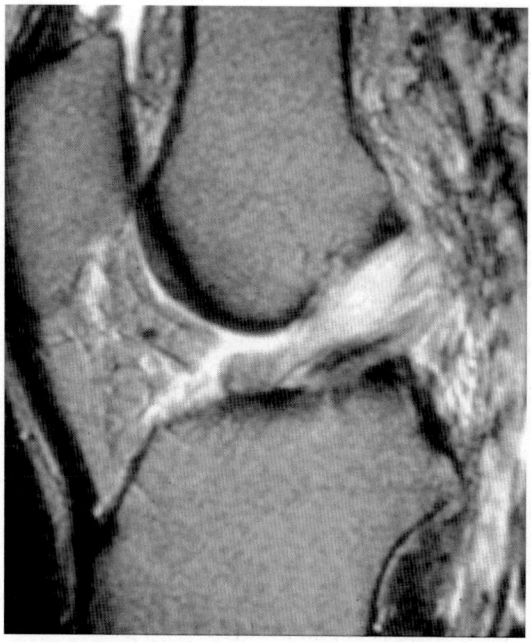

FIG. 9.18 **Anterior Cruciate Ligament (ACL) cyst.** This sagittal T2-weighted image with fat suppression through the intercondylar notch shows the ACL with a drumstick appearance and high signal within. This is the appearance of an ACL cyst.

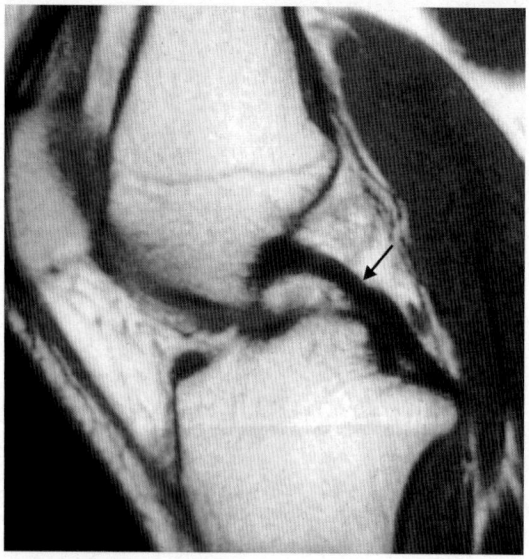

FIG. 9.19 **Normal Posterior Cruciate Ligament (PCL).** A sagittal T1-weighted image through the intercondylar notch shows the appearance of the normal PCL with its characteristic uniform low signal *(arrow).*

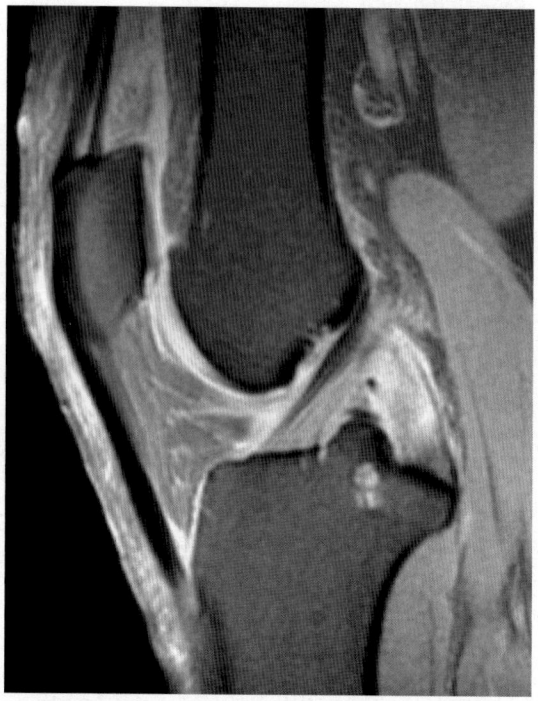

FIG. 9.20 **Torn Posterior Cruciate Ligament (PCL).** A sagittal proton density (PD)-weighted image through the intercondylar notch reveals the PCL to have a fat or thickened appearance with diffuse intermediate signal throughout. This is typical for a torn PCL.

and do not repair it when torn because it rarely is a cause of instability. A former fellow I worked with tried to publish an MR imaging sign for a torn PCL. After collecting a dozen cases with torn posterior cruciates, he got the operative reports from the patients' records. We were surprised to find that not one surgeon even mentioned the PCL in any of the cases! We called a few of the surgeons, and each gave the same answer—they virtually never repair the PCL because it does not lead to instability; hence they don't even bother to look at it during arthroscopy. While not all surgeons subscribe to this philosophy, many do. If yours does, it's a kind of freedom you have in looking at the posterior cruciate. You can tell them it's tied in a knot, and it won't matter.

A low-signal round structure is often seen just anterior or posterior to the PCL on the sagittal views. A loose body or a flap of a piece of torn meniscus can have this appearance (Fig. 9.21), but it is most commonly due to a meniscofemoral ligament, which extends obliquely across the knee from the medial femoral condyle to the

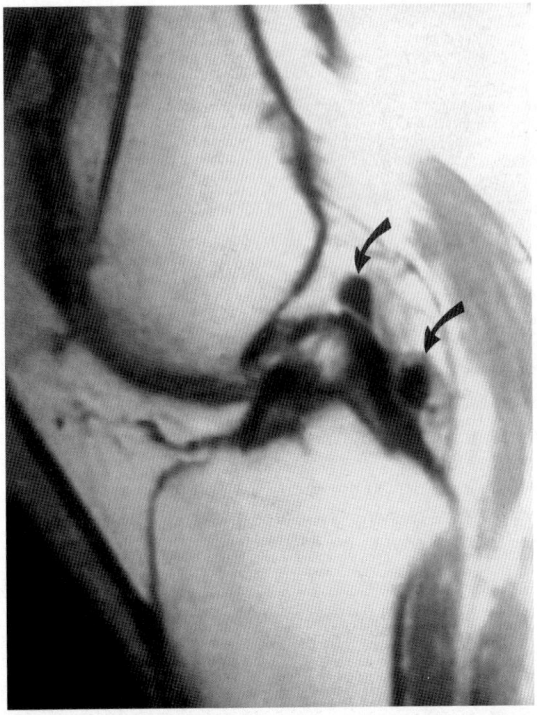

FIG. 9.21 **Loose Bodies.** A sagittal T1-weighted image through the intercondylar notch in this patient shows two rounded low-signal structures *(arrows),* which are loose bodies. A meniscofemoral ligament of Wrisberg could have the appearance of either of these loose bodies.

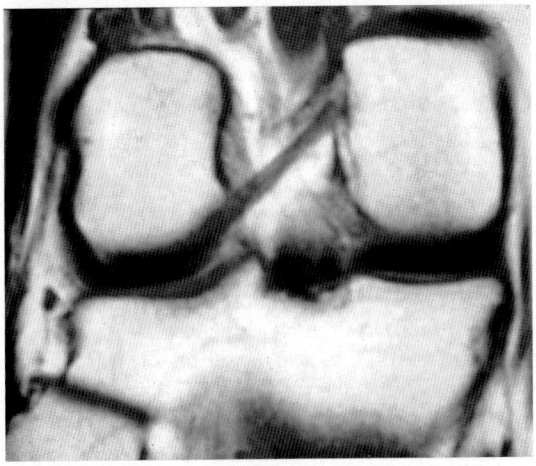

FIG. 9.22 **Ligament of Wrisberg.** This coronal T1-weighted image shows an obliquely oriented structure (arrow) extending from the medial femoral condyle to the lateral meniscus. This is a normal ligament of Wrisberg.

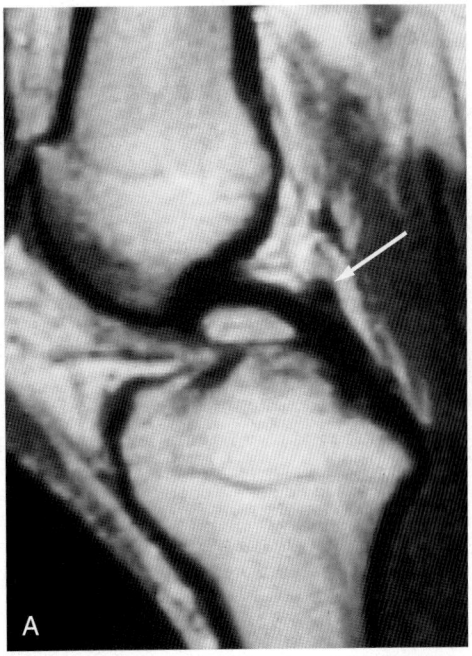

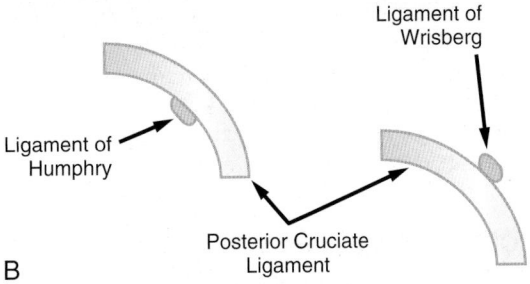

FIG. 9.23 **Ligament of Wrisberg.** (A) A sagittal T1-weighted image through the intercondylar notch shows a rounded low-signal structure posterior to the posterior cruciate ligament, which is the meniscofemoral ligament of Wrisberg *(arrow).* (B) This drawing shows the relationship of the ligaments of Wrisberg and Humphry to the posterior cruciate ligament.

posterior horn of the lateral meniscus (Fig. 9.22). If it passes in front of the PCL, it is called the ligament of Humphry, and if it passes behind the PCL, it is the ligament of Wrisberg (Fig. 9.23). One or the other is present in up to 72% of all knees on MRI. In fewer than 5% of cases, both will be present.

The insertion of the ligament of Humphry or Wrisberg onto the lateral meniscus can produce a pseudotear similar to that caused by the transverse ligament on the anterior horn of the lateral meniscus (Fig. 9.24).

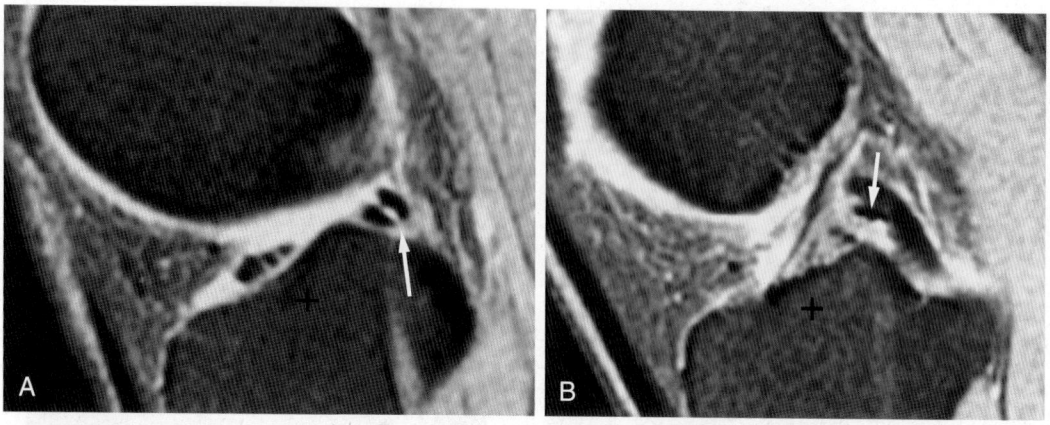

FIG. 9.24 **Pseudotear From Ligament of Humphry Insertion.** (A) A sagittal proton density fat-suppressed image through the lateral meniscus reveals an apparent tear of the posterior horn *(arrow)*, which is the insertion of the ligament of Humphry onto the meniscus. (B) On the image through the intercondylar notch, a ligament of Humphry *(arrow)* is seen anterior to the posterior cruciate ligament (PCL). The ligament of Humphry could be followed on adjacent images, from anterior to the PCL to its insertion on the posterior horn of the lateral meniscus.

Prior to calling a tear on the upper aspect of the posterior horn of the lateral meniscus, care must be taken to look for a meniscofemoral ligament to be certain it is not a pseudotear from the ligament's insertion. Similarly, prior to calling a loose body in front of or behind the PCL, care must be taken to try and follow the structure across to the lateral meniscus to determine if it is a meniscofemoral ligament.

COLLATERAL LIGAMENTS

The MCL originates on the medial femoral condyle and inserts on the tibia. It is closely applied to the joint and is intimately associated with the medial joint capsule and the medial meniscus. The MCL is uniformly low in signal on all imaging sequences. Injuries to the MCL usually occur from a valgus stress, a blow to the lateral part of the knee. A grade 1 injury represents a mild sprain and is diagnosed on MR imaging by noting fluid or hemorrhage in the soft tissues medial to the MCL. The ligament is otherwise normal. A grade 2 injury is a partial tear and is seen as high signal in and around the MCL on T2 coronal sequences; the ligament is intact, although the deep or superficial fibers may show minimal disruption (Fig. 9.25). A grade 3 injury is a complete disruption of the MCL. It can be best appreciated on T2 images (Fig. 9.26). It is unusual for a surgeon to operate on an MCL, even if it is a complete disruption. MCL partial tears, and even complete tears, heal quite nicely simply with immobilization.

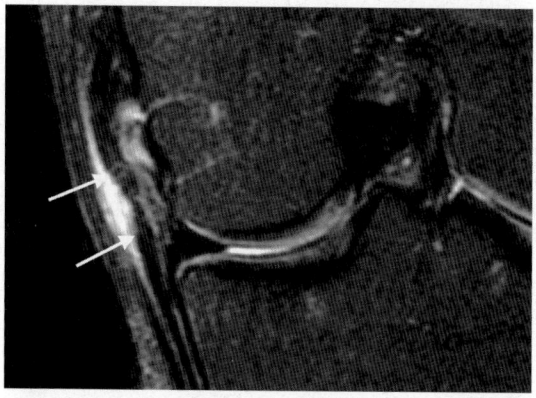

FIG. 9.25 **Grade 2 Sprain of The Medial Collateral Ligament (MCL).** A T2-weighted coronal image reveals high signal in the soft tissues adjacent to the MCL *(arrows)*, which represents edema and hemorrhage from a sprain of the MCL. The MCL is somewhat attenuated *(area between the arrows)*, indicative of a grade 2 sprain.

A meniscocapsular separation occurs when the medial meniscus is torn from its attachment to the joint capsule. It occurs most commonly at the site of the MCL and often occurs concomitantly with an MCL injury. It is easily recognized on a T2 coronal image by noting joint fluid extending between the medial meniscus and the capsule. It is essential to use T2 sequences because a T1-weighted image may not detect the fluid between the meniscus and the capsule (Fig. 9.27). They can be overlooked at arthroscopy if they involve only the superficial fibers of the capsule because they are then essentially extracapsular. It is

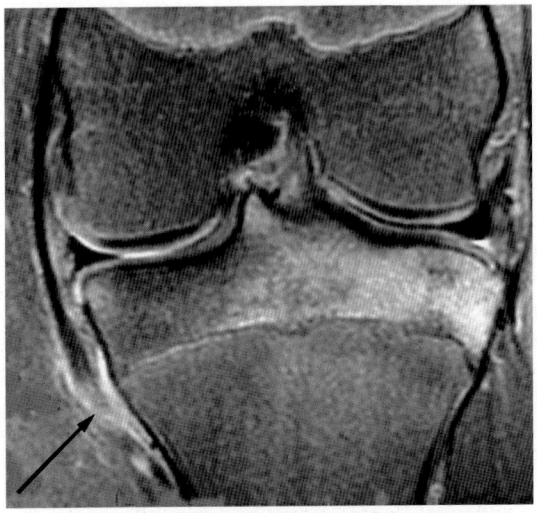

FIG. 9.26 **Torn Medial Collateral Ligament (MCL).** A coronal T2WI shows a tear of the MCL distally *(arrow)*.

an important diagnosis to make because it involves a very vascular portion of the meniscus; hence it will readily heal with immobilization or with suturing by the surgeon. If overlooked and continued activity occurs, it can lose the vascular interface and never heal.

The lateral collateral ligament consists of three parts. The most posterior structure is the tendon of the biceps femoris, which inserts onto the head of the fibula. Next, anterior to the biceps is the true lateral collateral ligament, also called the fibulocollateral ligament, which extends from the lateral femoral condyle to the head of the fibula (Fig. 9.28). The biceps and the fibulocollateral ligament usually join and insert onto the head of the fibula in a conjoined manner. Anterior to the fibulocollateral ligament is the iliotibial band, which extends into the fascia more anteriorly and inserts onto Gerdy's tubercle on the anterolateral tibia. The lateral collateral ligament complex is infrequently torn but can have significant long-term consequences of pain and instability in athletes if not treated aggressively. This is called posterolateral corner instability.

The posterolateral corner is basically the soft tissues in and around the lateral collateral ligament complex. These structures are injured in hyperextension and about 95% of the time are associated with a PCL and/or an ACL tear.[10] If an ACL and/or PCL tear is present with a tear of two or more of the following structures, posterolateral corner instability should be suggested: fibulocollateral ligament, biceps tendon, iliotibial band, popliteofibular ligament, popliteus tendon, and arcuate ligament (Fig. 9.29). Some of these structures are hard to identify and take a lot of experience; therefore one can simply suggest posterolateral corner injury if an ACL and/or PCL is torn and part of the lateral collateral ligament complex has a definite tear. This is a significant injury, and usually the surgeon appreciates a phone call, as many surgeons feel the posterolateral corner needs to be repaired promptly.

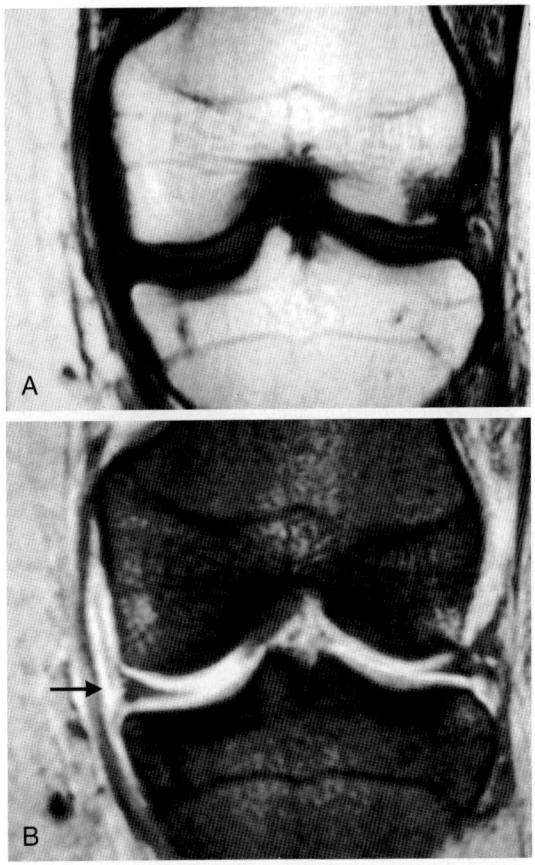

FIG. 9.27 **Meniscocapsular Separation.** (A) A T1-weighted coronal image reveals a contusion of the lateral femoral condyle *(arrow)* indicative of a valgus strain, which is often associated with a medial collateral ligament (MCL) tear. The MCL appears normal on this image; however, the linear low signal in the soft tissues just adjacent to the MCL is suggestive of fluid. This would indicate a partial tear or sprain of the MCL. (B) A coronal gradient-echo image in the same knee reveals fluid between the medial meniscus and the MCL *(arrow)*, which is diagnostic for a meniscocapsular separation. Faint high signal in the MCL and adjacent to it indicate a partial tear. A T2 or T2* sequence in the coronal plane are necessary to see these abnormalities.

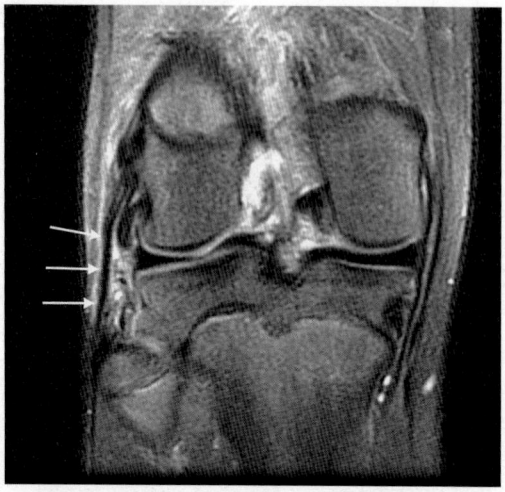

FIG. 9.28 **Normal Lateral Collateral Ligament.** This coronal fast spin-echo (FSE) T2 with fat suppression shows a normal fibulocollateral ligament (lateral collateral ligament) *(arrows)* extending from the lateral femoral condyle to the fibular head.

PATELLA AND CARTILAGE

The patellar cartilage commonly undergoes degeneration, causing exquisite pain and tenderness. This is called chondromalacia patella. It can be diagnosed on sagittal images but is generally more reliably identified on axial images. T2, T2*, or short tau inversion recovery (STIR) sequences are typically used to diagnose chondromalacia patella.

Chondromalacia begins with focal swelling and degeneration of the cartilage. This can be seen as high-signal foci in the cartilage. As it progresses, it causes thinning and irregularity of the articular surface of the cartilage, and finally underlying bone is exposed (Fig. 9.30).

A normal structure that is seen in over half of the population is the medial patellar plica. It is an embryologic remnant from when the knee was divided into three compartments. It is a thin fibrous band that extends from the medial capsule toward the medial facet of the patella (Fig. 9.31). A suprapatellar and infrapatellar plica can also be present. The medial patellar plica can, on rare occasions, thicken and cause clinical symptoms indistinguishable from a torn meniscus, which has been termed plica syndrome (Fig. 9.32). T2 images and a joint effusion are necessary to visualize a plica in most instances. An abnormal plica can be easily removed arthroscopically.

An abnormality that can clinically mimic plica syndrome, as well as mimic a torn meniscus, is bursitis. Several bursae typically are identified medially, which can become symptomatic. The first is the pes anserine bursa. Three tendons, the sartorius, gracilis, and semitendinosus (remembered by the mnemonic "Some Girls Stand"), insert onto the anteromedial aspect of the tibia in a fan-shaped manner that has been likened to a goose's foot, hence the name pes anserinus. A bursa lies beneath the insertion site, which can become inflamed and cause medial joint line or patellar pain that can be confused with plica syndrome or a torn medial meniscus (Fig. 9.33). A second, much more common, medial bursa is the semimembranosus tibial collateral ligament bursa (an unwieldy name, to say the least!). It occurs at the medial joint line and often mimics a meniscal cyst. It has a characteristic comma shape as it drapes over the semimembranosus tendon (Fig. 9.34). Making the diagnosis of pes anserinus or semimembranosus tibial collateral ligament bursitis with MR imaging can prevent an unnecessary arthroscopy procedure—one in which the bursa would be overlooked since they are extracapsular structures. Another medial-sided bursa that can become inflamed is an MCL bursa. It lies deep to the MCL, but can protrude anteriorly or posteriorly (Fig. 9.35).

BONY ABNORMALITIES

The most frequently encountered bony abnormality seen with MR imaging is a contusion. A contusion represents microfractures from trauma. They are also called bone bruises. They are easily identified on T1-weighted sequences as subarticular areas of inhomogeneous low signal. With T2-weighting, a contusion will show increased signal for several weeks, depending on its severity (Fig. 9.36). It can be difficult to see increased signal with T2* images because of the susceptibility artifacts of the bone inherent with T2* images. Contusions can progress to osteochondritis dissecans if they are not treated with diminished weight bearing; hence an isolated bone contusion, with no other internal derangement, is a serious finding that requires protected weight bearing.

A commonly seen contusion is one that occurs on the posterior part of the lateral tibial plateau (Fig. 9.37). It is invariably associated with a torn ACL.[11] A kissing contusion on the lateral femoral condyle is typically seen. When one or both of these contusions are present, an ACL tear is a virtual certainty. The only exception to this rule is in teenagers who are flexible enough to twist the knee and suffer the contusions while not tearing the ACL.

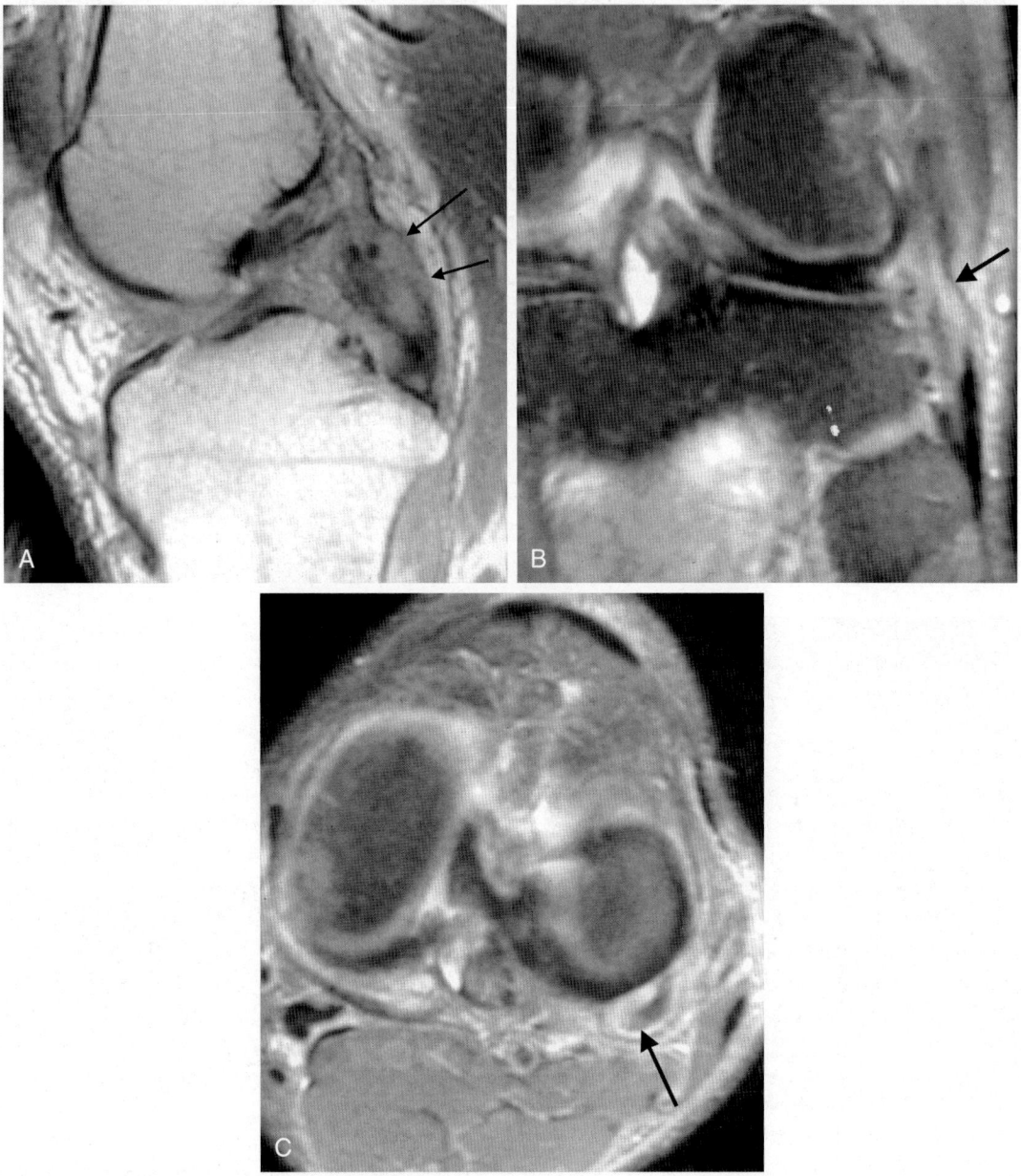

FIG. 9.29 **Posterolateral Corner Injury.** (A) This sagittal proton density image shows the posterior cruciate ligament (PCL) to be fat and increased in signal *(arrows),* indicative of a torn PCL. (B) A coronal fast spin-echo (FSE) T2 with fat suppression reveals a tear of the lateral collateral ligament *(arrow).* (C) An axial FSE T2 with fat suppression shows an injury to the popliteus tendon *(arrow)* with thickening and increased signal. This constellation of injuries indicates posterolateral corner instability.

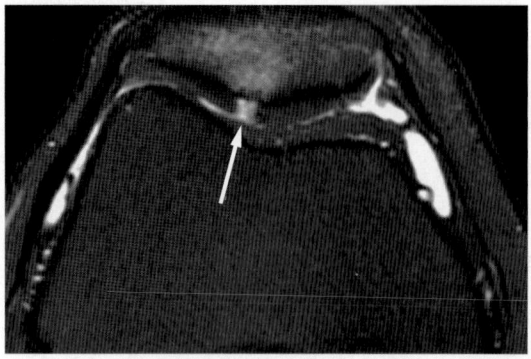

FIG. 9.30 **Chondromalacia Patella.** An axial T2-weighted image through the patella shows a focal chondral defect at the apex of the patella *(arrow).*

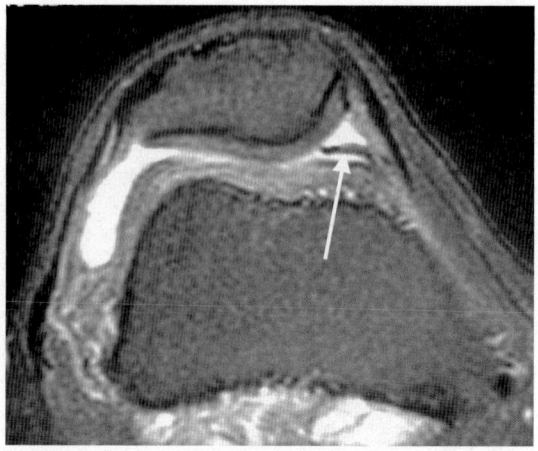

FIG. 9.32 **Thickened Medial Patellar Plica.** This axial fast spin-echo (FSE) T2-weighted image with fat suppression shows a thickened medial patellar plica *(arrow).* This patient presented with a painful clicking knee, symptoms typical for either a torn meniscus or plica syndrome.

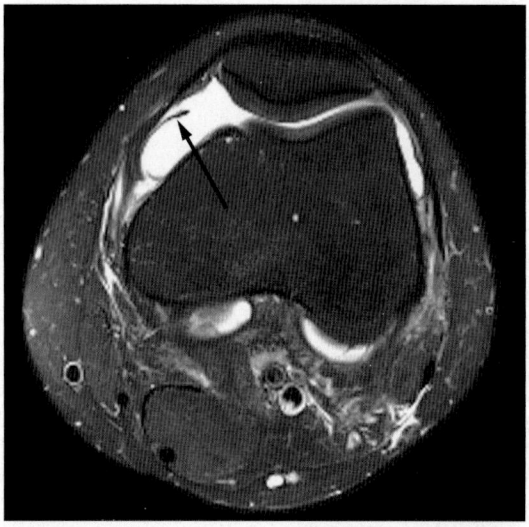

FIG. 9.31 **Plica.** An axial T2-weighted image through the patella shows a low-signal linear structure *(arrow)* extending from the medial capsule towards the medial facet of the patella. This is a normal medial patellar plica. Without the joint effusion or the T2 weighting, the plica would not be visualized.

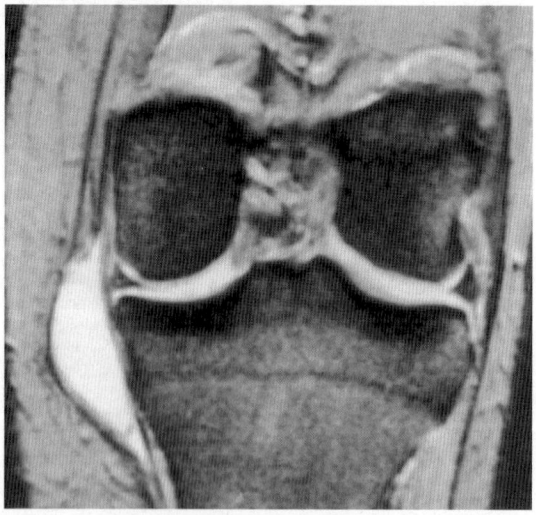

FIG. 9.33 **Pes Anserinus Bursitis.** A coronal T2* gradient echo image shows a fluid collection below the medial joint line near the insertion of the pes anserinus tendons. This is pes anserinus bursitis.

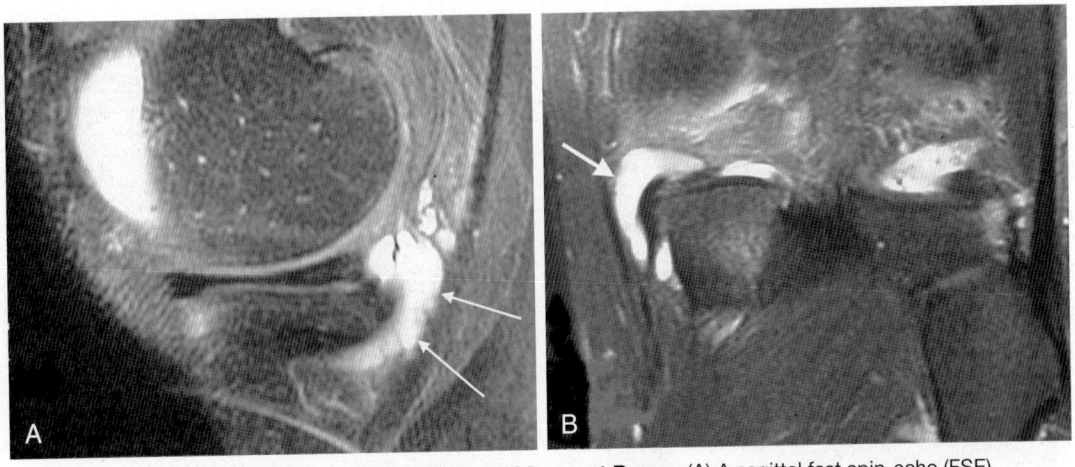

FIG. 9.34 **Semimembranosus Tibial Collateral Ligament Bursa.** (A) A sagittal fast spin-echo (FSE) T2-weighted image with fat suppression through the medial aspect of the knee shows a fluid collection *(arrows)* at the joint line that is adjacent to the posterior horn of the medial meniscus. This is characteristic of a semimembranosus medial collateral ligament bursa. (B) A coronal FSE T2-weighted image with fat suppression shows this bursa *(arrow)* at the joint line with a comma-shaped appearance.

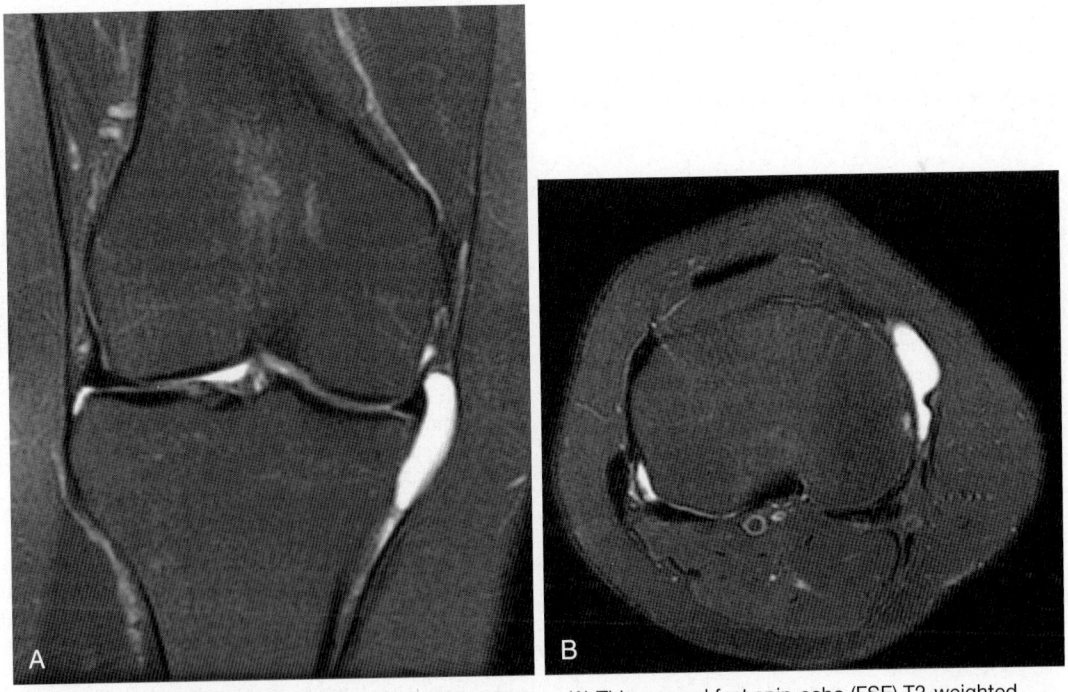

FIG. 9.35 **Medial Collateral Ligament (MCL) Bursa.** (A) This coronal fast spin-echo (FSE) T2-weighted image shows a fluid collection deep to the MCL, which is an MCL bursa. (B) An axial image shows the bursa deep to the MCL and protruding anteriorly.

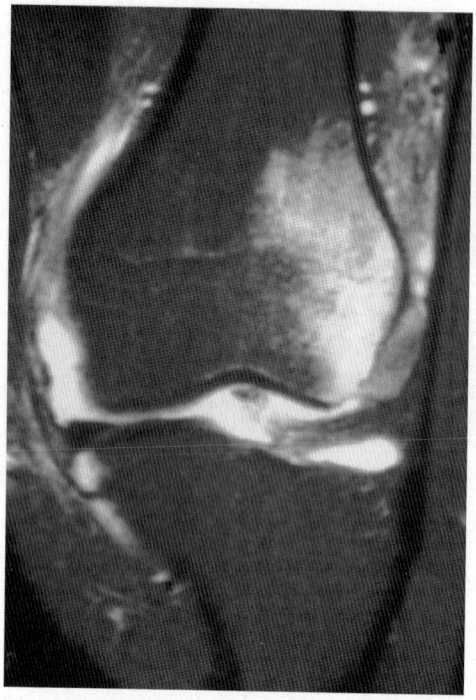

FIG. 9.36 **Contusion.** A coronal fast spin-echo (FSE) T2-weighted image with fat suppression shows a focus of high signal in the lateral femoral condyle, which is a characteristic appearance for a severe bone contusion. This occurred from a patella dislocation.

MR imaging is useful in examining fractures about the knee. Tibial plateau fractures can be imaged precisely with computed tomography; however, MR imaging allows the soft tissues, including internal derangements, to be seen in addition to any bony abnormalities.

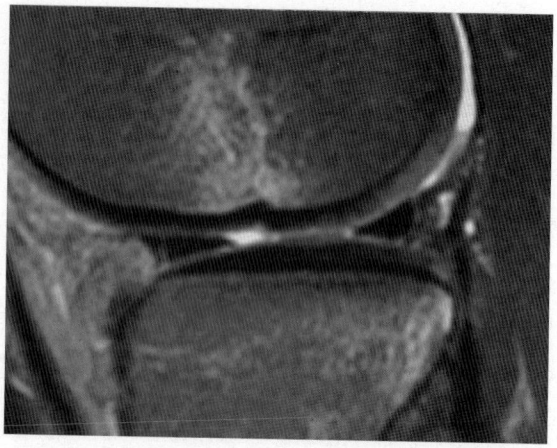

FIG. 9.37 **Contusions.** A sagittal fast spin-echo (FSE) T2-weighted image through the lateral compartment shows irregular high signal in a subarticular location in the posterior tibial plateau and in the anterior part of the lateral femoral condyle. These findings are characteristic for bone contusions. This distribution of contusions in the posterior lateral tibial plateau and anterior in the lateral femoral condyle is almost always associated with a torn anterior cruciate ligament.

REFERENCES

1. Ruwe P, Wright J, Randall R, Lynch J, Jokl P, McCarthy S. Can MR imaging effectively replace diagnostic arthroscopy? *Radiology*. 1992;183:335–339.
2. Crues JI, Mink J, Levy T, Lotysch M, Stoller D. Meniscal tears of the knee: accuracy of MR imaging. *Radiology*. 1987;164:445–448.
3. Mink JH, Deutsch AL. Magnetic resonance imaging of the knee. *Clin Orthop Relat Res*. 1989;244:29–47.
4. Helms CA. The meniscus: recent advances in MR imaging of the knee. *AJR*. 2002;179(5):1115–1122.
5. De Smet A, Norris M, et al. MR diagnosis of meniscal tears of the knee: importance of high signal in the meniscus that extends to the surface. *AJR*. 1993;161:101–107.
6. Helms CA, Laorr A, et al. The absent bow tie sign in bucket-handle tears of the menisci in the knee. *AJR*. 1998;170(1):57–61.
7. Anderson J, Helms CA. Conner: new observations on meniscal cysts. *Skeletal Radiology*. 2010;39:1187–1191.
8. Lee J, Yao L, Phelps C, Wirth C, Czajka J, Lozman J. Anterior cruciate ligament tears: MR imaging compared with arthroscopy and clinical tests. *Radiology*. 1988;166:861–864.
9. Rodriquez Jr W, Vinson EN, Helms CA, Toth AP. MRI appearance of PCL tears. *AJR*. 2008;191:W155–W159.
10. Covey DC. Injuries of the posterolateral corner of the knee. *J Bone Joint Surg Am*. 2001;83-A:106–118.
11. Murphy B, Smith R, Uribe J, Janecki C, Hechtman K, Mangasarian R. Bone signal abnormalities in the posterolateral tibia and lateral femoral condyle in complete tears of the anterior cruciate ligament: a specific sign? *Radiology*. 1992;182:221–224.

CHAPTER 10

Magnetic Resonance Imaging of the Shoulder

Magnetic resonance (MR) imaging of the shoulder has been shown to have a high degree of accuracy, especially when performed with arthrography.[1,2] Although most texts divide the shoulder into either cuff or labral abnormalities, it is important to know that cuff and labral pathology often coexist, causing great confusion in the clinical presentation and the physical exam. Most surgeons are aware that failure to address a labral abnormality when fixing a torn cuff can result in failed surgery, and conversely, fixing a labral abnormality and ignoring a cuff problem may not address the patient's real problem. MRI can show both the cuff and the labrum to good advantage. Also, MRI of the shoulder may reveal one of the entities I will discuss in the last part of this chapter, such as suprascapular nerve entrapment, quadrilateral space syndrome, or Parsonage–Turner syndrome, any one of which can present clinically with findings similar to a cuff problem.

ANATOMY

The rotator cuff is comprised of the tendons of four muscles that converge on the greater and lesser tuberosities of the humerus: the supraspinatus, infraspinatus, subscapularis, and teres minor (Fig. 10.1). Of these, the supraspinatus is the one that most commonly causes clinically significant problems and is almost exclusively the one that is addressed surgically.

The supraspinatus tendon lies just superior to the scapula and inferior to the acromioclavicular joint and the acromion. In inserts onto the greater tuberosity of the humerus. One to two centimeters proximal to its insertion is a section of the tendon called the "critical zone." This area is reported to have decreased vascularity and is therefore less likely to heal following trauma. It is also the area of the tendon that undergoes fibrillar and myxoid degeneration (also called tendinosis), presumably from aging and trauma, although this has not been proven. The critical zone of the supraspinatus tendon is where many rotator cuff tears occur, although the majority occur at the bone/tendon interface.

The glenoid labrum is a fibrocartilaginous ring that surrounds the periphery of the bony glenoid of the scapula. It serves as an attachment site for the capsule and broadens the base of the glenohumeral joint to allow increased stability. Tears of the glenoid labrum most commonly occur from, and result in, humeral head instability and dislocations.

IMAGING PROTOCOL

There are many variations in the imaging protocol that are all acceptable for showing normal and pathologic findings in the shoulder. The rotator cuff, that is, the supraspinatus tendon, is best seen on oblique coronal images that are aligned parallel to the supraspinatus muscle (Fig. 10.2). T2-weighted sequences, or acceptable variations, are mandatory. A commonly used protocol is an oblique coronal fast spin-echo (FSE) T2-weighted sequence with fat suppression. The slice thickness should be no greater than 5 mm, and 3 mm is preferable. As with most joint imaging, a small field of view (16–20 cm) is recommended. A dedicated shoulder coil or a surface coil placed anteriorly over the shoulder is necessary, although no particular type of shoulder coil appears to be clearly superior.

The glenoid labrum is best seen on axial T2-weighted images. T1-weighted images do not give any additional information and can be eliminated. If a joint effusion is present, the labrum is easily identified. Without fluid in the joint, it can be more difficult to clearly see the labrum; therefore many radiologists will perform an MR arthrogram. Either saline alone, or saline mixed with a small amount of gadolinium (a ratio of 1:250 is recommended), can be injected into the joint followed by MR imaging. MR arthrography is a routine part of shoulder imaging in many centers.

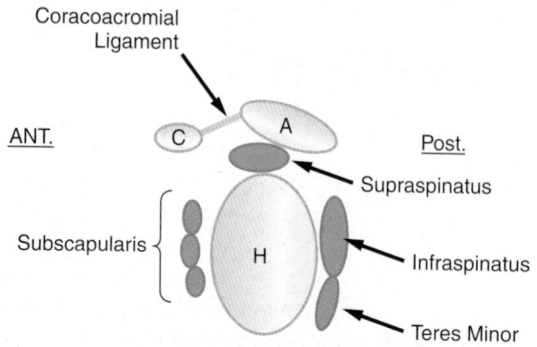

FIG. 10.1 **Schematic of Shoulder Anatomy.** This drawing shows the rotator cuff muscles in a sagittal plane (*A*, Acromion; *C*, coracoid; *H*, humeral head; anterior is on the left).

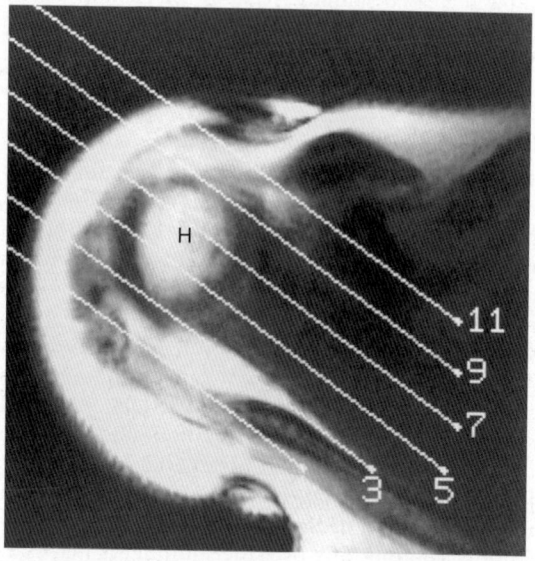

FIG. 10.2 **Scout View for Oblique Coronal Images.** This axial image through the supraspinatus shows the cursors angled along the plane of the supraspinatus muscle (anterior on top; *H*, Humeral head).

The oblique sagittal sequence is one of the most useful and is performed in our protocol as a standard T1-weighted sequence without fat suppression (to identify fatty atrophy) and as an FSE T2-weighted sequence with fat suppression. This is very useful in identifying cuff tears, fluid collections about the shoulder, and muscle edema. With T2 weighting, fluid in the subacromial bursa can occasionally be seen to better advantage than on the oblique coronal images.

ROTATOR CUFF

The etiology of rotator cuff disease has for decades been thought to be due to impingement or wear and tear on the cuff due to entrapment from the acromion and A-C joint osteophytes. Coracoacromial arch decompression was one of the most common procedures for shoulder pain, whereby the coracoacromial ligament was cut, the anterolateral portion of the acromion was removed, and A-C joint osteophytes were resected. More recently, coracoacromial arch decompression has largely been abandoned, with most shoulder specialists agreeing that impingement is not a true entity and that intrinsic degeneration is the most likely source of most rotator cuff problems.[2,3] Treating intrinsic degeneration requires debriding the abnormal tissue and repairing the cuff.

In examining the rotator cuff, the anterior-most oblique coronal images will show the critical zone of the supraspinatus tendon. A useful landmark for noting the supraspinatus tendon is the bicipital groove, which has the anterior-most fibers of the supraspinatus just lateral to the groove. This is where most cuff tears begin and can be easily overlooked if the shoulder is internally rotated, which is common[4] (Fig. 10.3).

The normal supraspinatus tendon is said to be uniformly low in signal on all pulse sequences. Unfortunately, this is not always the case. In fact, it usually has some intermediate to high signal in the critical zone, which has caused much confusion in the evolution of interpreting shoulder MR imaging exams. We imaged around 20 "normal" volunteers (residents and fellows) in the early days of learning shoulder MR imaging, and only found one or two that had uniform low signal throughout the critical zone. This was very distressing because the literature at that time said any high signal in the critical zone meant it was abnormal. We know now that there are many causes for intermediate to high signal on T1-weighted images in the normal shoulder. We no longer even obtain an oblique coronal T1-weighted sequence, as it does not add any additional information to the oblique coronal FSE T2-weighted sequence.

If signal in the critical zone is brighter on the T2-weighted images, it is abnormal and represents a partial tear if it is fluid bright. A partial tear can also be present if the cuff has focal thinning of the tendon (Fig. 10.4).

Myxoid or fibrillar degeneration of the supraspinatus tendon are commonly found in autopsy specimens, which increases with age. The majority of asymptomatic shoulders in patients over the age of

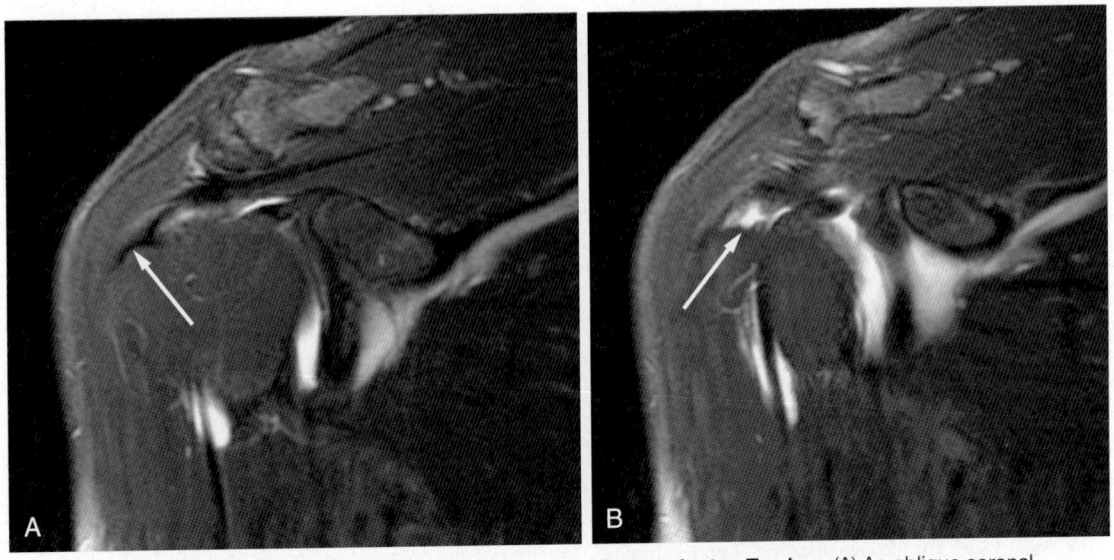

FIG. 10.3 **Internal Rotation Hiding Partial Tear of the Supraspinatus Tendon.** (A) An oblique coronal fast spin-echo (FSE) T2WI shows an apparently normal supraspinatus inserting onto the greater tuberosity *(arrow)*. (B) One slice anteriorly, the bicipital groove can be identified with the anterior fibers of the supraspinatus just lateral to the groove lifted off of the greater tuberosity *(arrow)*. This is a partial tear of the rotator cuff at its anterior-most portion.

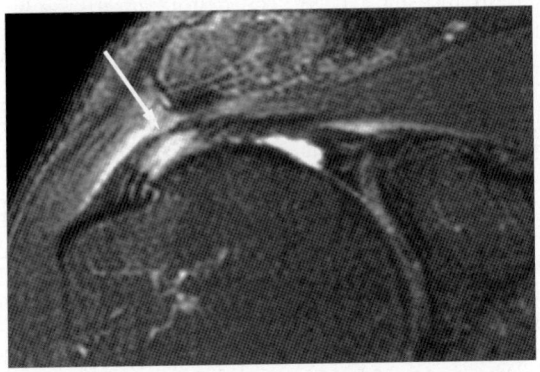

FIG. 10.4 **Partial Tear of the Supraspinatus.** An oblique coronal fast spin-echo (FSE) T2WI with fat suppression shows thinning of the supraspinatus tendon *(arrow)*, which is a partial articular-sided cuff tear.

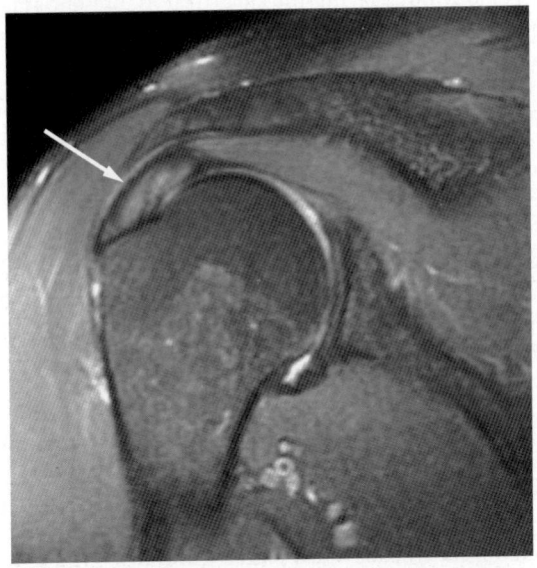

FIG. 10.5 **Tendinosis.** An oblique coronal fast spin-echo (FSE) T2WI shows intermediate signal in a supraspinatus tendon that has fusiform swelling. This is myxoid degeneration or tendinosis.

50 are felt to have some tendon degeneration in the supraspinatus, which has been termed "tendinosis." This is seen as intermediate to high signal in the critical zone on T1-weighted images that does not increase with T2 weighting.[5] Some tendon degeneration (tendinosis) can be seen in asymptomatic shoulders of all ages; hence it needs to be correlated with the clinical picture. If the signal gets brighter on T2-weighted images, it must be considered pathologic—a partial tear. If intermediate signal in the cuff tendons is accompanied by fusiform or focal thickening, myxoid degeneration is present (Fig. 10.5). Surgeons will debride this when it is prominent.

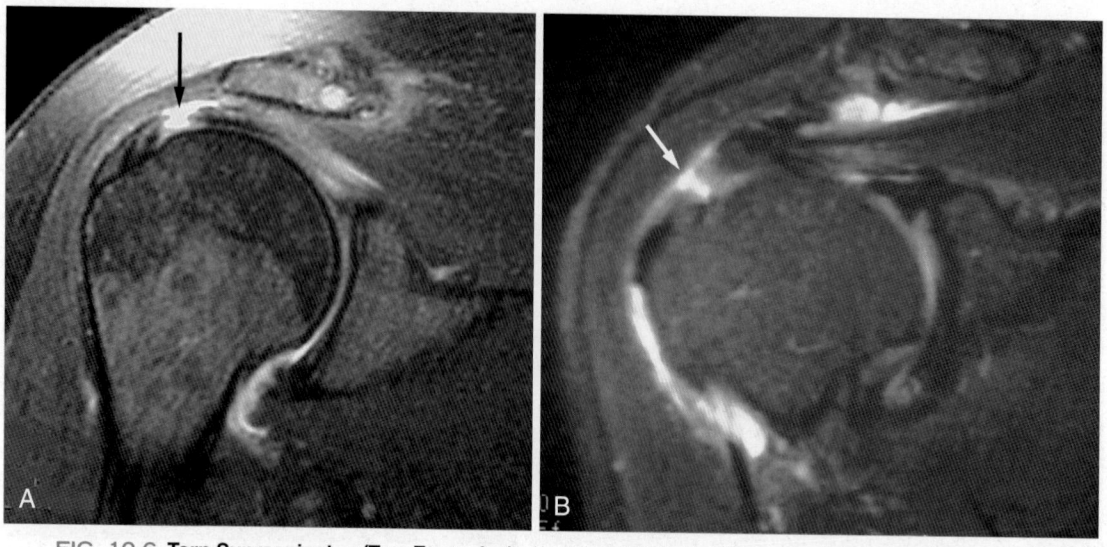

FIG. 10.6 **Torn Supraspinatus (Two Examples).** (A) This oblique coronal fast spin-echo (FSE) T2WI with fat suppression shows a gap in the supraspinatus tendon *(arrow)*. (B) This oblique coronal FSE T2WI with fat suppression shows a gap in the supraspinatus tendon *(arrow)*.

If disruption of the supraspinatus tendon can be seen, obviously a full-thickness tear is present (Fig. 10.6). In these cases, fluid is invariably present in the subacromial bursa. Care should be taken to look for retraction of the supraspinatus muscle, as marked retraction will obviate some types of surgery.

PARTIAL TEARS

Partial cuff tears have marked clinical significance, since most agree that they will not heal on their own if they are greater than 25% of the cuff thickness.[6] Although we generally can't be so precise as to what percentage of the cuff is involved, we can usually identify partial cuff tears. If there is an irregularity or thinning of the cuff on either the bursal side of the cuff or on the joint side, I will describe it as small, medium, or large (near full thickness). Bursal sided partial tears are exceedingly uncommon, 25–30 times less frequent than articular sided partial tears. The most common cuff tear encountered is an articular sided partial tear called a rim rent. It occurs at the insertion of the fibers of the cuff onto the greater tuberosity, most commonly anteriorly at the insertion of the supraspinatus (Fig. 10.7). Rim rent tears comprise 20%–40% of all cuff tears.[4]

BONY ABNORMALITIES

In about 5% of the population, the distal acromion fails to fuse with the scapula, leaving an unfused apophysis called an os acromiale (Fig. 10.8). This should fuse by age 25. The deltoid inserts on the acromion, and, if a mobile os acromiale is present, it can pull the acromion down like a flap with resultant cuff impingement. As the surgeon cannot see this at arthroscopy (or with open surgery), it is imperative to identify an os acromiale preoperatively so the surgeon can consider fusing it.

Abnormalities of the humeral head include sclerosis and cystic changes about the greater tuberosity that are commonly present in patients with rotator cuff tears. Bony impaction on the posterosuperior aspect of the humeral head can be seen in patients with anterior instability of the humeral head. This is called a Hill–Sachs lesion and is best identified on the superior-most two or three axial images (Fig. 10.9). The normal humeral head should be round on the superior slices—an irregularity posteriorly is abnormal. A Hill–Sachs lesion is almost always associated with a torn or detached anterior inferior labrum (called a Bankart deformity).

GLENOID LABRUM

Tears or detachment of the glenoid labrum result in glenohumeral joint instability. They are commonly caused by dislocations, but less traumatic episodes, such as repeated trauma from throwing, can result in labral tears. Torn or detached labra are often repaired arthroscopically with good results. Labrum

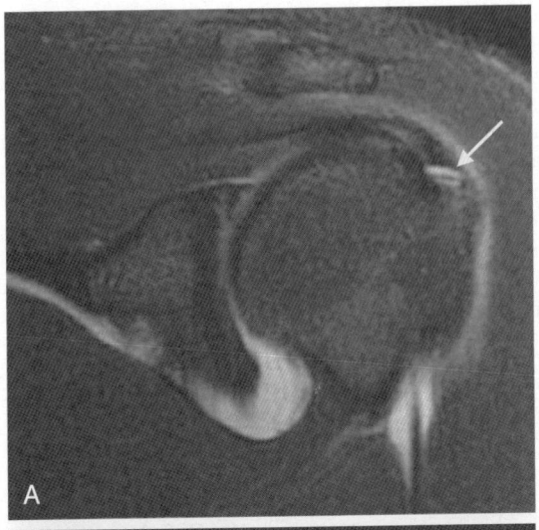

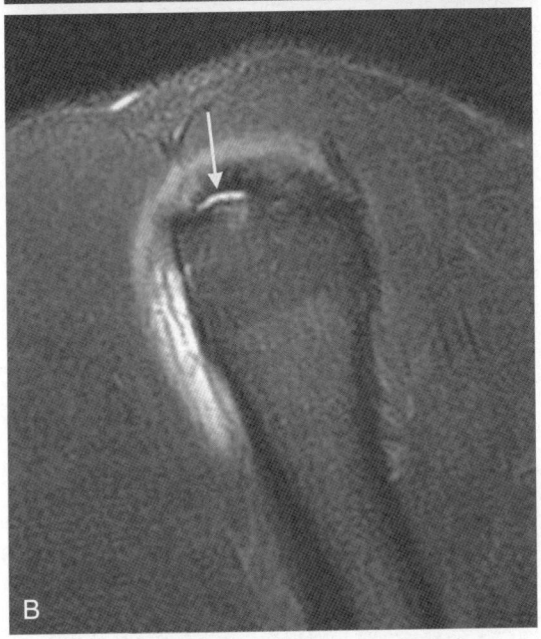

FIG. 10.7 **Rim Rent Tear.** (A) This oblique coronal fast spin-echo (FSE) T2-weighted image with fat suppression shows linear increased signal at the insertion of the supraspinatus *(arrow)*. (B) The oblique sagittal FSE T2-weighted image with fat suppression shows the same finding located anteriorly *(arrow)*. This is a partial tear on the articular side of the cuff.

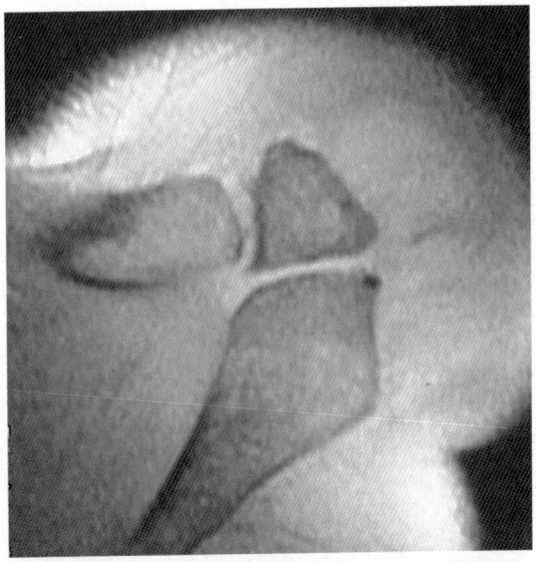

FIG. 10.8 **Os Acromiale.** An axial fast spin-echo (FSE) T2WI with fat suppression through the upper part of the shoulder shows an unfused apophysis of the acromion, which is an os acromiale.

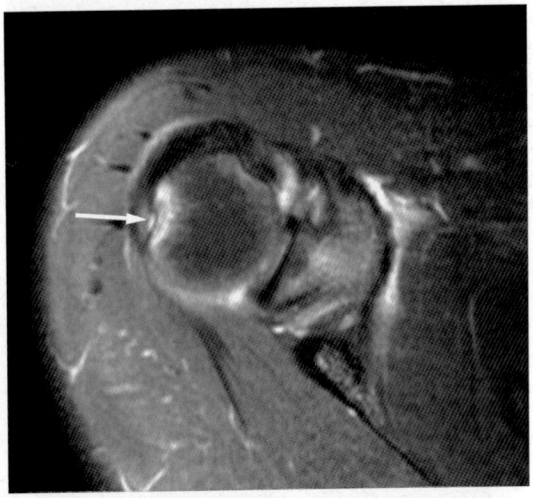

FIG. 10.9 **Hill–Sachs Lesion.** An axial fast spin-echo (FSE) T2WI with fat suppression through the superior portion of the humeral head shows a posterior impaction *(arrow)* caused by the glenoid labrum during an anterior dislocation of the humerus. This has been termed a Hill–Sachs lesion.

and rotator cuff abnormalities often coexist, and an abnormality of one can lead to an abnormality in the other.

The normal labrum is a triangular-shaped low-signal structure, as viewed on an axial image, with the anterior labrum usually larger than the posterior labrum (Fig. 10.10). The anterior labrum is said to be much more commonly involved with tears than the posterior, and the superior labrum is said to be rarely involved. In fact, the posterior and the superior labra are torn as often as the anterior labrum.

The superior labrum is best evaluated on the oblique coronal views. Tears of the superior labrum are called SLAP lesions (superior labrum anterior to posterior). They are said to be seen mostly in throwing athletes as a result of the insertion of the long head of the biceps tendon onto the labrum avulsing part of the labrum during a forceful throwing motion. In fact, they can be seen in any shoulder; however, since they cause a decrease in performance in the elite throwing athlete, these patients attract more attention.

If no joint effusion is present, a labral tear can be difficult to see unless it is extremely large. If joint fluid extends between the bony glenoid and the base of the labrum, a detached labrum is present. In the anteroinferior labrum, this is called a Bankart deformity (Fig. 10.11). Tears in the body of the labrum are diagnosed by noting fluid extending into the labrum or by truncation of the labrum. The attachment of the glenohumeral ligaments to the labrum can strip off, resulting in instability, just as with a torn or detached labrum. This is termed a labroligamentous disruption (Fig. 10.12). Therefore

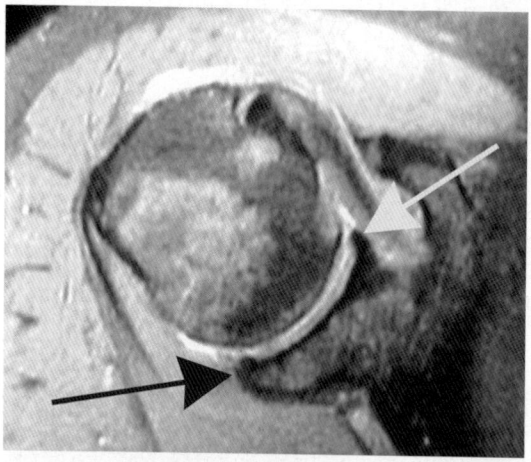

FIG. 10.10 **Normal Labrum.** An axial T2* gradient-echo image shows a normal anterior *(white arrow)* and posterior *(black arrow)* glenoid labrum. The anterior labrum is usually larger than the posterior.

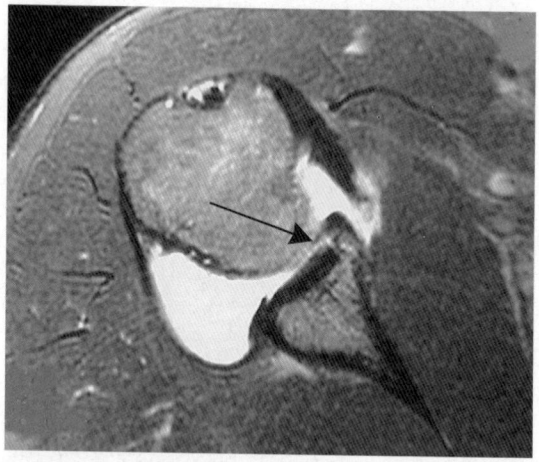

FIG. 10.11 **Detached Labrum.** An axial fast spin-echo (FSE) T2WI with fat suppression shows a tear of the anterior labrum *(arrow)*.

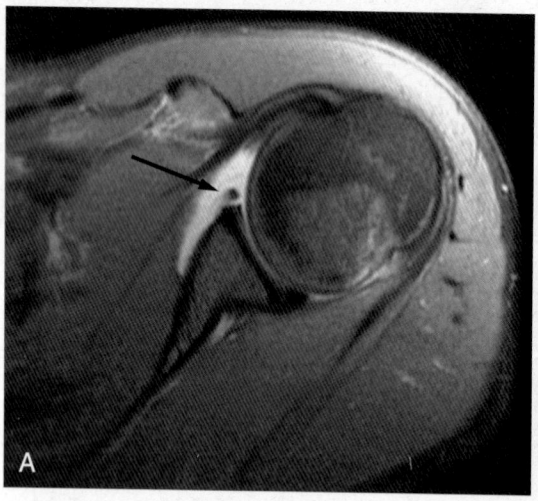

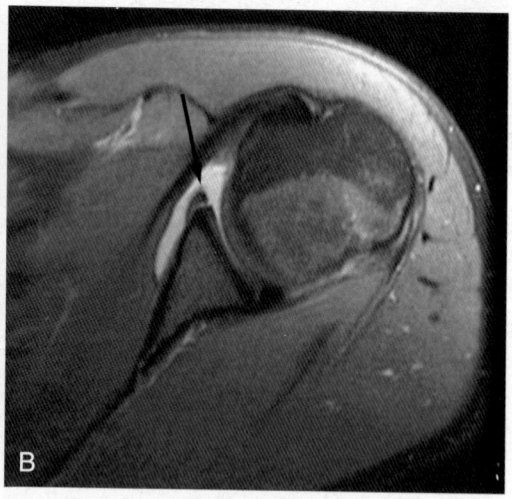

FIG. 10.12 **Labroligamentous Tear.** (A) An axial fast spin-echo (FSE) T2WI with fat suppression through the inferior glenoid shows detachment of the inferior glenohumeral ligament from the anterior labrum *(arrow)*. (B) One slice more inferiorly shows the stripping of the ligament extending down the labrum *(arrow)*.

a shoulder dislocation can result in one of three types of abnormalities of the labrum: (1) a detachment, (2) a tear, or (3) a labroligamentous tear.

Several variations of normal exist in the labrum, which can be confused for pathologic conditions. The most common one is seen in the superior labrum at the biceps attachment. This is a sublabral recess (Fig. 10.13), and it can be very difficult at times to differentiate from a SLAP tear. It should only be seen near the anterior portion of the superior labrum where the biceps attaches, and should be thin and smooth in configuration. It is found in up to 40% of shoulders, and quite frankly I often find cases in which I cannot confidently tell if it is a sublabral recess or a SLAP tear.

Another commonly seen variant, found in 10%–20% of shoulders, is a sublabral foramen. Like the sublabral recess, it has the appearance of a detached labrum (Fig. 10.14); however, it is differentiated from a detached labrum by its location in the anterosuperior quadrant of the glenoid—a location that is virtually immune from isolated labral pathology. A much less common variant is the Buford complex. It consists of an absent anterosuperior labrum with a thickened, cord-like middle glenohumeral ligament (Fig. 10.15). It is found in only about 1%–3% of shoulders.

BICEPS TENDON

The long head of the biceps tendon runs in the bicipital groove between the greater and lesser tuberosities and inserts onto the superior labrum. It can have a partial tear or a complete tear, or it can undergo myxoid degeneration similar to the cuff. In tenosynovitis, fluid can be seen in the tendon sheath surrounding an otherwise normal tendon. Because fluid in the glenohumeral joint can normally fill the biceps tendon sheath, this diagnosis is difficult to make with MR imaging alone. If the tendon is enlarged and/or has signal within it, tendinosis is present (Fig. 10.16). If the tendon is not seen on one or more of the axial images, it is disrupted (Fig. 10.17) or dislocated.

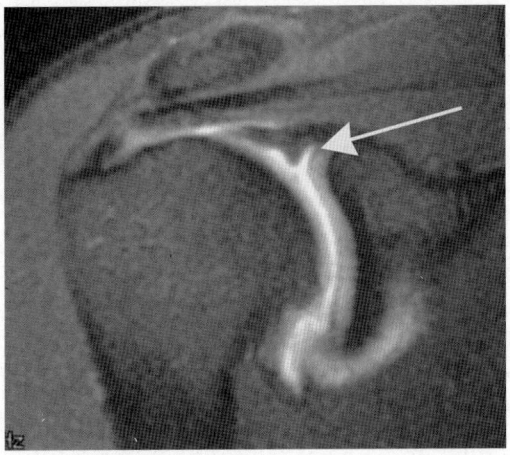

FIG. 10.13 **Sublabral Recess.** A coronal T1-weighted gadolinium arthrogram with fat suppression shows fluid between the superior labrum and the cartilage *(arrow)* of the bony glenoid, which is thin and smooth. This is a sublabral recess.

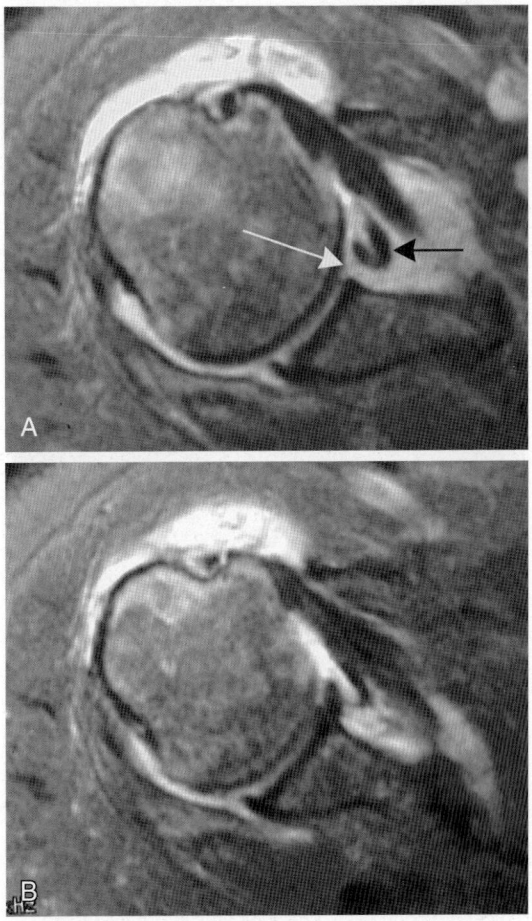

FIG. 10.14 **Sublabral Foramen.** (A) An axial fast spin-echo (FSE) T2WI with fat suppression through the glenohumeral joint at the level of the coracoid shows a space between the anterior labrum and the bony glenoid *(white arrow)*, which is a sublabral foramen. A detached labrum could have this appearance, but this is in the anterosuperior part of the joint. The middle glenohumeral ligament *(black arrow)* is seen as a separate structure anterior to the labrum. (B) A few slices inferiorly, the labrum is seen attached firmly to the anterior glenoid.

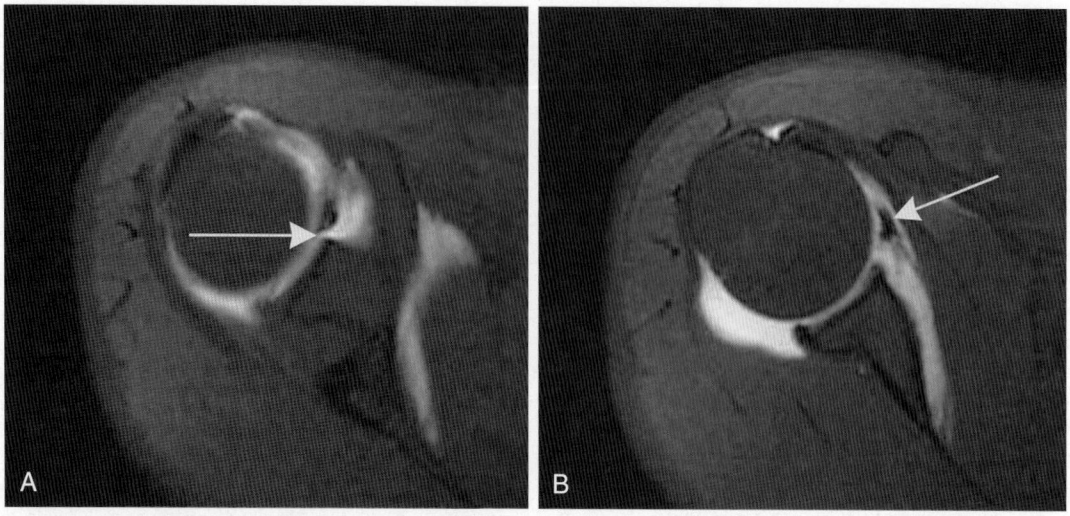

FIG. 10.15 **Buford Complex.** (A) An axial fast spin-echo (FSE) T2-weighted image with fat suppression through the upper part of the joint shows the anterior labrum appearing to be separated from the bony glenoid *(arrow)*. (B) Lower in the joint, the anterior labrum is firmly attached to the glenoid, but a thick, cord-like middle glenohumeral ligament is present *(arrow)*. This is a Buford complex. In (A), the anterior labrum is absent, and a thick middle glenohumeral ligament is simulating the anterior labrum.

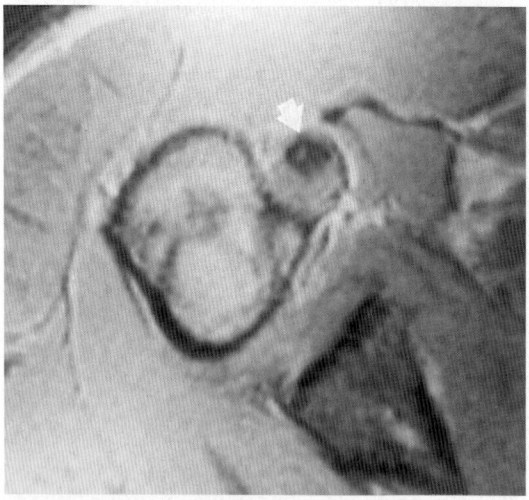

FIG. 10.16 **Biceps Tendinosis.** An axial gradient-echo image shows the bicipital groove to be empty *(arrow)*, with no biceps tendon seen. This indicates a torn, retracted biceps tendon.

When dislocation occurs, the tendon can be seen to lie anteromedial to the bicipital groove (Fig. 10.18), and it is inferred that the superior fibers of the subscapularis are torn.

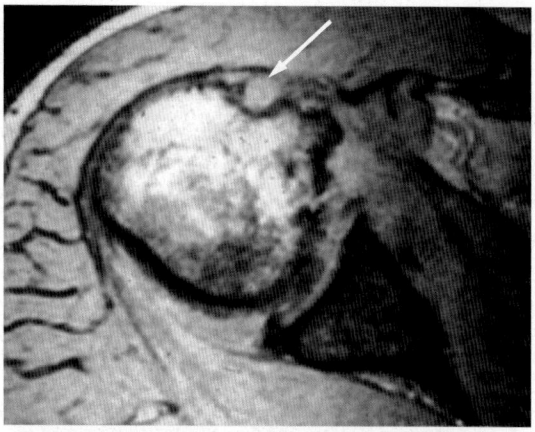

FIG. 10.17 **Ruptured Biceps Tendon.** An axial gradient-echo image shows the biceps tendon sheath filled with fluid *(arrow)* but with no tendon. This indicates a torn biceps tendon.

SUPRASCAPULAR NERVE ENTRAPMENT

The suprascapular nerve is made up of branches from the C4, C5, and C6 roots of the brachial plexus. It runs superior to the scapula, from anterior to posterior, just medial to the coracoid process. It gives off a branch that innervates the supraspinatus muscle as it courses posteriorly in the suprascapular notch. It then innervates the

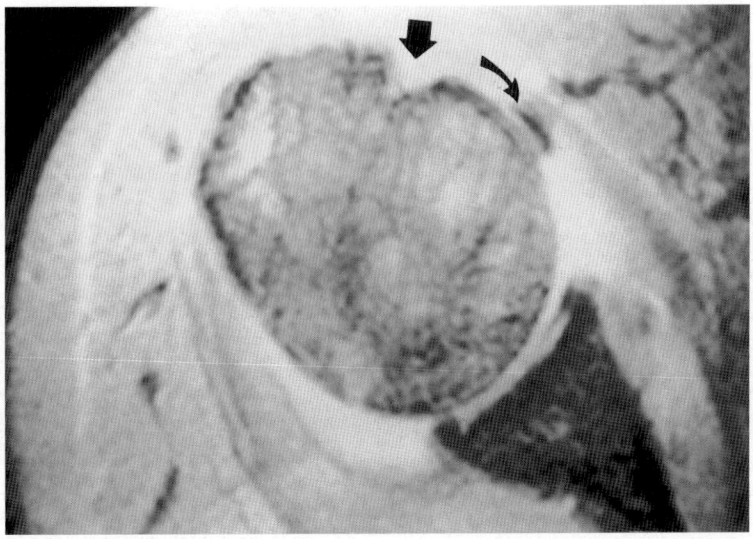

FIG. 10.18 **Dislocated Biceps Tendon.** This axial gradient-echo image shows an empty bicipital groove *(arrow)*, suggesting a torn biceps tendon; however, the biceps tendon is dislocated and can be seen anterior to the labrum *(curved arrow)*.

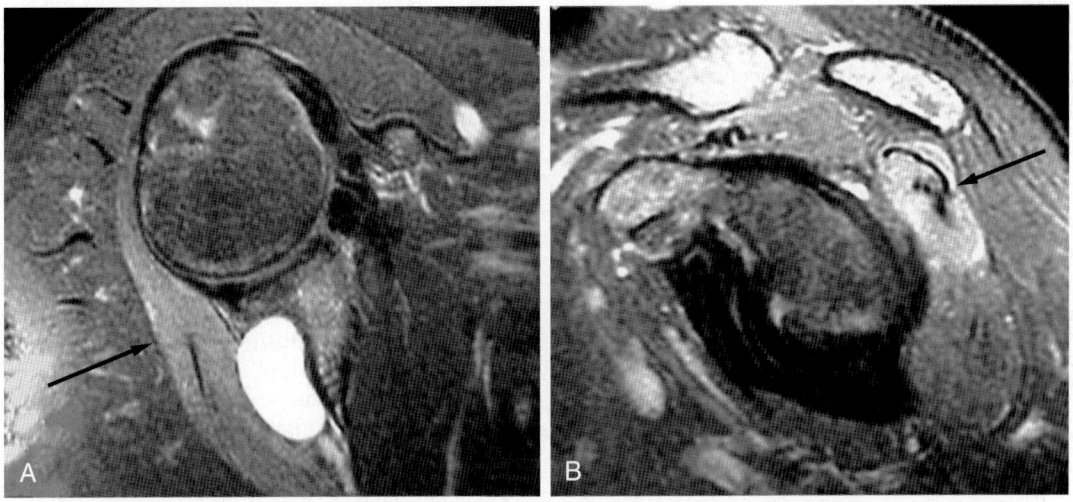

FIG. 10.19 **Ganglion in Spinoglenoid Notch.** (A) An axial fast spin-echo (FSE) T2-weighted image with fat suppression reveals a high-signal mass posterior to the scapula in the spinoglenoid notch. Note the neurogenic edema in the infraspinatus muscle *(arrow)*. (B) A sagittal image shows the infraspinatus edema *(arrow)* as well as atrophy (compare the size of the infraspinatus to the adjacent teres minor and note the difference). This is a ganglion that has impressed the suprascapular nerve, causing shoulder pain and atrophy of the infraspinatus muscle.

infraspinatus as it runs inferiorly through the spinoglenoid notch in the posterior scapula. A not uncommon finding is a ganglion in the spinoglenoid notch that impresses the infraspinatus portion of the nerve with resultant pain. Atrophy and/or edema of the infraspinatus muscle is seen on MRI (Fig. 10.19).[7] These are always associated with a torn or detached posterior labrum. This has been reported almost exclusively in

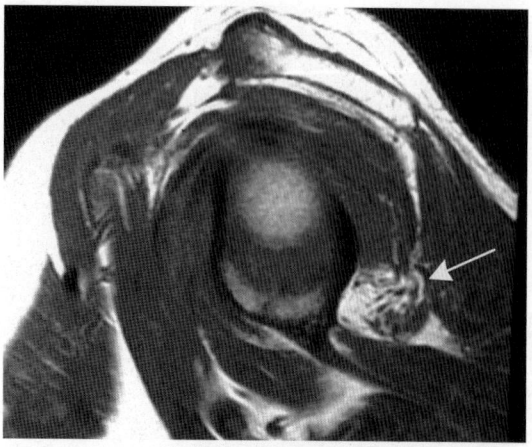

FIG. 10.20 **Quadrilateral Space Syndrome.** This oblique sagittal T1-weighted image shows fatty atrophy of the teres minor muscle *(arrow)*, which is diagnostic of quadrilateral space syndrome.

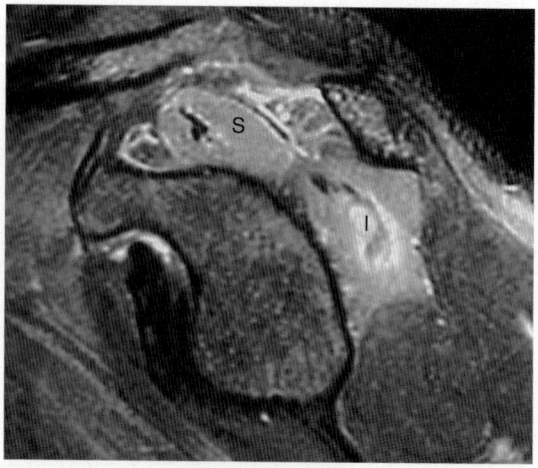

FIG. 10.21 **Parsonage–Turner Syndrome.** An oblique sagittal T2-weighted image with fat suppression shows edema in the supraspinatus *(S)* and the infraspinatus *(I)* muscles, consistent with involvement of the suprascapular nerve. The sudden onset with no history of trauma is characteristic for Parsonage–Turner syndrome.

males who are athletic, particularly weightlifters. It is important to see on preoperative MRI, as the ganglion is extracapsular and cannot be seen at arthroscopy. These patients can clinically mimic having a rotator cuff tear; hence MRI is critical to making this diagnosis.

QUADRILATERAL SPACE SYNDROME

My search pattern for a shoulder MRI begins with the oblique sagittal T1-weighted images to look for fatty atrophy in any of the cuff muscles. If the infraspinatus is smaller than the other muscles and/or has fatty infiltration, the aforementioned suprascapular nerve entrapment secondary to a ganglion in the spinoglenoid notch is the likely diagnosis. If the teres minor has fatty atrophy (Fig. 10.20), the only diagnosis I'm aware of is quadrilateral space syndrome. This most commonly occurs from fibrous bands or scar tissue in the quadrilateral space impinging on the axillary nerve. The quadrilateral space lies between the teres minor superiorly, the teres major inferiorly, the long head of the triceps medially, and the diaphysis of the humerus laterally. The axillary nerve traverses the quadrilateral space and innervates the teres minor and deltoid muscles; however, the deltoid is never involved in quadrilateral space syndrome. We have found quadrilateral space syndrome in about 1% of our shoulder MRIs. These patients can present clinically similar to a rotator cuff tear, and I have seen several patients who have had needless surgery for presumed cuff pathology when the real problem was quadrilateral space syndrome. Generally, no surgery is necessary, as physical therapy is usually successful in breaking up the fibrous bands or scar tissue that cause this entity.

PARSONAGE–TURNER SYNDROME

After I look at the oblique sagittal T1-weighted images for fatty atrophy, I look at the oblique sagittal FSE T2-weighted fat-suppressed images for muscle edema. In about 1% of cases, neurogenic edema is found in muscle groups, which corresponds to a particular nerve (i.e., supraspinatus/infraspinatus = suprascapular nerve; teres minor/deltoid = axillary nerve). This is characteristic for Parsonage–Turner syndrome (Fig. 10.21). It becomes pathognomonic once the clinical presentation is provided. If there is no history of trauma or of an insidious onset, and if the onset is sudden, with severe pain, followed in a day or two with profound weakness, the edema pattern is virtually pathognomonic for Parsonage–Turner syndrome.

The etiology of Parsonage–Turner syndrome is unknown, but it seems to have an association with prior vaccinations, viral illness, or general anesthesia in about one-third of cases. It is bilateral in about 10%–15% of cases. It affects all ages of both sexes and is self-limited. It can affect either the axillary or suprascapular nerve, or both simultaneously. For that matter, it can affect any of the brachial plexus nerves, including the long thoracic and phrenic. I have seen unnecessary shoulder, brachial plexus, and cervical spine surgery performed before the correct diagnosis of Parsonage–Turner syndrome was made.

Parsonage–Turner syndrome was first described in the radiology literature in 1998, indicating we all missed it on MRI for over 15 years.[8] That's because we did not routinely fat-suppress our shoulder images until the early 1990s, and the edema in the muscles was not conspicuous enough to be picked up on non–fat suppressed sequences.

REFERENCES

1. Palmer W, Brown J, et al. Rotator cuff: evaluation with fat-suppressed MR arthrography. *Rad*. 1993;188:683–688.
2. Budoff JE, Nirschl RP, Guidi EJ. Debridement of partial-thickness tears of the rotator cuff without acromioplasty. Long-term follow-up and review of the literature. *JBJS*. 1998;80:733–748.
3. Papadonikolakis A, McKenna M, Warme W, Martin BL, Matsen 3rd FA. Published evidence relative to the diagnosis of impingement syndrome of the shoulder. *JBJS*. 2011;93:1827–1832.
4. Vinson EN, Helms CA, Higgins LD. Rim-rent tears of the rotator cuff: a common and easily overlooked partial tear. *AJR*. 2007;189:943–946.
5. Kjellin I, Ho CP, Cervilla V, et al. Alterations in the supraspinatus tendon at MR imaging: correlation with histopathologic findings in cadavers. *Radiology*. 1991;181: 837–841.
6. Fukuda H. The management of partial-thickness tears of the rotator cuff. *J Bone Joint Surg Br*. 2003;85:3–11.
7. Fritz R, Helms C, Steinbach L, Genant H. Suprascapular nerve entrapment: evaluation with MR imaging. *Radiology*. 1992;182:437–444.
8. Helms CA, Martinez S, et al. Acute brachial neuritis (Parsonage-Turner-syndrome) - MR imaging appearance - report of three cases. *Radiology*. 1998;207:255–259.

CHAPTER 11

Lumbar Spine: Disc Disease and Stenosis

Imaging the lumbar spine for disc disease and stenosis has evolved in the past 30 years from predominantly myelography-oriented exams to plain computed tomography (CT) and magnetic resonance (MR) imaging exams. Although few differences between CT and MR imaging have been noted concerning diagnostic accuracy in the lumbar spine, MR imaging will give more information and a more complete anatomic depiction than will CT.[1,2] There are a host of things that can be seen on an MR imaging study that cannot be seen with CT. For example, MR imaging can determine if a disc is degenerated by showing loss of signal on T2-weighted images (Fig. 11.1). CT cannot give this information, but it hardly matters since no treatment is currently given solely for a degenerated disc. In fact, degenerative discs have been reported in asymptomatic children who deny a past history of back pain.[3] Nevertheless, MRI has evolved as the imaging procedure of choice for the lumbar spine.

IMAGING PROTOCOLS

To achieve a high degree of accuracy, it is imperative that the proper imaging protocol be observed. Thin-section axial images (4 or 5 mm) should be obtained from the midbody of L-3 to the midbody of S-1. Angling of the plane of imaging to be parallel to the discs is not necessary (Fig. 11.2), and contiguous images without skip areas are considered mandatory (Fig. 11.3). Even though sagittal images will be obtained, a host of entities are more easily identified on the axial images than on the sagittal. These include migrated free disc fragments, spondylolysis (pars breaks), conjoined nerve roots, the facets, the neuroforamen, the lateral recesses, and intraspinal synovial cysts. We looked at 103 consecutive spine MRI studies[4] in which we obtained our standard axial and sagittal T1- and T2-weighted sequences; the axial cuts were contiguous, stacked images without gaps or angling. In addition, we obtained axial images that were angled parallel to the discs and covered only the disc spaces, thereby leaving a gap between one level and the next (Fig. 11.2). The angled axial images were combined with the sagittal images and evaluated for free disc fragments and pars breaks, and then compared to the original interpretations, which had the stacked axials and the sagittals. Our standard imaging protocol found 15 cases of spondylolysis and 8 free disc fragments. The angled axial protocol only showed 8 cases of spondylolysis and 3 free fragments, even though the sagittal images were available. We missed three-quarters of the free fragments! These patients would likely have all had failed surgery with the angled axial protocol. There's no reason I've ever heard of for angling the axial cuts and leaving gaps, yet about a third of all the consult spine cases I look at use this protocol. I think it's the number one cause of missed diagnoses in spine imaging.

Both T1- (or proton density) weighted and T2- (or T2*-) weighted images should be obtained in both the sagittal and the axial planes. Coronal images have not been shown to add additional information and are not typically included.

DISC DISEASE

Terminology plays a large role in how radiologists describe disc bulges or protrusions. Since the advent of CT in the 1970s, disc bulges have been described by their morphology. A broad-based disc bulge was said to be a bulging annulus fibrosus, while a focal disc bulge was called a herniated nucleus pulposus (HNP) (Fig. 11.4). This is no longer the accepted terminology.

Although no universally accepted classification of disc disease is present, most agree on something like the following: a broad-based disc bulge is called a bulge; a focal bulge is called a protrusion; a piece of disc that has migrated from the parent disc is a free fragment or sequestration. The term HNP is no longer considered acceptable. More significantly, most surgeons do not care what name is applied to a disc bulge—they do not treat a bulging annulus any differently than a protrusion. They treat the patient's symptoms and have to decide if the disc bulge is

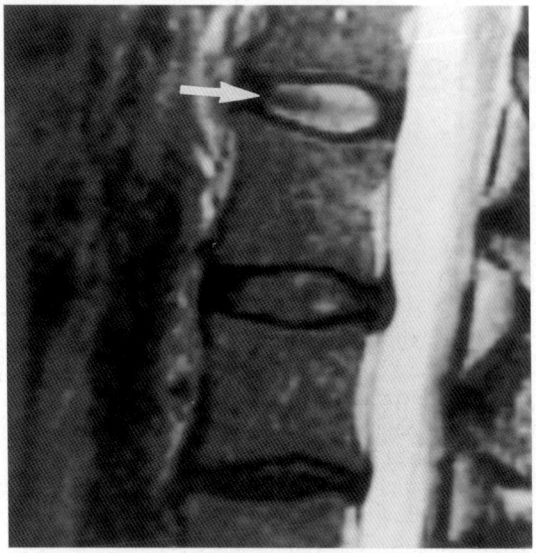

FIG. 11.1 **Desiccated Disc.** A sagittal T2-weighted image shows the L2-3 and L3-4 discs to be abnormally low in signal indicating disc desiccation and degeneration. Compare with the normal L1-2 disc *(arrow),* which has high signal.

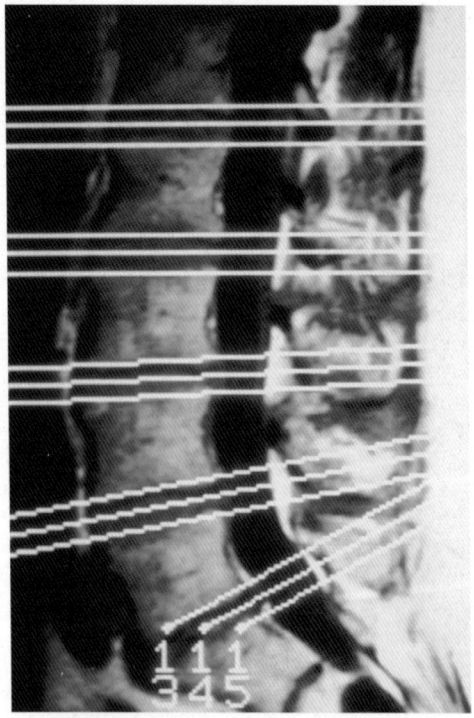

FIG. 11.2 **Inadequate Technique—Skip Areas.** A computed tomography (CT) scout film with cursors placed through the disc spaces. This allows large gaps or skip areas that can result in multiple missed diagnoses, including missed free fragments of discs.

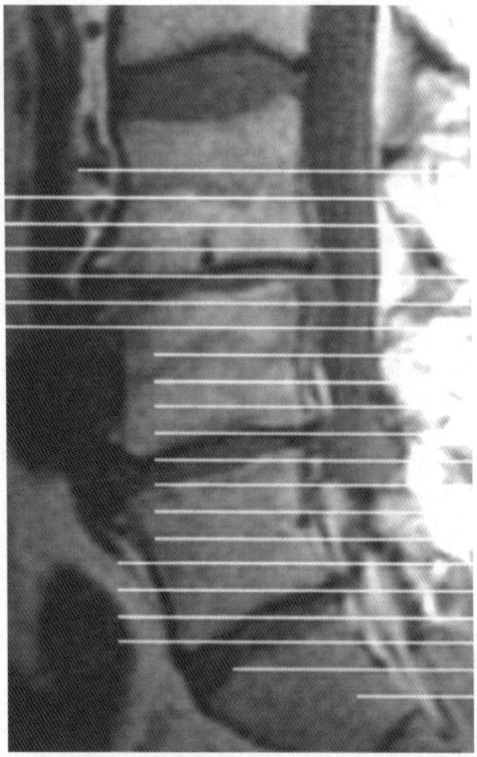

FIG. 11.3 **Proper Magnetic Resonance (Mr) Imaging Technique.** This MR imaging scout with cursors placed contiguously from the body of L-3 to S-1 allows complete coverage of the lower lumbar spine in the axial plane.

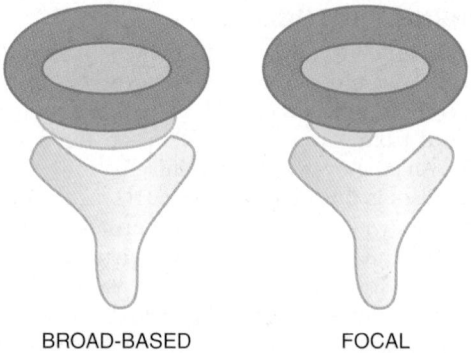

FIG. 11.4 **Schematic of Types of Disc Bulges.** The broad-based disc bulge (left) is typical for a bulging annulus fibrosus. A focal disc bulge (right) is more consistent with a protrusion.

responsible for those symptoms. It has been shown in multiple studies that from 40% to 50% of asymptomatic people have disc bulges or protrusions;[5] hence, just seeing a disc bulge on CT or MR imaging does not mean it is clinically significant.

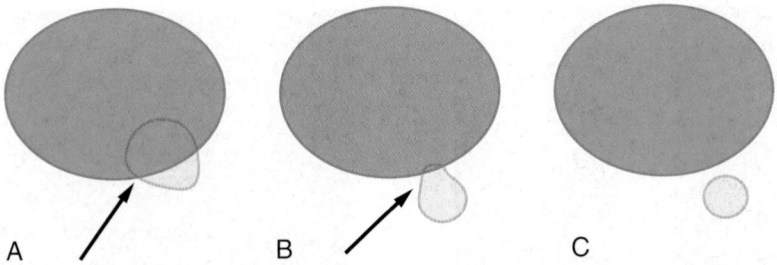

FIG. 11.5 **Disc Protrusions.** (A) shows a focal disc protrusion with a wide neck or base *(arrow)*. This has been termed a *protrusion*. (B) shows a focal disc protrusion with a narrow neck or base *(arrow)*. This has been termed an *extrusion*. (C) shows a piece of disc that has broken off as a free fragment. This has been termed an *extruded* disc.

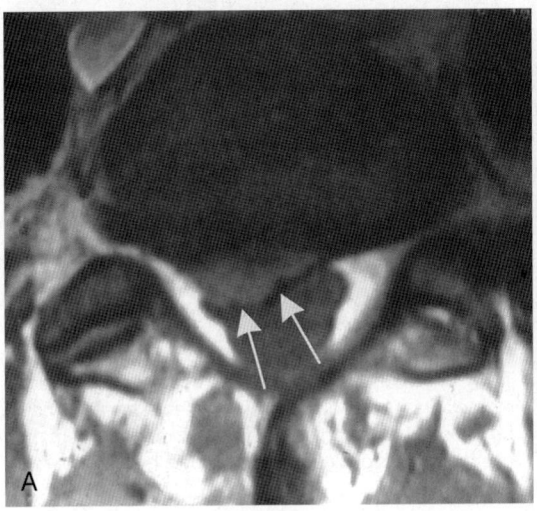

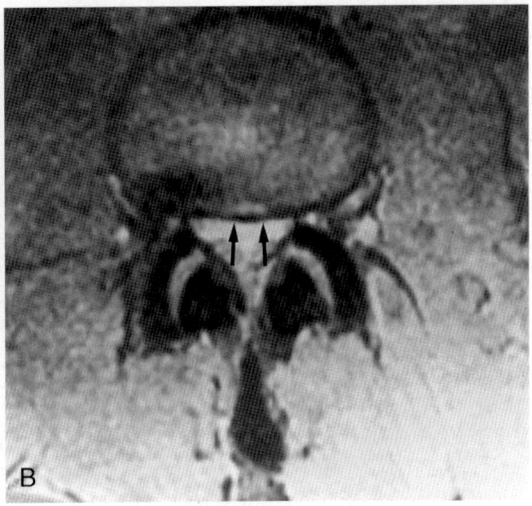

FIG. 11.6 **Disc Protrusions.** An axial T1WI (A) shows a focal disc protrusion *(arrows)*. An axial T2WI (B) shows a broad-based disc bulge *(arrows)*. Since these are both showing impression of the thecal sac, they could each cause symptoms.

One of the most widely used classifications has the terms *protrusion*, *extrusion*, and *extruded* as the basis for describing the type of disc bulge present. I have seen this terminology cause misadventures for patients because it was either used incorrectly by the radiologist or not understood by the surgeon. In this classification, a *protrusion* is a focal disc bulge with a wide neck or base (Fig. 11.5A), an *extrusion* is a focal bulge with a narrow neck or base (Fig. 11.5B), and an *extruded* disc is a free disc fragment (Fig. 11.5C). Surgeons don't treat a patient with a protrusion any differently than one with an extrusion—it's an artificial distinction based solely on the neck width of the bulge. If that's all it were, so what, but it's much more significant because of the term *extruded*, which is a free fragment. Missing a free disc fragment is one of the leading causes of failed back surgery, and identifying it will guide the surgeon to search for it and remove it. I have seen several cases in which the terms *extrusion* and *extruded* were misused or not understood, and patients had free fragments left behind (the surgeon didn't realize the term *extruded* meant a free fragment), and in others, the surgeon searched for a free fragment when there was none because the term *extruded* was incorrectly applied. Since there is no clinical or surgical difference between having a protrusion or an extrusion, and surgical mistakes can occur when this terminology is employed, I do not let my residents and fellows use these terms.

MR imaging has a high degree of accuracy in delineating disc protrusions and showing if neural tissue is impressed (Fig. 11.6). MR imaging can also show if

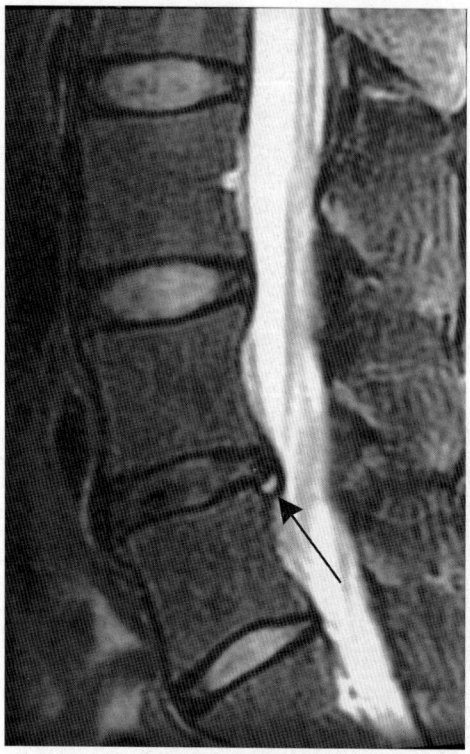

FIG. 11.7 **Annular Tear.** This sagittal fast spin-echo (FSE) T2 image shows a focus of increased signal *(arrow)* in the annulus, which is called an HIZ (high-intensity zone), which indicates an annular tear.

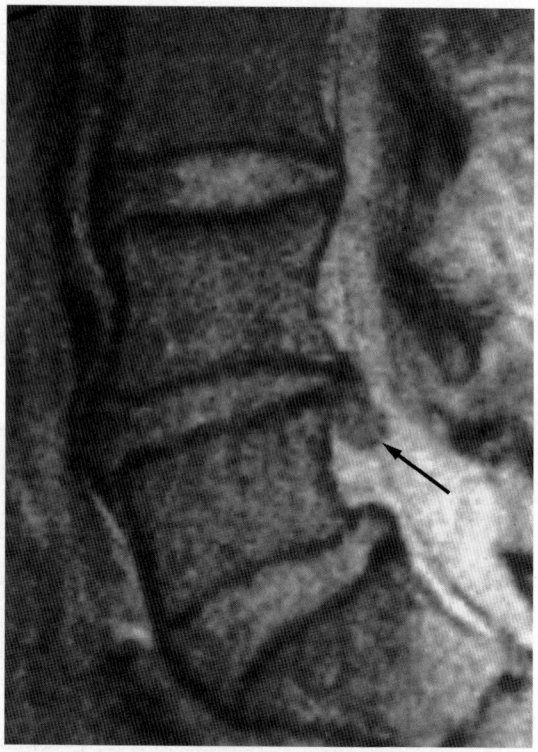

FIG. 11.8 **Sequestration or Free Fragment.** This sagittal T2WI shows disc material located caudal to the parent disc *(arrow)*. This is a sequestration or free fragment. It may still be attached and technically is not a "free" fragment, but it has the same significance whether it is attached or not.

annular fibers of the disc are disrupted (Fig. 11.7)—a so-called HIZ (high-intensity zone). Although CT cannot diagnose annular tears, clinicians do not currently treat them surgically. The annulus is innervated by the sinuvertebral nerve, which goes to the dorsal root ganglion and can mimic a focal disc protrusion at that level. They can cause back pain and even sciatica (buttock and leg pain), but typically resolve with conservative management.

Free Fragments

A type of disc abnormality that is critical to diagnose is the free fragment or sequestration. Missed free fragments are one of the most common causes of failed back surgery.[6] The preoperative diagnosis of a free fragment means the surgeon needs to explore more cephalad or caudally during the surgery in order to remove the free fragment. As free fragments can be very difficult to diagnose clinically, imaging is critical in the evaluation of the spine for any patient contemplating surgery. At times, it can be difficult to be absolutely certain as to whether or not a disc that lies above or below the disc space is still attached to the parent disc or is really "free." So long as disc material is above or below the level of the disc space, it really does not matter if it is attached or not. The key element is recognizing that disc material is present away from the level of the disc space (caudally or cranially) so the surgeon will be aware that he may have to increase his exposure to find and account for the additional disc material, whether it is attached to the parent disc or not.

Free fragments are diagnosed on MR imaging by noting disc material cephalad or caudal to the disc space (Fig. 11.8). Free fragments may migrate either cranially or caudally, with no apparent preference.

Axial images often show the free fragment more conspicuously than the sagittal images (Fig. 11.9); therefore contiguous axial images without large skip

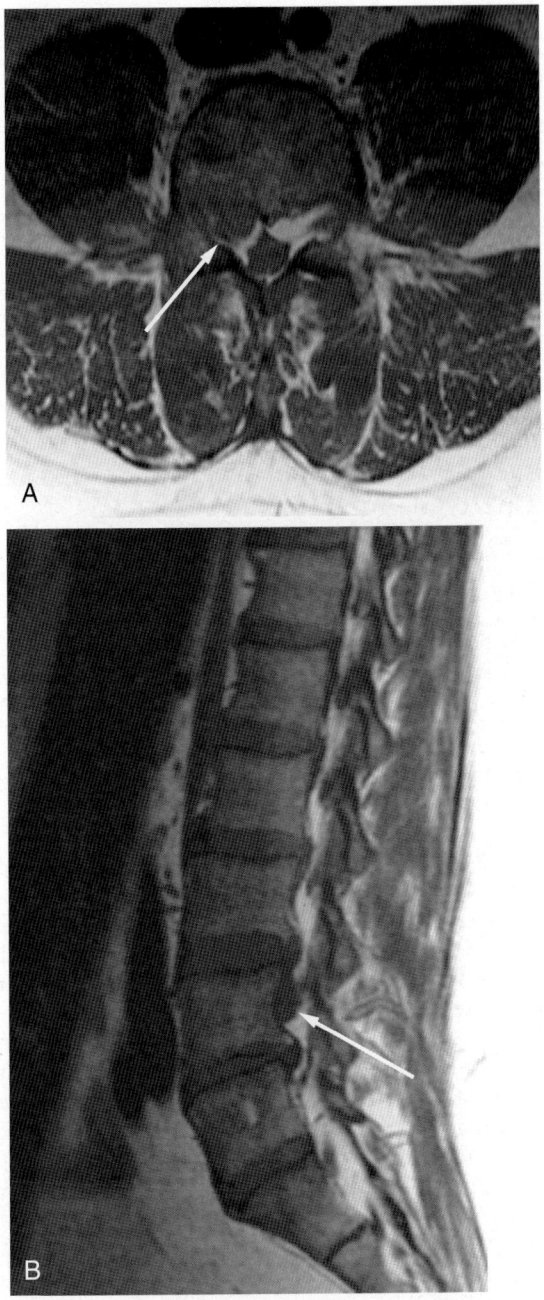

FIG. 11.9 **Free Fragment More Evident on Axial Images.** The axial image (A) reveals an obvious large free disc fragment *(arrow)*. It is not as conspicuous on the sagittal image (B). The free fragment can be seen posterior to the L-4 vertebral body *(arrow)*.

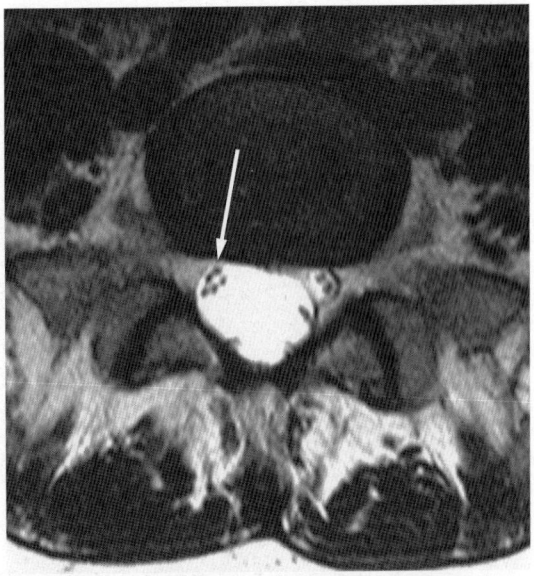

FIG. 11-10 **Conjoined Root.** An axial T2WI image shows several nerve root components clustered in the thecal sac on the right *(arrow)*, while the left side has a single root that has already left the thecal sac. This is known as a conjoined root but is really just delayed exit of the nerve roots on one side as compared to the other.

areas or gaps are imperative in order to not miss free fragments.

A conjoined root, which is a normal variant of two roots exiting the thecal sac together or in an anomalous manner (seen in 1% to 3% of the population)[7] (Fig. 11.10), or a Tarlov cyst, a normal variant in which a nerve root sleeve is dilated, can have a similar appearance to a free fragment but can almost always be differentiated from disc material by their signal staying isointense to the thecal sac on both T1 and T2 sequences. It is critical to identify a conjoined root or a Tarlov cyst and not confuse them for a free fragment. A surgeon will often change his procedure and certainly his amount of surgical exploration if he thinks there is a free fragment present. Many surgeons have inadvertently damaged conjoined or anomalous nerve roots, thinking they were free fragments. Obviously, a free fragment should be removed, and a conjoined nerve root should be left alone—the imaging study is where that difference should be ascertained, not during surgery.

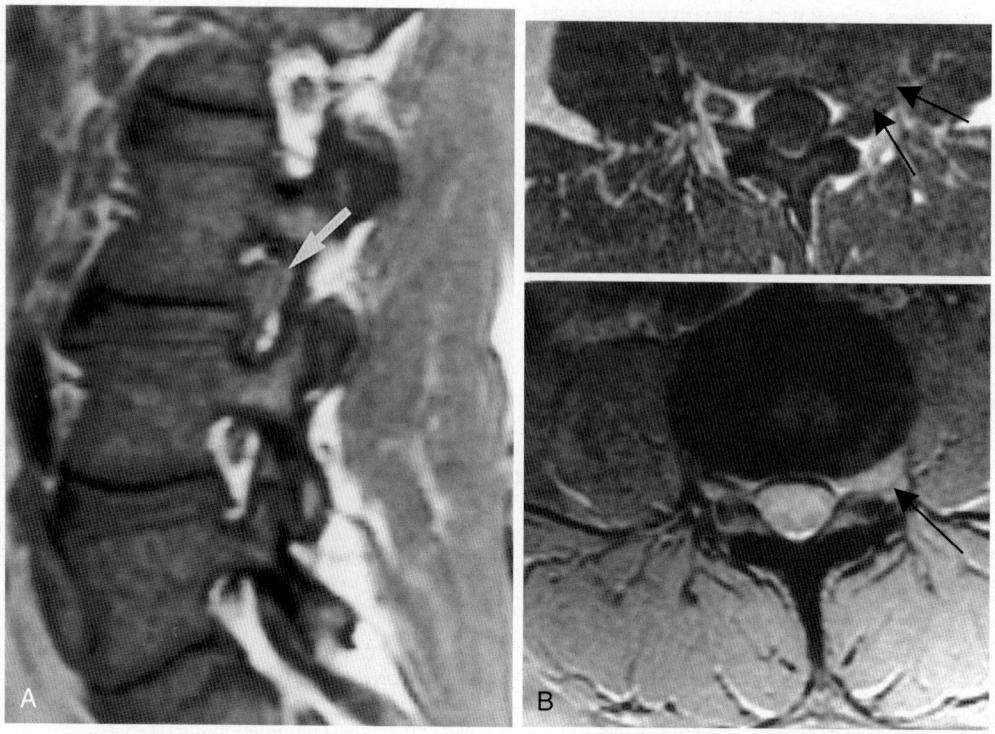

FIG. 11.11 **Lateral Disc.** (A) A sagittal T1-weighted magnetic resonance (MR) image through the left neuroforamen shows a low signal structure in the L-4 neuroforamen *(arrow)*, which is a lateral disc protrusion. (B) Axial T1 *(upper)* and T2* *(lower)* show the lateral disc *(arrows)* in the left neuroforamen.

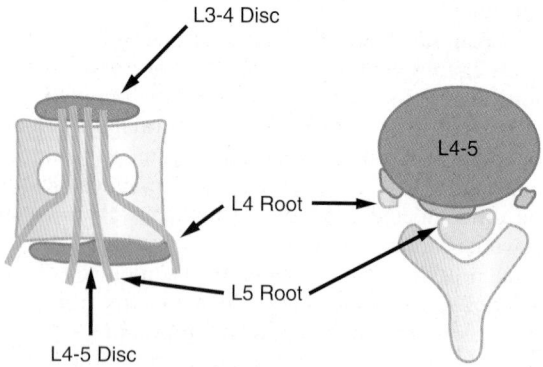

FIG. 11.12 **Schematic of Lateral Disc.** This schematic illustrates how a posterior L4-5 disc protrusion affects the L5 nerve root, yet a lateral L4-5 disc affects the L4 root.

Lateral Discs

Discs will occasionally protrude in a lateral direction, causing the nerve root that has already exited the central canal to be stretched (Fig. 11.11). Although not common (less than 5% of cases), these are frequently overlooked and are known to be a source of failed back surgery.[8] Since they affect the previously exited root, they can clinically mimic symptoms of a disc protrusion from one level more cephalad (Fig. 11.12). For example, in a patient with multilevel disc disease and symptoms referable to the L3-4 disc, the disc protrusion is usually a posterior L3-4 bulge that impresses the L4 nerve root. However, a lateral disc at L4-5 could impress the L4 nerve root and cause the same symptoms. If not noticed, surgery could be performed at the L3-4 disc—the wrong level. Unfortunately, I have seen this on several occasions. Also, it is important to notify the surgeon that the disc is lateral to the neuroforamen, as a standard surgical approach through the lamina might not allow removal of a lateral disc.

Lateral discs are best identified on axial images. Sagittal images will often show a lateral disc occluding a neuroforamen, but many times, a lateral disc will not extend into the foramen, and the sagittal images will appear normal.

STENOSIS

By definition, spinal stenosis is encroachment of the bony or soft tissue structures in the spine on one or more of the neural elements with resulting symptoms. These symptoms are often indistinguishable from those of disc disease, and, in fact, disc disease often coexists with spinal stenosis. Patients with spinal stenosis classically present with back pain and bilateral sciatica, intermittent claudication, pain with hyperextension and relief with flexion, and pain with standing that is relieved by lying down.

Spinal stenosis is classically divided into congenital and acquired types; however, even the most severe forms of congenital stenosis do not cause symptoms unless a component of acquired stenosis (usually degenerative disease of the facets and the discs) is present. A more useful classification of stenosis is on an anatomic basis: central canal, neuroforaminal, and lateral recess. It is important to realize that stenosis and disc disease are often present concomitantly, and it can be very difficult to clinically differentiate the two. As with disc disease, it is imperative that any imaging findings be matched with the clinical picture. It is not unusual to have a patient with severe stenosis on an imaging study and no clinical symptoms.

It should be noted that a disc protrusion alone should not be considered a cause of stenosis, even though, technically speaking, narrowing of the central canal or foramen has occurred. An isolated disc protrusion is simply disc disease. A bulging disc can be a component of stenosis when it is accompanied by facet and ligamentum flavum hypertrophy, but not by itself. I often have residents report that a large focal disc protrusion has caused central canal or foraminal stenosis, but that is not the terminology that surgeons use.

Central Canal Stenosis

Although at one time, measurements were considered very useful in the determination of central canal stenosis, they are no longer felt to be a valid indicator of disease. Instead, simply noting whether the thecal sac is compressed or round will reliably serve for determining central canal stenosis (Fig. 11.13). A subjective assessment as to whether the compression (usually in an anteroposterior direction) is mild, moderate, or severe is all that is necessary for evaluating the central canal. It is quite common to note moderate or severe central canal stenosis with flattening of the thecal sac in a patient who is asymptomatic.

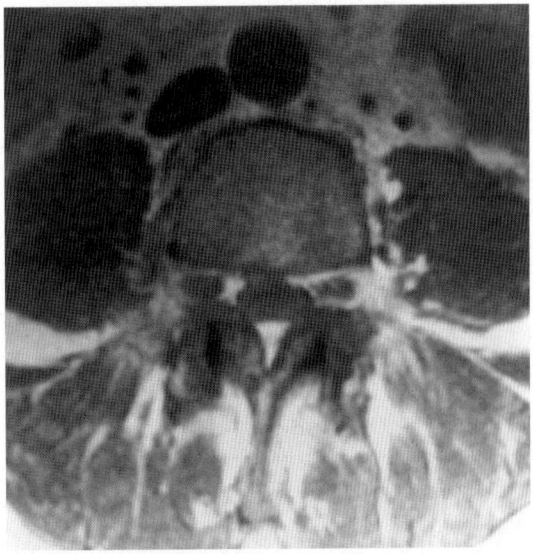

FIG. 11.13 **Central Canal Stenosis.** An axial T2WI shows marked compression of the thecal sac in an anteroposterior direction, diagnostic of central canal stenosis.

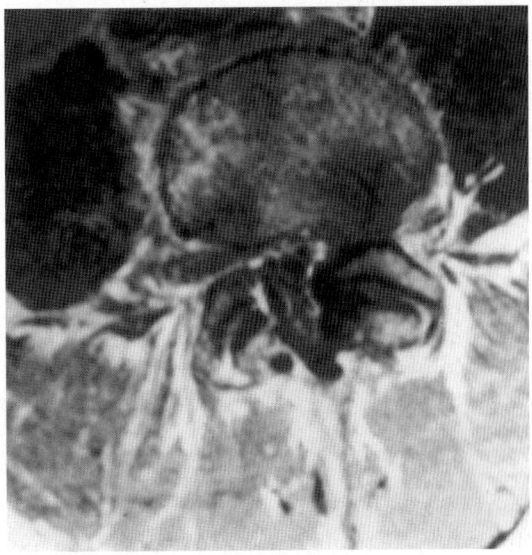

FIG. 11.14 **Facet Hypertrophy Causing Stenosis.** This magnetic resonance (MR) image shows marked facet degenerative disease, with hypertrophy of the facets causing lateral recess and central canal stenosis.

Conversely, mild stenosis can be a cause of symptoms in some people.

The most common cause of central canal stenosis is degenerative disease of the facets with bony hypertrophy which encroaches on the central canal

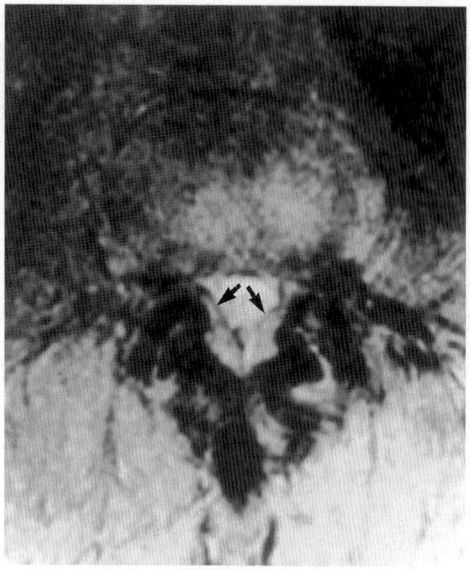

FIG. 11.15 **Ligamentum Flavum Hypertrophy.** Inward bulging of the ligamentum flavum *(arrows)* is shown on this MR image. Central canal stenosis from ligamentum flavum hypertrophy is common.

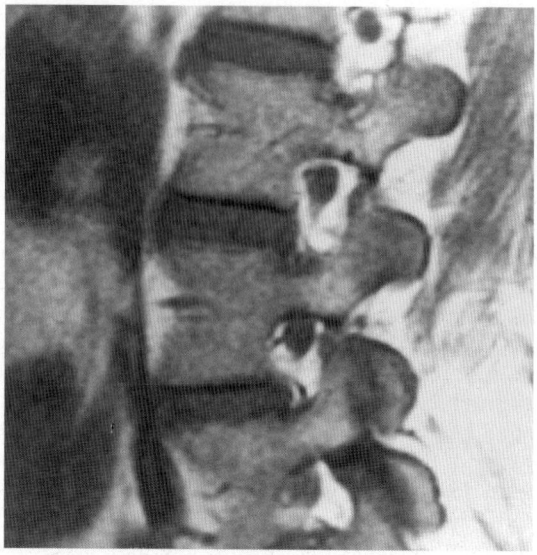

FIG. 11.16 **Normal Neuroforamen.** A sagittal T1-weighted image through the neuroforamen shows the nerve roots surrounded by fat with no evidence of foraminal stenosis. This does not exclude, however, a focus of foraminal stenosis that is medial or lateral to this sagittal image.

(Fig. 11.14). This is also the most common cause of lateral recess stenosis. When the facets undergo degenerative joint disease (DJD), they often have some slippage, which results in buckling of the ligamentum flavum. Although a misnomer, this has been termed ligamentum flavum hypertrophy and is a common cause of central canal stenosis (Fig. 11.15). Frequently, mild disc bulging is associated with minimal facet hypertrophy and ligamentum flavum hypertrophy. This combination can result in severe focal central canal stenosis.

Less common causes of central canal stenosis include bony overgrowth from Paget disease, achondroplasia, posttraumatic changes, and severe spondylolisthesis.

Neuroforaminal Stenosis

DJD of the facets with bony hypertrophy is the most common cause of neuroforaminal stenosis; however, encroachment on the nerve root in the neuroforamen can be seen with free disc fragments, postoperative scar, and from a lateral disc protrusion.

The neuroforamen is best evaluated on axial images just cephalad to the disc space. The disc space lies at the inferior portion of the neuroforamen, and the exiting nerve root lies in the superior or cephalad portion of the neuroforamen. Although the neuroforamen can be clearly seen on sagittal MR images (Fig. 11.16), care

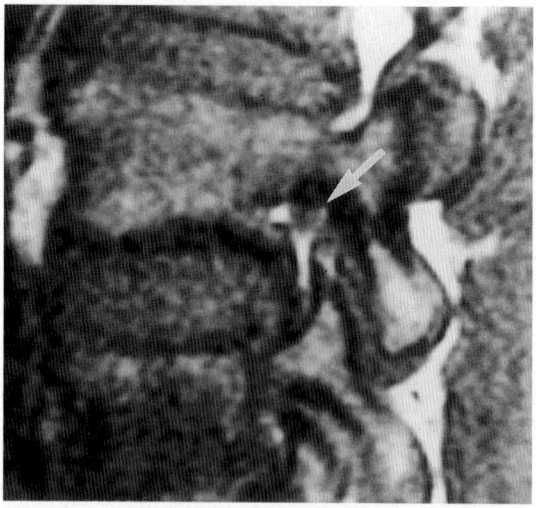

FIG. 11.17 **Neuroforaminal Stenosis.** Marked narrowing of the neuroforamen *(arrow)* is seen on this sagittal T1-weighted image.

must be taken to evaluate the entire neuroforamen and not just the 4 or 5 mm of one sagittal image. A normal appearing neuroforamen on a sagittal image does not exclude neuroforaminal stenosis (the axial images must be evaluated), whereas a stenotic foramen seen

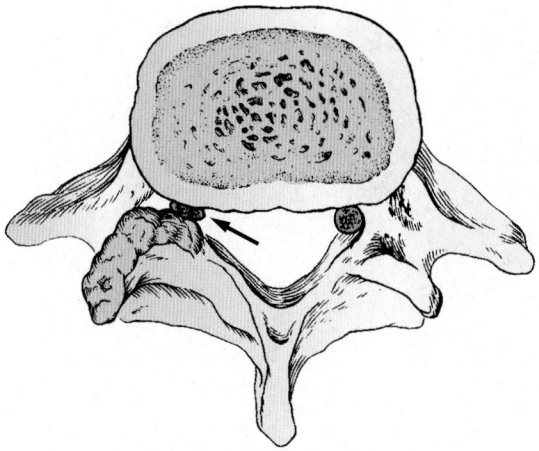

FIG. 11.18 **Lateral Recess Stenosis.** Hypertrophy of the right-sided facet with encroachment into the lateral recess *(arrow)* is seen on this drawing.

on a sagittal image (Fig. 11.17) can be counted on as being reliable for pathology.

Lateral Recess Stenosis

The lateral recesses are the bony canals in which the nerve roots lie after they leave the thecal sac and before they enter the neuroforamen. The lateral recesses are bounded by the neuroforamen caudally and cranially. They are triangular in shape when viewed on axial images, and the nerve root can be identified as a low-signal rounded structure on all imaging sequences. Hypertrophy of the superior articular facet from DJD is the most common cause of encroachment on the lateral recesses (Fig. 11.18), although, as with the neuroforamen, disc fragments and postoperative scarring can cause nerve root impingement.

POST-OPERATIVE CHANGES

Failed back surgery, unfortunately, is common. It can occur from many causes, including inadequate surgery (including missed free disc fragments), postoperative scarring, failure of bone grafting for fusion, and recurrent disc protrusion. CT is useful in evaluating bone grafts but is not reliable for differentiating postoperative scarring from disc material. MR imaging has been shown to be particularly useful in distinguishing scar from disc material. Most surgeons will reoperate for recurrent disc protrusions, but not for postoperative scar; therefore it's critical to distinguish scar from disc.

The use of intravenous gadolinium has traditionally been used to distinguish scar from disc. Scar tissue will be enhanced following administration of gadolinium, whereas disc material will have only some minimal peripheral enhancement, presumably due to inflammation or scarring. Many have found that by just looking at the morphology of the soft tissues, one can distinguish scar from disc material. A disc will cause a mass impression on the thecal sac, whereas scar will surround neural tissue (Fig. 11.19). Some centers have omitted the routine use of gadolinium in the postop spine with the exception of patients with possible infection.

BONY ABNORMALITIES

Spondylolysis and Spondylolisthesis

Defects in the bony pars interarticularis (spondylolysis) are commonly found in asymptomatic individuals, yet they can be a source of low back pain and instability. Prior to disc surgery or other back surgery, it is imperative that any spondylolysis be identified. Since spondylolysis can mimic back pain from other pathology, it is important to assess it preoperatively. If necessary, it can then be surgically addressed at the same time as the other surgery. Failure to note and evaluate spondylolysis is a known source of failed back surgery.

CT is superior to MR imaging at identifying spondylolysis.[9] Although MR imaging will show spondylolysis defects, they can be very difficult to see at times. As previously mentioned, this is the only area in which CT is reported to be clearly superior to MR imaging in evaluating the lumbar spine. Spondylolysis is identified on the axial images through the mid-vertebral body as a break in the normally intact bony ring of the lamina (Fig. 11.20). A protocol employing axial images only through the discs will routinely miss spondylolysis defects. Care must be used in calling spondylolysis on the sagittal views, as the normal pars often has a low signal area that resembles spondylolysis. If the pars appears normal on the sagittal view, it can be considered a reliable finding; however, if the pars appears abnormal on the sagittal view, the axial view must be used to determine if a break is really present or not.

Spondylolisthesis (forward slippage of one vertebral body on a lower one) occurs from either slippage of two vertebral bodies following bilateral spondylolysis or from DJD of the facets with slippage of the facets. Bilateral spondylolysis can result in a large amount of slippage, whereas facet DJD will usually result in only

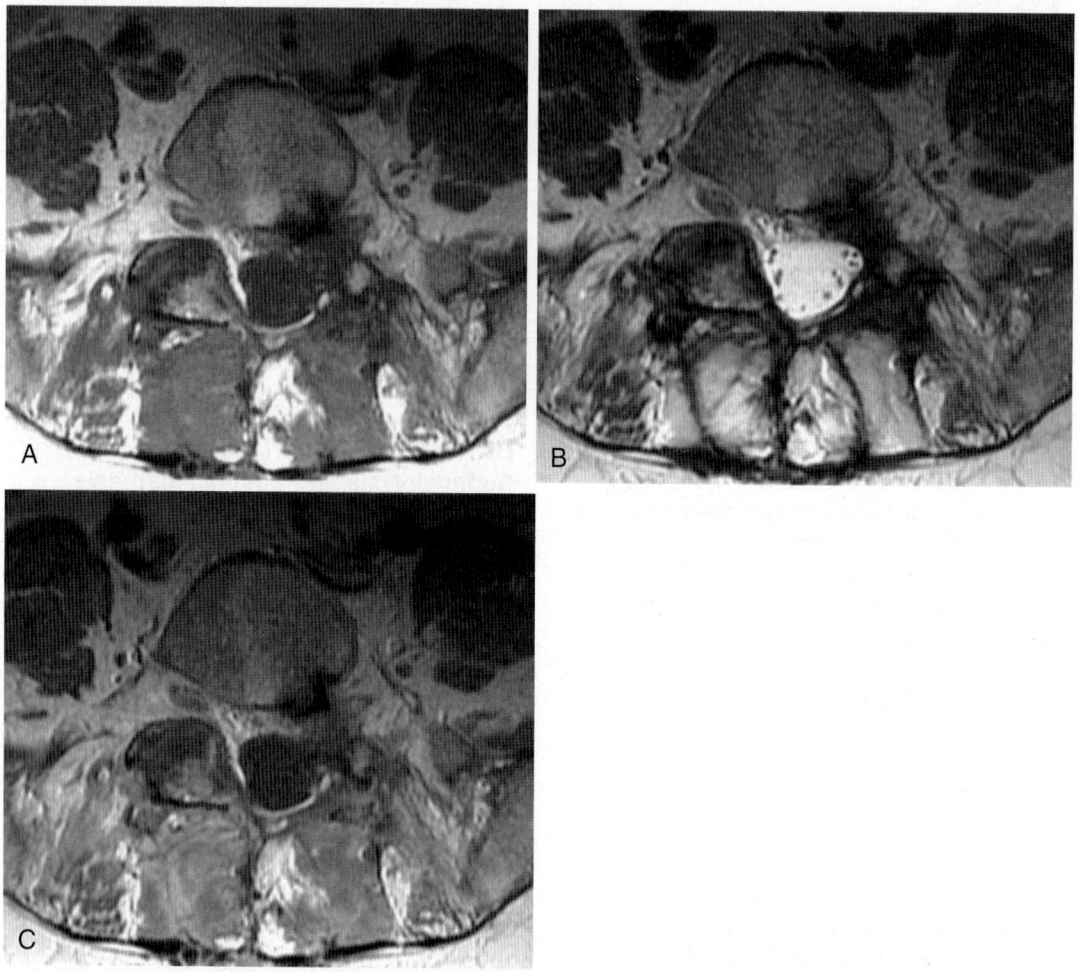

FIG. 11.19 **Postoperative Scar.** (A) A T1-weighted axial image shows a left-sided mass that could be either postop scar or a recurrent disc. (B) A T2WI image through the same level shows the soft tissue mass is wrapping around the thecal sac rather than impressing it. This is typical for scar, not recurrent disc protrusion. (C) Following administration of intravenous gadolinium (Gd-DTPA) intravenously, enhancement of the scar tissue adjacent to the thecal sac is seen. The diagnosis of postop fibrosis could be made without the administration of gadolinium.

minimal slippage. If spondylolisthesis is severe, it can result in central canal stenosis, neuroforaminal stenosis, or both.

End Plate Changes

Parallel bands of high or low signal adjacent to the vertebral body end plates are often seen in association with degenerative disc disease. A common appearance is of high-signal bands on T1-weighted images that remain high on T2-weighted images (Fig. 11.21). This represents fatty marrow conversion. It was seen in 16% of cases in the first report by Modic et al.[10] and was termed type 2 changes (generally referred to as "Modic type 2"). Modic type 1 changes are seen as low-signal bands parallel to the end plates on T1-weighted images that get brighter on T2-weighted images (Fig. 11.22). This represents an inflammatory or granulomatous response to degenerative disc disease. The type 1 changes were reported in 4% of cases and must be distinguished from disc space infection (Fig. 11.23). In disc space infection, the disc should get bright on the T2-weighted images, whereas it is unusual for a degenerative disc to have high signal on T2-weighted images. Modic type 3 changes

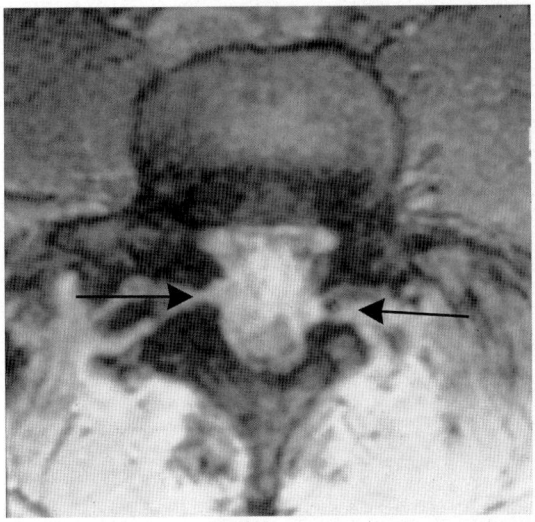

FIG. 11.20 **Spondylolysis.** An axial T2-weighted image through the midvertebral body reveals a break in the bony laminae bilaterally *(arrows)*, which indicates spondylolysis. An axial cut through the pedicles should have an intact bony ring around the central canal.

are parallel bands of low signal adjacent to the end plates on both T1- and T2-weighted images. Type 3 changes represent bony sclerosis seen on plain films.

Mimics

There are multiple entities that can mimic disc disease clinically and if not noted can result in unnecessary disc surgery. Many of these can be identified on the routine lumbar spine MRI, and include annular tears, pars breaks (spondylolysis), and facet disease. In addition, sacroiliac joint and sacral abnormalities can mimic disc disease and should be looked for on every spine MRI (Fig. 11.24). Tendinosis or partial tears at the

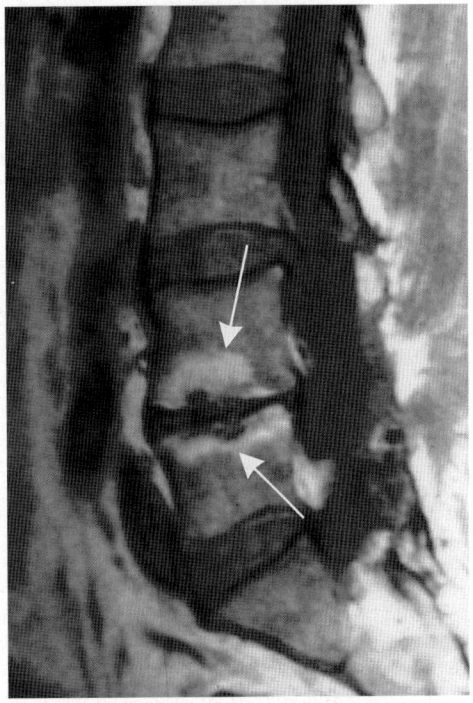

FIG. 11.21 **Type 2 Marrow Changes.** A sagittal T1-weighted image in a patient with degenerative disc disease shows bands of fatty marrow parallel to the L4-5 end plates *(arrows)*, which are type 2 marrow changes seen often with degenerative disc disease.

hamstring insertion on the ischial tuberosity is often misdiagnosed as sciatica with resultant L-spine MRI. I have seen several patients that had focal disc protrusions that were surgically removed as the putative cause of sciatica when in fact the "sciatica" was secondary to an abnormality at the hamstring insertion—the disc was an incidental, asymptomatic bulge. Disc surgery

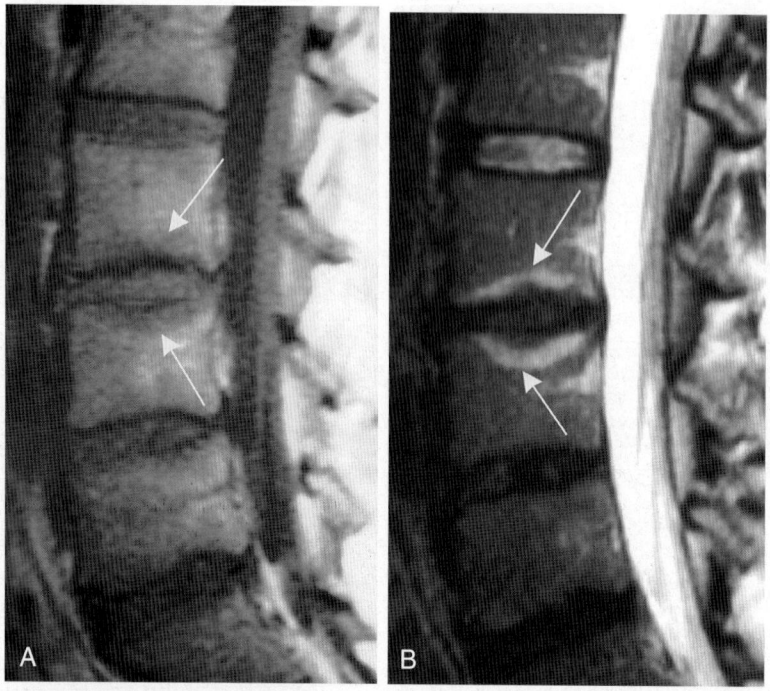

FIG. 11.22 **Type 1 Marrow Changes.** (A) A sagittal T1-weighted image in a patient with degenerative disc disease at L3-4 shows faint bands of low signal parallel to the L3-4 end-plates *(arrows)*. (B) A sagittal fast spin-echo (FSE) T2-weighted image with fat suppression shows bands of high signal adjacent to the L3-4 end plates. This represents granulation tissue seen with degenerative disc disease and has been called type 1 marrow change. It can be differentiated from a disc infection by the low signal of the disc on the T2-weighted image.

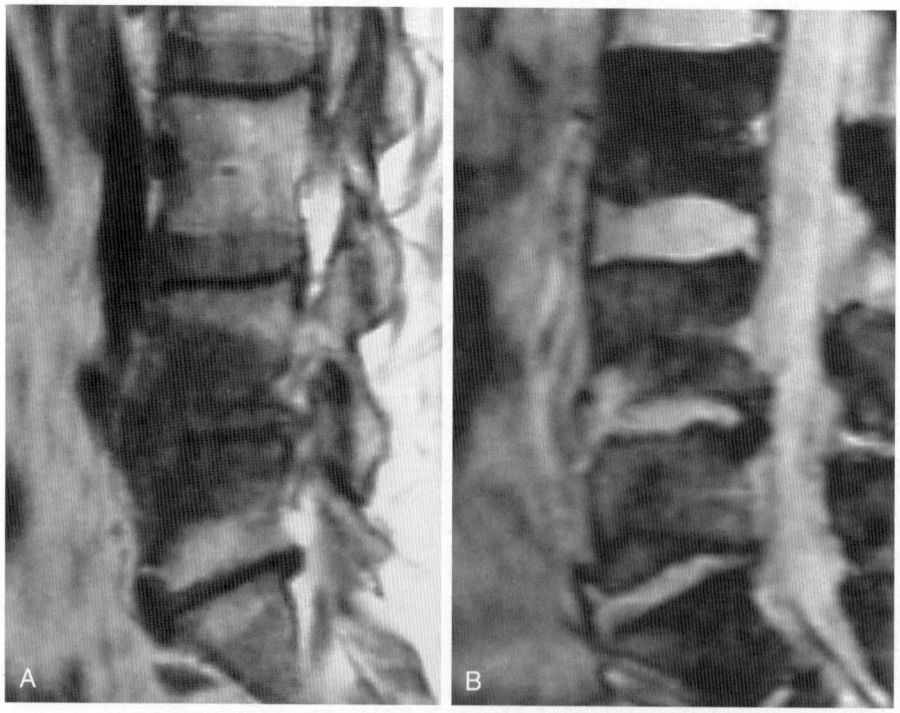

FIG. 11.23 **Disc Infection.** (A) A sagittal T1-weighted image shows bands of low signal in the vertebral bodies adjacent to the L4-5 end plates. On a T2-weighted (gradient-echo) image (B), the vertebral body/end plate signal increase is faintly seen, as it is a gradient-echo sequence. However, note the high signal in the disc, which makes this consistent with a disc infection rather than type 2 signal of a degenerative disc.

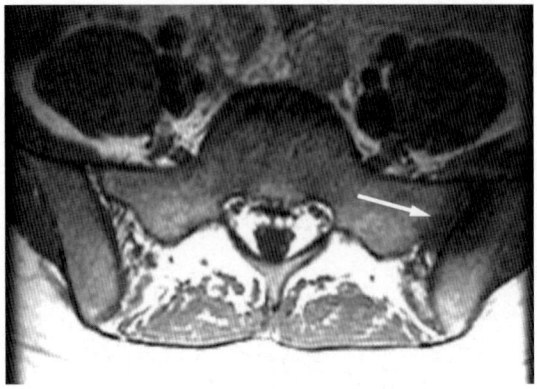

FIG. 11.24 **Sacroiliitis Presenting as Disc Disease.** This young adult presented with low back pain and what was thought to be sciatica on clinical exam. This axial T1WI, which was the most caudal image on the routine lumbar spine magnetic resonance image (MRI), shows low signal surrounding the left sacroiliac (SI) joint *(arrow)*, which turned out to be sacroiliitis secondary to psoriasis.

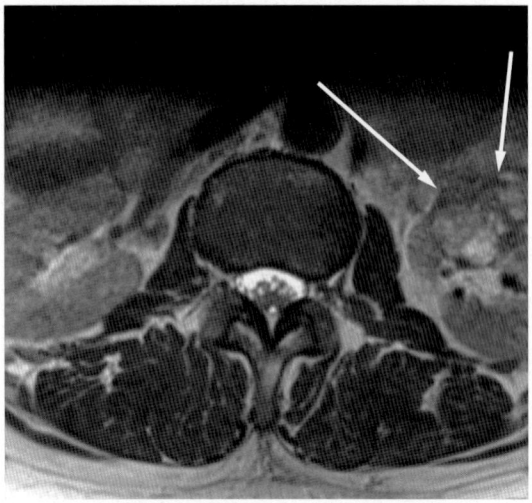

FIG. 11.25 **Renal Cell Carcinoma Seen on Routine Lumbar Spine Magnetic Resonance Imaging (MRI).** This elderly man presented with left-sided back pain that was thought to be from disc disease. The most cranial axial T2WI shows a left-sided renal mass *(arrows)*, which was a renal cell carcinoma. The remainder of his lumbar spine MRI was normal.

in those cases, obviously, was unnecessary and did not improve their pain.

Lastly, a lumbar spine MRI typically includes at least part of the kidneys. A renal cell carcinoma can cause back pain that can be mistakenly attributed to a disc protrusion, and, if overlooked on the L-spine MRI, can result in a tragic outcome for the patient (Fig. 11.25).

REFERENCES

1. Jackson R, Becker G, Jacobs R, Montesano P, Cooper B, McManus G. The neuroradiographic diagnosis of lumbar herniated nucleus pulposus (I): a comparison of computed tomography, myelography, CT-myelography, discography, and CT-discography. *Spine*. 1989;14:1356–1361.
2. Jackson R, Cain J, Jacobs R, Cooper B, McManus G. The neuroradiographic diagnosis of lumbar herniated nucleus pulposus (II): a comparison of computed tomography, myelography, CT-myelography, and magnetic resonance imaging. *Spine*. 1989;14:1362–1367.
3. Tertti M, Salminen J, Paajanen H, Terho P, Kormano M. Low-back pain and disk degeneration in children: a case-control MR imaging study. *Radiology*. 1991;180:503–507.
4. Singh K, Helms CA, Fiorella D, et al. Disc space targeted axial MR images in the lumbar spine: a potential source of diagnostic error. *Skeletal Radiol*. 2007;36:1147–1153.
5. Jensen MC, Brant-Zawadzki MN, Obuchowski N, et al. Abnormal magnetic-resonance scans of the lumbar spine in asymptomatic subjects. *NEJM*. 1994;331:69–73.
6. Onik G, Mooney V, Maroon J, et al. Automated percutaneous discectomy: a prospective multi-institutional study. *Neurosurgery*. 1989;26:228–233.
7. Helms CA, Dorwart RH, Gray M. The CT appearance of conjoined nerve roots and differentiation from a herniated nucleus pulposus. *Radiology*. 1982;144:803–807.
8. Winter DDB, Munk PL, Helms CA, Holt RG. CT and MR of lateral disc herniation: typical appearance and pitfalls of interpretation. *J Can Assoc Radiol*. 1989;40:256–259.
9. Grenier N, Kressel HY, Schiebler ML, Grossman RI. Isthmic spondylolysis of the lumbar spine: MR imaging at 1.5 T. *Radiology*. 1989;170:489–494.
10. Modic M, Masaryk T, Ross J, Carter J. Imaging of degenerative disk disease. *Radiology*. 1988;168:177–186.

CHAPTER 12

Magnetic Resonance Imaging of the Foot and Ankle

I have always found topics on the foot and ankle to be exceedingly boring. This is mainly because I was never called on to use any of the information I learned; hence I quickly forgot all that I was told. I learned early in my residency that during lectures on the foot and ankle, I could find better use of my time—like running or playing golf. That has changed now that magnetic resonance (MR) imaging is being used in the foot and ankle. MR imaging is playing an increasingly important role in examining the foot and ankle. Orthopedic surgeons and podiatrists are learning that critical diagnostic information can be obtained in no other way and are relying on MR imaging for many therapeutic decisions.

When most of us first encounter an ankle MR image, we get out a cross-sectional atlas and start trying to determine where all the tendons, muscles, vascular structures, and so on lie. I can assure you this will be unnecessary after reading this chapter. Although the anatomy of the foot and ankle can be complex, the significant anatomy, that is, the anatomy that must be learned because it is affected by disease, is fairly straightforward and easily learned.[1] There is no need to memorize tendons, ligaments, and muscles that are only rarely seen to be abnormal; therefore this chapter will dwell only on the pathologically significant areas.

I must admit, imaging the foot and ankle is getting more complex—it seems there is a new article every month on the utility of MRI in this area. Foot and ankle imaging is one of the fastest growing studies in musculoskeletal imaging.

TENDONS

One of the more common reasons to perform an MR imaging exam on the foot and ankle is to examine the tendons. Although multiple tendons course through the ankle, only a few are routinely affected pathologically. These are primarily the flexor tendons, located posteriorly in the ankle. The extensor tendons, located anteriorly, are rarely abnormal.

Tendons can be directly traumatized or be injured from overuse. Either etiology can result in *tenosynovitis*, which is seen on MR imaging as fluid in the tendon sheath with the underlying tendon appearing normal; or *tendinosis*, which is seen as focal or fusiform swelling of the tendon with signal within the tendon that does not get bright on T2 images. This represents myxoid degeneration and can progress to a partial or complete tear. A partial tear has thinning or attenuation or has T2 high signal within it. A complete tear or rupture has a gap in the tendon. It is often diagnosed on axial images by noting absence of a tendon on one or more images.

It is important to distinguish between tendinosis and a partial tear or complete disruption because surgical repair is often warranted for the latter two and not for the former. It is often difficult to make the distinction clinically.

Complete tendon disruption can be difficult to see on sagittal or coronal images because of the tendency for tendons to course obliquely to the plane of imaging. An exception to this is the Achilles tendon, which is usually best seen on a sagittal image. The imaging protocol for the foot and ankle must include axial images with T1 (or proton density) and T2 (or T2*) sequences. It is not recommended that both ankles be studied together. An extremity coil around one ankle with a small field of view will give the highest image quality. Both sagittal and coronal images with T1 and T2 weighting are also performed.

Achilles Tendon

The Achilles tendon does not have a sheath associated with it; therefore tenosynovitis does not occur. Tendinosis and partial tears are commonly seen in the Achilles. Complete disruption is commonly seen in athletes and in males around the age of 40; however, it is such an easy clinical diagnosis that MR imaging is usually not necessary. Complete tears are also commonly associated with other systemic disorders that cause tendon weakening, such as rheumatoid arthritis, collagen vascular diseases, crystal deposition diseases, and hyperparathyroidism.

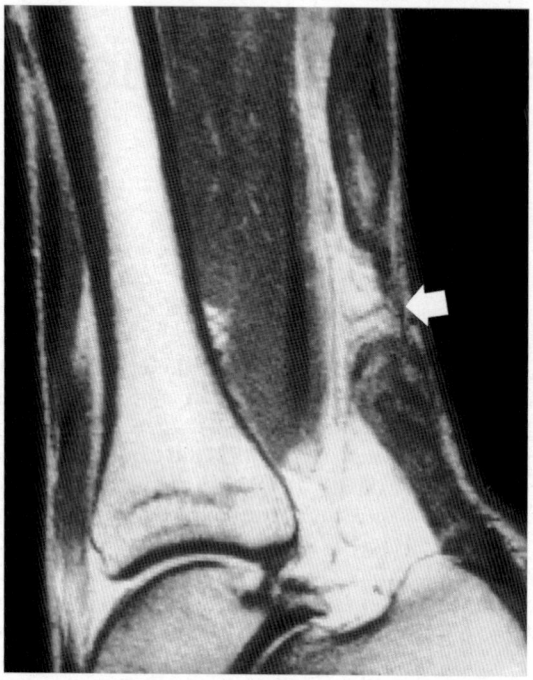

FIG. 12.1 **Torn Achilles Tendon.** A sagittal T1-weighted image reveals the Achilles to be torn with a 2-cm gap. Only a thin remnant of the tendon remains intact across the gap *(arrow)*. Note the high signal in the swollen ends of the separated tendon, indicative of hemorrhage and/or tendinosis.

Achilles tendon disruption can be treated surgically or by placing the patient in a cast with equinus positioning (marked plantar flexion) for several months. It is very controversial as to which treatment is superior, with both methods of treatment seemingly working well. I have known two surgeons who were dogmatic in their approach to always recommending surgery for torn Achilles tendons until they ruptured their own and opted for nonsurgical treatment.

MR imaging is being used by some surgeons to help decide if surgery should be performed. If a large gap is present (Fig. 12.1), some surgeons feel surgery should be performed to reappose the torn ends of the tendon, whereas if the ends of the tendon are not retracted, nonsurgical treatment is preferred. No papers have been published to show that this is, in fact, scientifically valid.

Posterior Tibial Tendon

The flexor tendons are easily remembered and identified by using the mnemonic "Tom, Dick, and Harry," with Tom representing the posterior Tibial tendon (PTT), Dick the flexor Digitorum longus, and Harry the flexor Hallucis longus (Fig. 12.2). The posterior tibial tendon is the most medial and the largest, with the exception of the Achilles, of the flexor tendons. The PTT inserts onto the navicular, second to fourth cuneiforms, and the bases of the second to fourth metatarsals. As it sweeps under the foot, it provides some support for the longitudinal arch; hence, problems in the arch or plantar fascia can sometimes lead to stress on the PTT with resulting tendinosis or even rupture. Posterior tibial tendinosis and rupture are commonly encountered in rheumatoid arthritis.

Rupture of the PTT results clinically in a flat foot due to the loss of arch support given by this tendon. The spring ligament runs just deep to the PTT and then goes underneath the neck of the talus, which it supports in a sling-like fashion. When the PTT tears, the stress is then placed on the spring ligament to support the talus and the arch. The spring ligament has a high incidence of disruption when the PTT tears. Once the PTT and the spring ligament tear, the next structure to fail is the subtalar joint ligaments—the sinus tarsi. We looked at 20 patients with PTT tears and found that 92% of the cases had abnormal spring ligaments (thickened or torn), and 75% had an abnormal sinus tarsi.[2] It's clear these structures are linked, and injury or stress to one can affect the others.

Differentiation of partial tears from tendon rupture can be difficult clinically, and MR imaging has become very valuable for making this distinction.[3] Most surgeons will operate on a disrupted PTT, whereas nonoperative therapy is often preferred for partial tears.

Posterior tibial tendinosis is seen on axial T1- or T2-weighted images as swelling and/or signal within the normally low-signal tendon on one or more images (Fig. 12.3). The increased signal should not be fluid bright on the T2 images. Tendon disruption is diagnosed by noting the absence of low-signal tendon on one or more axial images (Fig. 12.4). This typically occurs just at or above the level of the tibiotalar joint.

The spring ligament is identified on axial and coronal images just deep to the PTT. When it is stressed, it typically gets scarred and thickened (Fig. 12.5). A tear can be diagnosed by noting a gap in the ligament.

Flexor Hallucis Longus

The flexor hallucis longus (FHL) tendon is easily identified near the tibiotalar joint because it is usually the only tendon at that distal level that has muscle still attached. In the foot, the FHL is easily identified beneath the sustentaculum talus, which it uses as a pulley to plantar flex the foot.

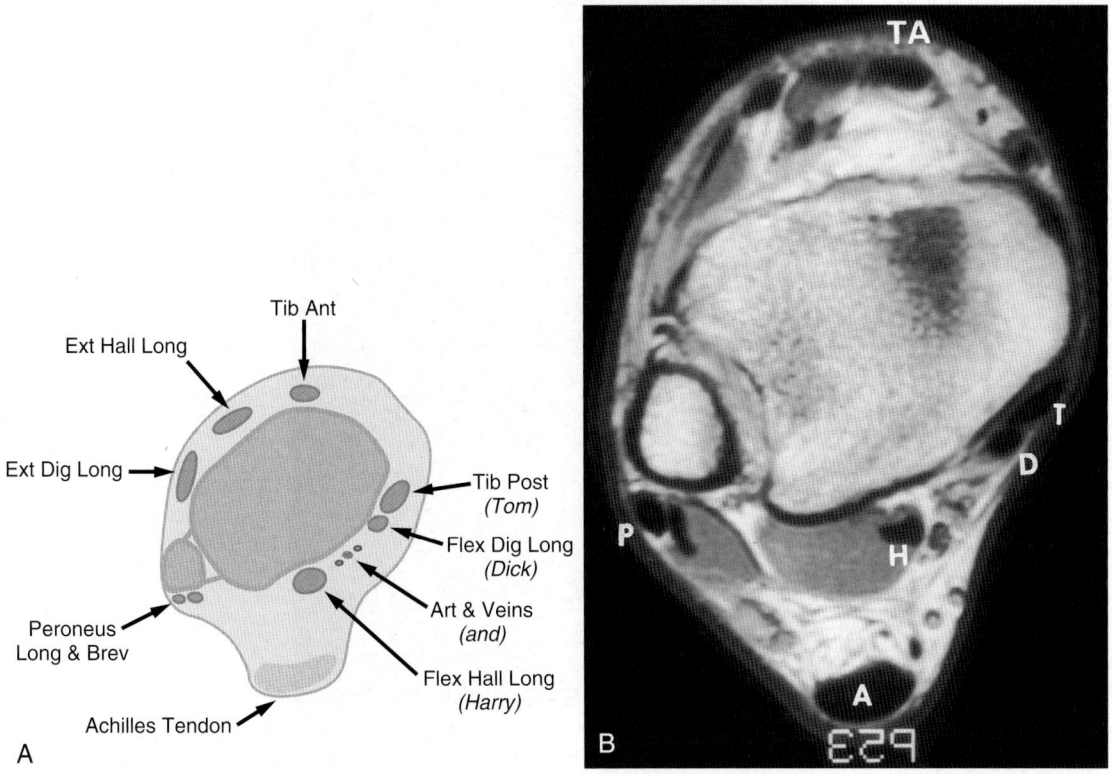

FIG. 12.2 **Normal Ankle Anatomy.** (A) This drawing of the tendons around the ankle at the level of the tibiotalar joint shows the relationship of the flexor tendons posteriorly and the extensor tendons anteriorly. (B) An axial T1-weighted image through the ankle just above the tibiotalar joint shows the normal anatomy. (*A*, Achilles tendon; *D*, flexor digitorum tendon; *H*, flexor hallucis tendon; *P*, peroneal tendons; *T*, posterior tibial tendon; *TA*, tibialis anterior tendon).

The FHL is known as the Achilles tendon of the foot in ballet dancers because of the extreme flexion position they frequently employ. Ballet dancers often will have tenosynovitis of the FHL, seen on MR imaging as fluid in the sheath surrounding the tendon. Care must be taken to have clinical correlation, as up to 20% of normal people have a communication between the ankle joint and the FHL tendon sheath; therefore fluid can be seen in the FHL tendon sheath from a connection to an ankle joint, which has an effusion. Rupture of the FHL is rare.

Peroneal Tendons

The peroneus longus and brevis tendons can be seen posterior to the distal fibula to which they are bound by a thin fibrous structure, the superior retinaculum. The fibula serves as a pulley for the tendons to work as the principal evertor of the foot. The tendons course close together adjacent to the lateral aspect of the calcaneus until a few centimeters below the lateral malleolus where they separate, with the peroneus brevis inserting onto the base of the fifth metatarsal and the peroneus longus crossing under the foot to the base of the first metatarsal. Avulsion of the base of the fifth metatarsal from a pull by the peroneus brevis is known as a "dancer's fracture" or a Jones fracture.

Disruption of the superior retinaculum, often seen in skiing accidents, can result in displacement of the peroneal tendons (Fig. 12.6), which must be surgically corrected. It often occurs with a small bony avulsion, called a flake fracture, off of the fibula caused by the avulsed superior retinaculum.

Entrapment of the peroneal tendons in a fractured calcaneus or fibula can occur and is easily diagnosed with MR or CT. This can be a difficult diagnosis to make clinically. Complete disruption of the peroneals is uncommon but is easily noted with MR.

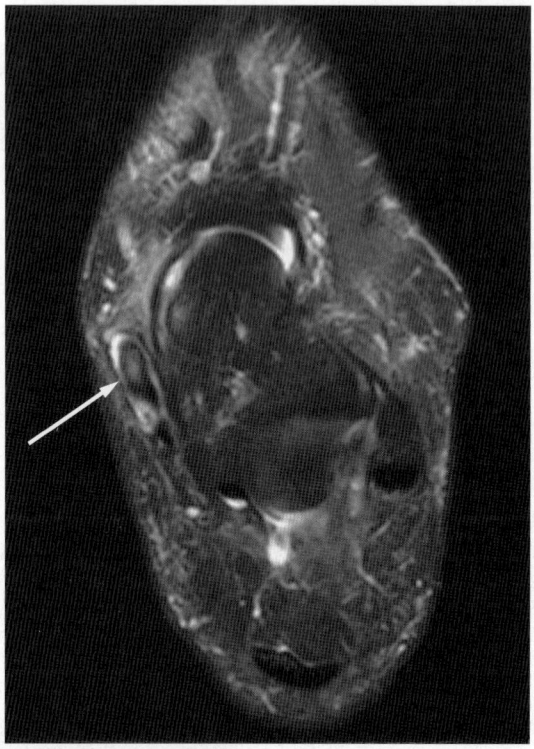

FIG. 12.3 **Posterior Tibial Tendon Tendinosis.** A T2W axial image through the ankle shows the posterior tibial tendon *(arrow)* swollen and containing high signal. This is the appearance of marked tendinosis.

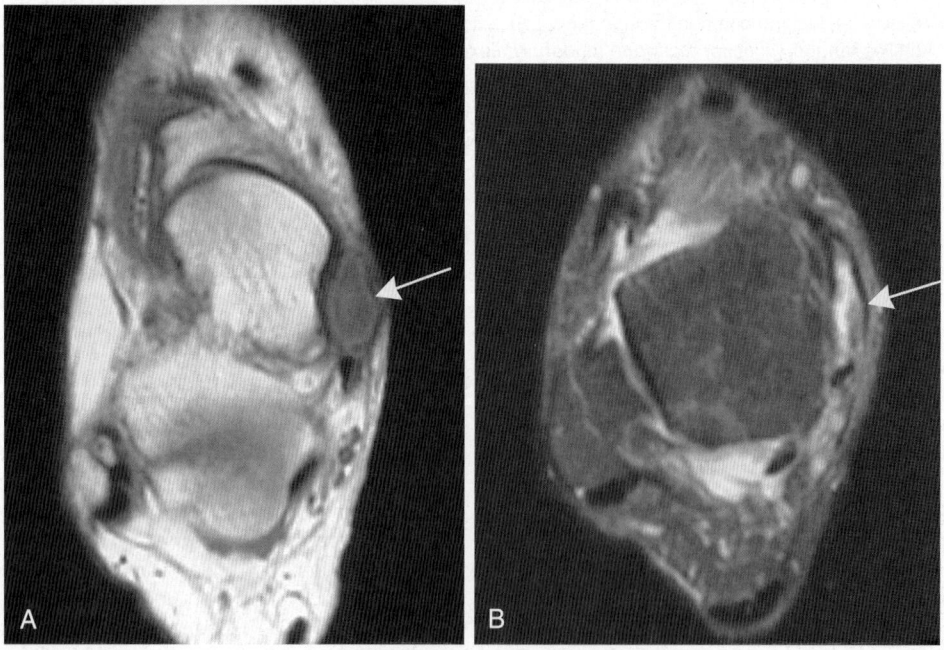

FIG. 12.4 **Torn Posterior Tibial Tendon.** An axial T1- (A) and T2-weighted (B) images through the ankle in this patient with chronic pain reveal a distended posterior tibial tendon sheath *(arrows)* with no low-signal tendon identified within. This is a tear of the posterior tibial tendon.

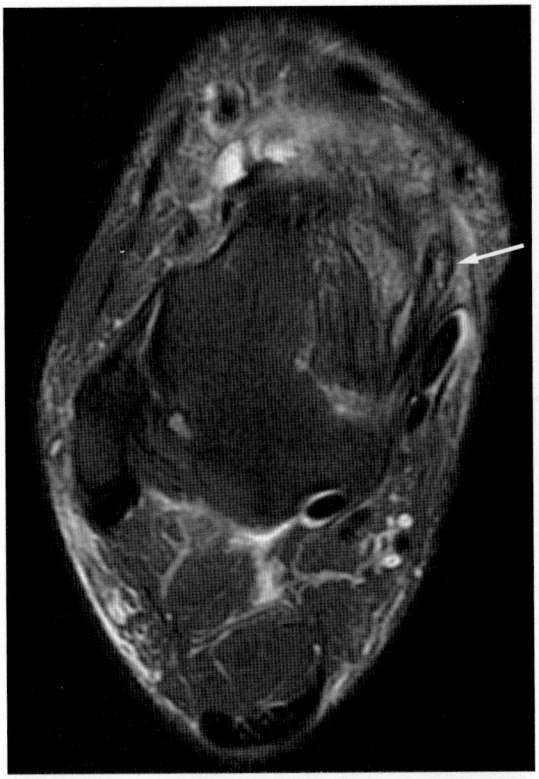

FIG. 12.5 **Abnormal Spring Ligament.** An axial T2-weighted image through the ankle shows a markedly thickened spring ligament *(arrows)* with high signal within it just deep to the posterior tibial tendon.

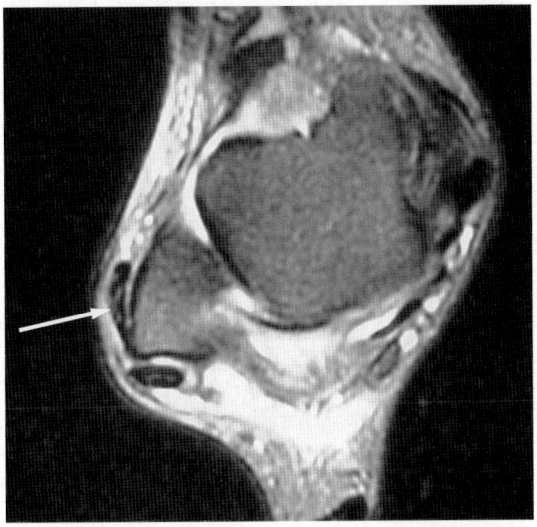

FIG. 12.6 **Dislocated Peroneus Longus Tendon.** An axial T2WI in this rock climber who injured his ankle in a fall shows a low-signal rounded structure *(arrow)* lateral to the lateral malleolus. This is a dislocated peroneus longus tendon.

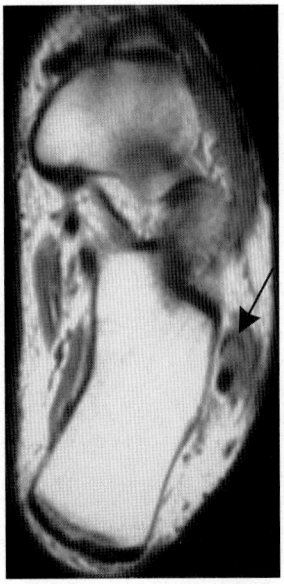

FIG. 12.7 **Longitudinal Split Tear of the Peroneus Brevis.** This axial T1-weighted image shows the peroneus brevis *(arrow)* with a *V* or chevron shape, which is characteristic for a longitudinal split tear of the brevis.

Longitudinal split tears of the peroneus brevis are commonly seen in patients following an inversion ankle sprain with associated dorsiflexion. The peroneus brevis gets trapped against the fibula by the peroneus longus, and a longitudinal split tear of the peroneus brevis results. These patients have chronic lateral ankle pain, often associated with ankle instability due to the lateral collateral ligament disruption that also occurs with the inversion trauma. A split tear of the peroneus brevis is easily identified on MRI by noting either a chevron or *V* shape to the tendon distal to the fibula (Fig. 12.7), or noting a division of the tendon into two parts. There is an 80% association with lateral ligament tears, so close attention should be paid to the ligaments when a split tear of the peroneus brevis is found.

AVASCULAR NECROSIS

Avascular necrosis (AVN) commonly occurs in the foot and ankle. The talar dome is the second most common location of osteochondritis dissecans (the knee is the most common site). MR imaging is useful in identifying and staging osteochondritis dissecans (which, for whatever reason, is now called an osteochondral lesion, OCL). Even when not apparent on plain films, MR imaging can show an OCL as a focal area of low signal in the subarticular portion of the talar dome on

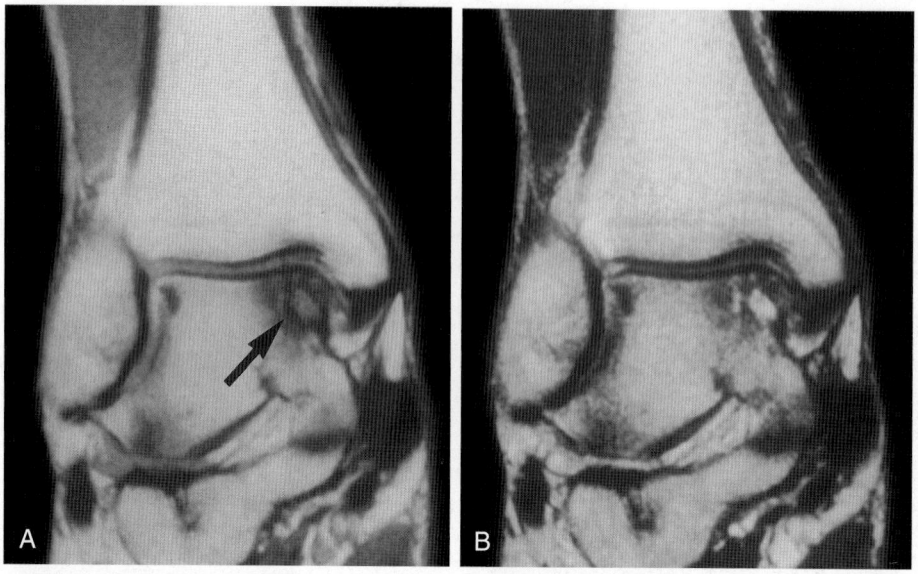

FIG. 12.8 **Unstable Osteochondritis Dissecans of the Talus.** (A) A proton-density coronal image through the talus shows a focus of low signal in the medial subarticular part of the talus *(arrow)*. This is a characteristic appearance for osteochondritis dissecans. (B) A T2-weighted image shows high signal throughout the focus of osteochondritis dissecans, which indicates an unstable fragment.

T1-weighted images. On T2 images, if high signal is seen surrounding the OCL fragment in the bone at the bed of the fragment or throughout the fragment (Fig. 12.8), it is most likely an unstable fragment. These signs seem to be less useful in adolescents than in adults. If the fragment has become displaced and lies in the joint as a loose body, MR imaging can sometimes be useful in localizing it; however, loose bodies in any joint can be exceedingly difficult to find.

Diffuse low signal throughout a tarsal bone on T1- and T2-weighted images is typical for AVN. If the T2-weighted images have increased signal throughout, it may or may not be reversible. This occasionally occurs in the tarsal navicular (Fig. 12.9). MR imaging can be useful in making this diagnosis when plain films are normal or equivocal. AVN in the tarsal navicular can result from continued weight bearing on a fracture that was not diagnosed. This is often seen in athletes, especially basketball players, and can be a career-ending injury in a professional athlete.

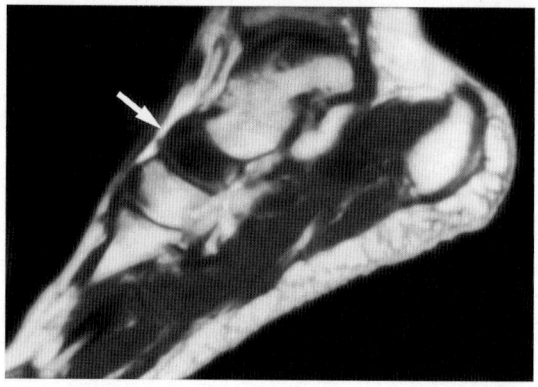

FIG. 12.9 **Avascular Necrosis of the Tarsal Navicular.** A T1-weighted sagittal image of the ankle in this patient with pain on the dorsum of the foot shows diffuse low signal throughout the tarsal navicular. This is a characteristic appearance for avascular necrosis and will often precede any plain-film findings.

TUMORS

There are a few tumors that have a predilection for the foot and ankle.[4] Up to 16% of synovial sarcomas occur in the foot. Desmoid tumors are commonly seen in the foot. Giant cell tumors of tendon sheath are often found in the tendon sheaths of the foot and ankle (Fig. 12.10). They are characterized by marked low signal in the synovial lining and in the tendons on T1 and T2 images, similar to the appearance of pigmented villonodular synovitis (PVNS) in a joint.

The differential diagnosis for calcaneal tumors is similar to that of the epiphyses: giant cell tumor, chondroblastoma, infection—and in addition, a unicameral bone cyst (Fig. 12.11). This differential works over 95%

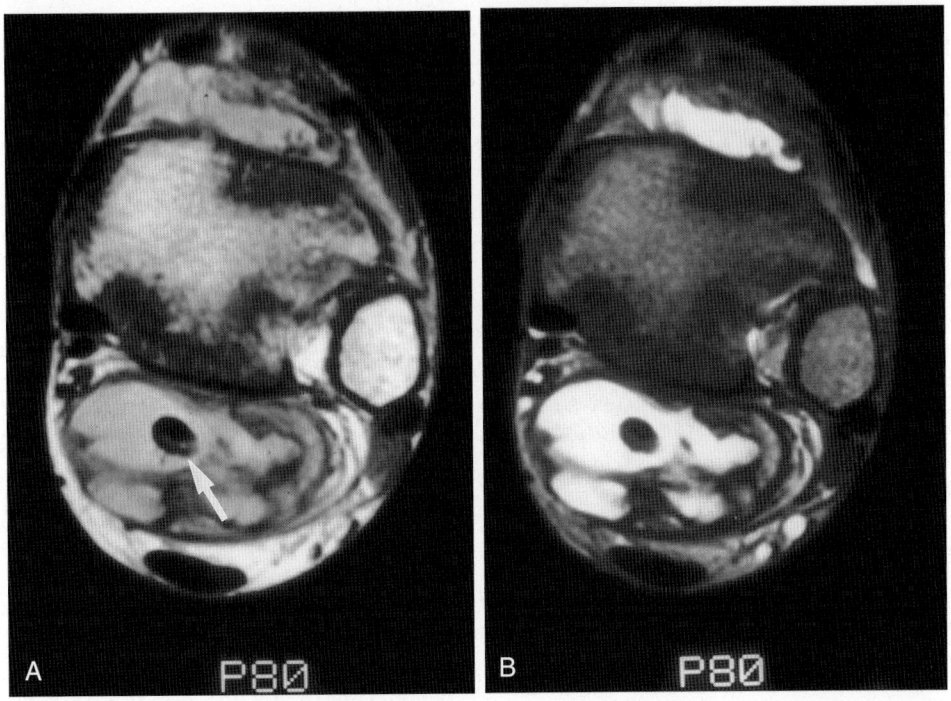

FIG. 12.10 **Giant Cell Tumor of Tendon Sheath.** Axial proton density (A) and T2-weighted (B) images reveal a mass surrounding the flexor hallucis longus tendon *(arrow)*, which is confined by the tendon sheath. Although high-signal fluid is present, large amounts of low signal material is lining the distended tendon sheath. This low signal is hemosiderin, which is typically found in a giant cell tendon of tendon sheath. pigmented villonodular synovitis (PVNS) in a joint has an identical appearance.

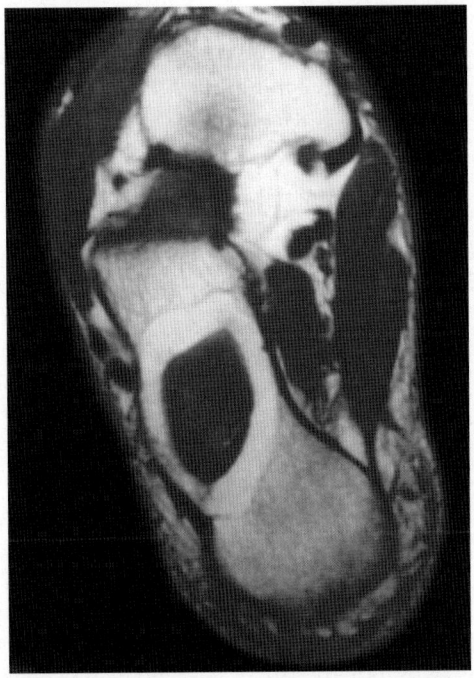

FIG. 12.11 **Calcaneal Unicameral Bone Cyst.** A T1-weighted axial image through the calcaneus reveals a typical unicameral bone cyst. Note that some fatty material is present in the periphery, and fluid is present in the central portion. Biopsy of the peripheral portion could lead to an erroneous diagnosis of an intraosseous lipoma. Unicameral bone cysts will occasionally have fatty elements within as well as serous fluid.

of the time for epiphyseal lesions; however, it may be less than 50% inclusive in the calcaneus—but it's a good starting point.

Soft tissue tumors in the medial aspect of the foot and ankle can press on the posterior tibial nerve, resulting in tarsal tunnel syndrome.[5] Clinically, patients with tarsal tunnel syndrome present with pain and paresthesia in the plantar aspect of the foot. In the aforementioned mnemonic, "Tom, Dick, and Harry," the "and" is for Artery, nerve, and vein. It is the position of the posterior tibial nerve. The nerve is easily compressed in the tarsal tunnel, which is bounded medially by the flexor retinaculum—a strong fibrous band that extends across the medial ankle joint for about 5 to 7 cm in a superior to inferior direction. Ganglions and neural tumors, both of which can look similar on T1- and T2-weighted images, often lie in the tarsal tunnel (Fig. 12.12) and compress the posterior tibial nerve, resulting in pain and paresthesia on the plantar aspect of the foot extending into the toes. Tarsal tunnel syndrome often occurs secondary to trauma, fibrosis, or idiopathically, all of which may not respond to surgical intervention; hence, MR imaging is valuable in delineating a treatable lesion (i.e., a mass) in many cases. An MR imaging exam for tarsal tunnel syndrome is becoming increasingly requested as surgeons learn how valuable it can be in identifying the source of the symptoms.

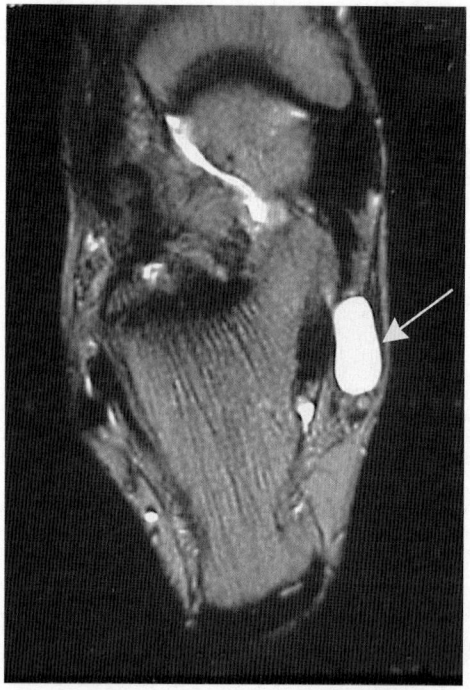

FIG. 12.12 **Ganglion Causing Tarsal Tunnel Syndrome.** A T2-weighted axial image of the ankle in a patient complaining of pain and paresthesia on the plantar aspect of the foot shows a high signal mass *(arrow)* lying adjacent to the flexor hallucis longus tendon. This is the position of the posterior tibial nerve that can be impinged by a mass, such as in this case, resulting in tarsal tunnel syndrome. This was a ganglion.

Anomalous muscles in the foot or ankle are reported to be present in up to 6% of the population. These can be mistaken for a tumor and biopsied unnecessarily. MR imaging will show these "tumors" to have imaging characteristics identical to normal muscle (Fig. 12.13) and to be sharply circumscribed. Accessory soleus and peroneus quartus muscles are the most common accessory muscles encountered around the foot and ankle.

LIGAMENTS

MR imaging is not the best way to diagnose acute ankle ligament abnormalities. The clinical evaluation is usually straightforward, and no diagnostic imaging of any type is necessary. Nevertheless, in clinically equivocal cases, when the exam is ordered for other reasons, or in cases of chronic lateral ankle pain, the ligaments can be clearly evaluated with high-quality MR imaging.[6]

The deltoid ligament lies medially as a broad band beneath the medial flexor tendons. It can be seen extending from the medial malleolus to the talus and calcaneus. It has multiple parts, which are not easily separated with MR imaging. It is considered injured when it has increased T2 signal or disruption of the linear fibers. Surgery to repair a torn deltoid is uncommon, whereas reconstruction of the lateral ligament complex is commonly performed.

The lateral collateral ligament complex is responsible for over 90% of all ankle ligament injuries. It is made up of two parts: a superior group, the anterior and posterior tib–fib ligaments that make up part of the syndesmosis (Fig. 12.14), and an inferior group, the anterior and posterior talofibular ligaments and the calcaneofibular ligament (Fig. 12.15). The anterior and posterior tib–fib ligaments can be seen on axial images at the level of the dome of the talus. The anterior and posterior talofibular ligaments are seen on the axial images just below the tibiotalar joint and emanate from a concavity in the distal fibula called the malleolar fossa (Fig. 12.15B). The most commonly torn ankle ligament is the anterior talofibular ligament. It is easily identified when a joint effusion is present because it makes up the anterior capsule of

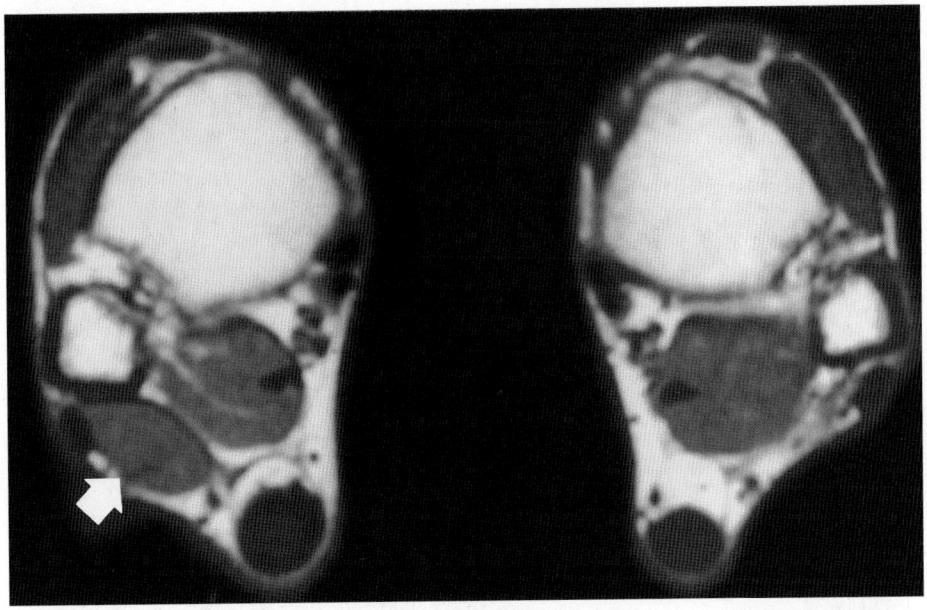

FIG. 12.13 **Anomalous Muscle.** An axial T1-weighted image of both ankles in this patient complaining of a mass in the right ankle shows an anomalous muscle *(arrow)*, a peroneus quartus, lateral to the flexor hallucis longus muscle, which is responsible for the mass the patient feels.

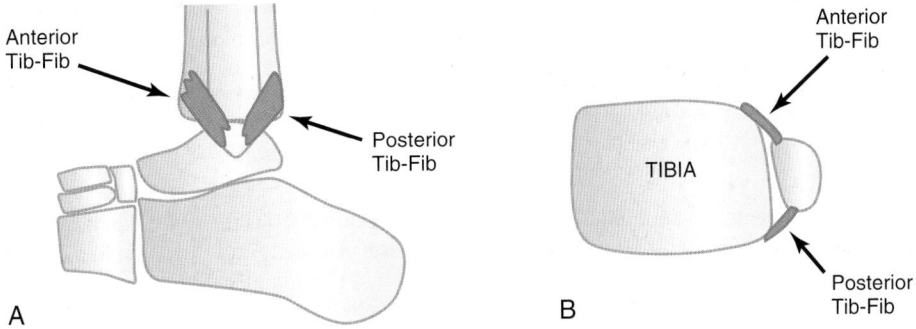

FIG. 12.14 **Schematic of Lateral Collateral Ligaments.** This drawing of the ankle in a lateral view (A) shows how the anterior and posterior tib–fib ligaments extend off of the fibula and course superiorly to the tibia. A drawing in the axial plane (B) shows that the fibula has a flat or convex surface at the origin of these ligaments.

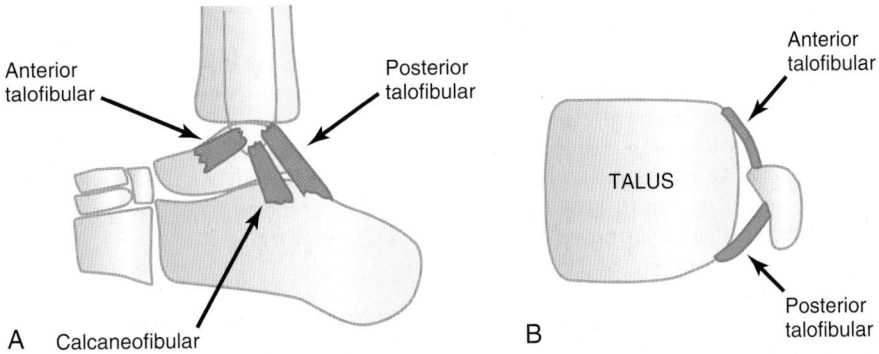

FIG. 12.15 **Schematic of Lateral Collateral Ligaments.** This drawing of the ankle in a lateral view (A) shows how the anterior and posterior talofibular ligaments and the calcaneofibular ligament extend off of the fibula and course inferiorly. These ligaments arise off of the fibula more distally than the anterior and posterior tib–fib ligaments. A drawing in the axial plane (B) shows that the anterior and posterior talofibular ligaments arise from the level of the distal fibula, which has a concave medial surface, the malleolar fossa.

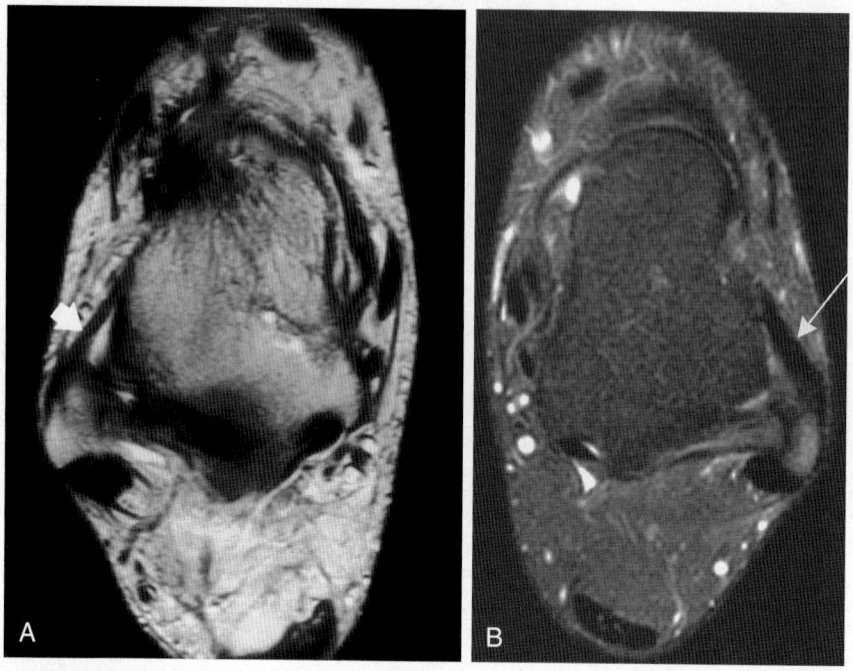

FIG. 12.16 **Anterior Talofibular Ligament.** (A) An axial T2-weighted image through the distal fibula at the level of the malleolar fossa (the concave medial surface of the fibula) shows an intact anterior talofibular ligament *(arrow)*, which makes up part of the joint capsule at this level. Note the high-signal joint fluid adjacent to the ligament. (B) This axial T2-weighted image at the level of the malleolar fossa reveals a thickened anterior talofibular ligament *(arrow)*. The marked thickening of the ligament indicates a chronic process with scarring.

the joint (Fig. 12.16). The anterior talofibular ligament is usually torn without other ligaments being involved; however, if the injury is severe enough, the next ligament to tear is the calcaneofibular ligament. Even with very severe trauma, the posterior talofibular ligament rarely tears. The anterior talofibular ligament always tears before the calcaneofibular ligament. A torn anterior talofibular ligament will be absent in some chronic tears but can be thickened (Fig. 12.16B); it can be attenuated or have a gap, also (Fig. 12.17).

Sinus Tarsi Syndrome

An entity that has a high association with torn lateral collateral ligaments in the ankle is sinus tarsi syndrome. Clinically, these patients have lateral ankle pain and a feeling of hindfoot instability. Up to 80% of these patients have torn lateral collateral ligaments, and up to one-third of patients who tear their lateral collateral ligaments have been reported to have sinus tarsi syndrome.[7] In the past, diagnosis has relied on clinical suspicion and injection of xylocaine into the sinus tarsus, which causes resolution of the pain. Treatment is varied but can include a joint fusion.

The sinus tarsi is the space that lies between the talus and the calcaneus and opens up in a cone-like configuration in the lateral aspect of the ankle beneath the lateral malleolus. It is filled with fat and several ligaments that give hindfoot stability. The most lateral of these ligaments are slips of ligaments from the lateral extensor retinaculum. Medial to these are the cervical ligament, and the most medial ligament is the interosseous ligament (Fig. 12.18). In sinus tarsi syndrome, the fat in the sinus tarsus is obliterated, and one or more of the ligaments are disrupted (Fig. 12.19). Visualization of the ligaments is not necessary—replacement of the normal fat with scar tissue makes the diagnosis. This syndrome is causing an increasing amount of MR imaging requests as surgeons and podiatrists recognize that a definitive diagnosis of sinus tarsi syndrome can be made with imaging.

BONY ABNORMALITIES

Tarsal coalition is a common cause of a painful flat foot. It occurs most commonly at the calcaneonavicular joint and the middle facet of the talocalcaneal

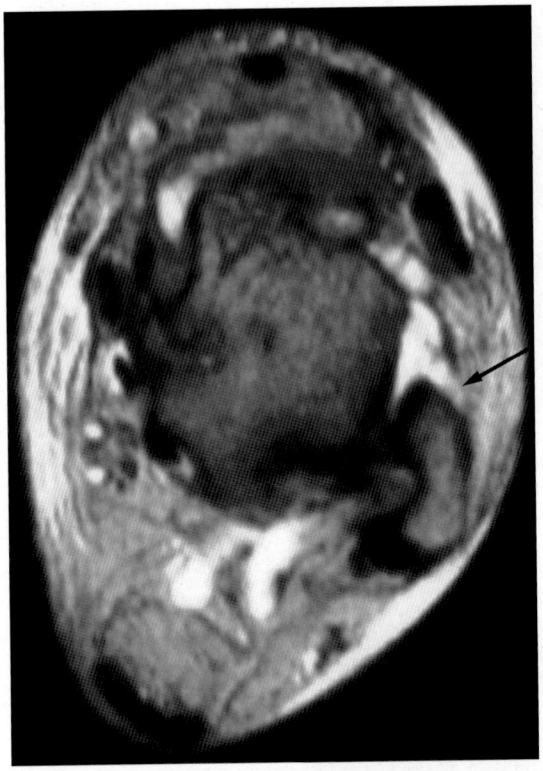

FIG. 12.17 **Torn Anterior Talofibular Ligament.** The anterior talofibular ligament is attenuated and has a gap *(arrow)* in this athlete who suffered a sprained ankle several days before this magnetic resonance imaging (MRI).

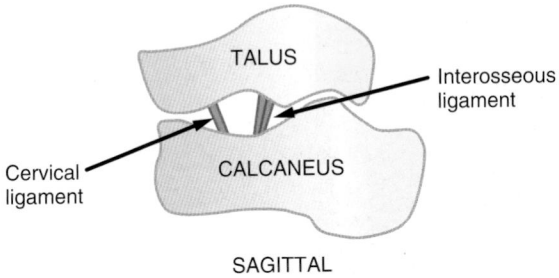

FIG. 12.18 **Schematic of the Sinus Tarsi.** A sagittal schematic of the sinus tarsi show the positions of the cervical and the interosseous ligaments. The cervical ligament lies more anteriorly and laterally in relation to the interosseous ligament.

joint (Fig. 12.20). Up to 50% of patients with tarsal coalition have bilateral coalition. It can be difficult (or impossible) to see the coalition on plain films; however, CT and MR imaging will show bony coalition with a high degree of accuracy. Coalitions most commonly are fibrous or cartilaginous. In these cases, secondary findings, such as joint space irregularity at the affected joint or degenerative joint disease (DJD) at nearby joints that are subjected to accentuated stress, can be seen. For now, MR imaging does not appear to have superiority to CT for diagnosing tarsal coalition.

Fractures of the foot and ankle are usually well documented with plain films. Stress fractures, however, can be difficult to radiographically or clinically diagnose and can mimic more sinister abnormalities. MR imaging will show stress fractures as linear low signal on T1-weighted images with high signal on T2 weighting (Fig. 12.21).

MR imaging has had mixed reviews when used for diagnosing osteomyelitis in the foot. In diabetics with foot infections, it is important to diagnose osteomyelitis, as the treatment is often much more aggressive, including amputation, than if the bone is not involved. If the marrow appears normal, MR imaging is useful in predicting no osteomyelitis; however, if high T2 signal is present in the marrow, osteomyelitis may or may not be present. High T2 signal can be caused by edema, hyperemia, trauma, reactive change from adjacent soft tissue infection, and even from red marrow, as well as from osteomyelitis. The only definitive MR findings for osteomyelitis are cortical disruption (Fig. 12.22), a bony abscess (not a common finding), or a sinus track (an even less common finding). However, if the low signal in the marrow on T1 images, which was high signal on T2 images, is as low as the adjacent soft tissues and muscle, osteomyelitis is almost certainly present. The other causes of high T2 signal in the marrow will have T1 low signal that is gray and higher in signal than the adjacent soft tissues. This finding is extremely helpful for diagnosing osteomyelitis when the presence of cortical disruption is not obvious.

CHRONIC LATERAL ANKLE PAIN

Chronic lateral ankle pain is, after the diabetic foot with infection, the bane of most foot and ankle specialists. There are many causes of chronic lateral ankle pain, including DJD, loose bodies, and an OCL of the talus; however, there are four common entities that are easily identified with MRI (Table 12.1). Newer surgical techniques are evolving to treat these; however, when several of these occur simultaneously (which is not uncommon), it can be very difficult to determine from the clinical exam where the abnormality lies. MRI is very useful in helping determine

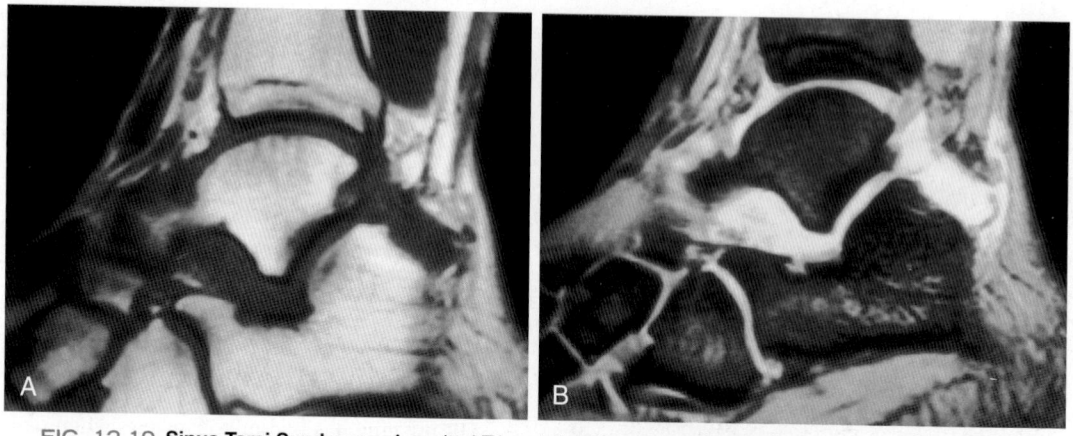

FIG. 12.19 **Sinus Tarsi Syndrome.** A sagittal T1-weighted image (A) shows obliteration of the normal fat in the sinus tarsi. No ligaments are visualized. A sagittal T2-weighted image (B) reveals no evidence of the normal cervical or interosseous ligaments. The high signal throughout the sinus tarsi represents scar or fibrosis. These findings are classic for sinus tarsi syndrome.

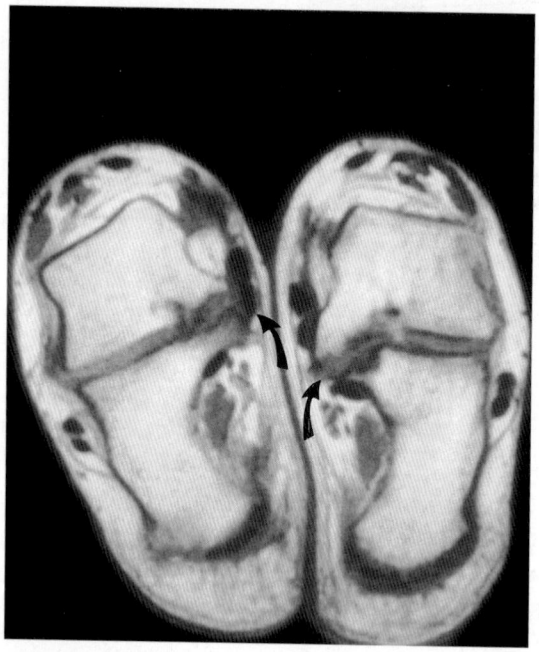

FIG. 12.20 **Tarsal Coalition.** An axial T1-weighted image in a patient with painful flat feet shows bilateral talocalcaneal coalition *(arrows)*, which is primarily fibrous. The joint space is irregular and widened bilaterally. In cases of suspected coalition, both ankles should be imaged because coalition often occurs bilaterally.

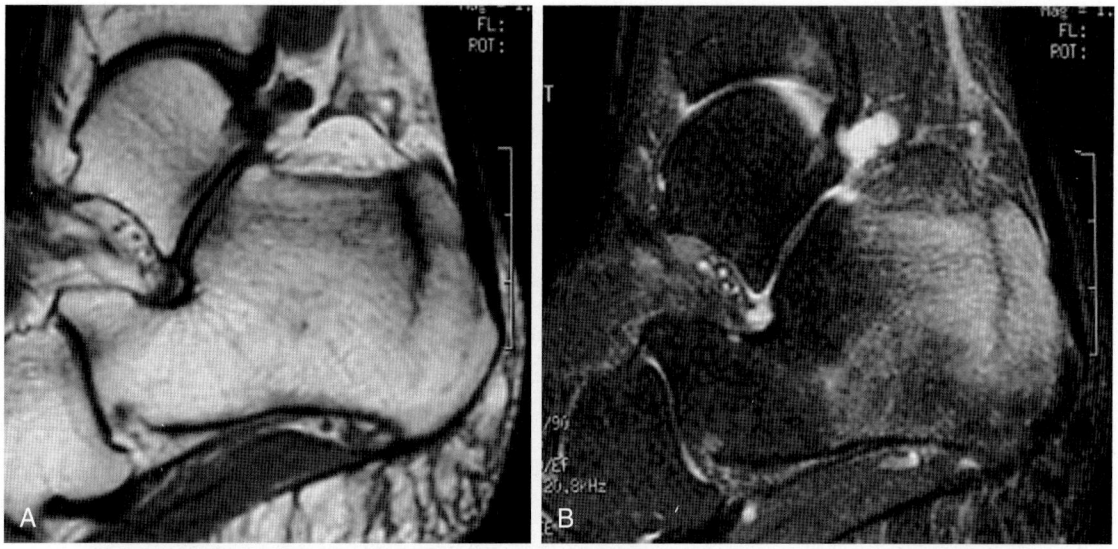

FIG. 12.21 **Calcaneal Stress Fracture.** (A) A sagittal T1-weighted image through the calcaneus shows linear low signal, which has surrounding high signal on the T2-weighted image (B), which is characteristic for a stress fracture.

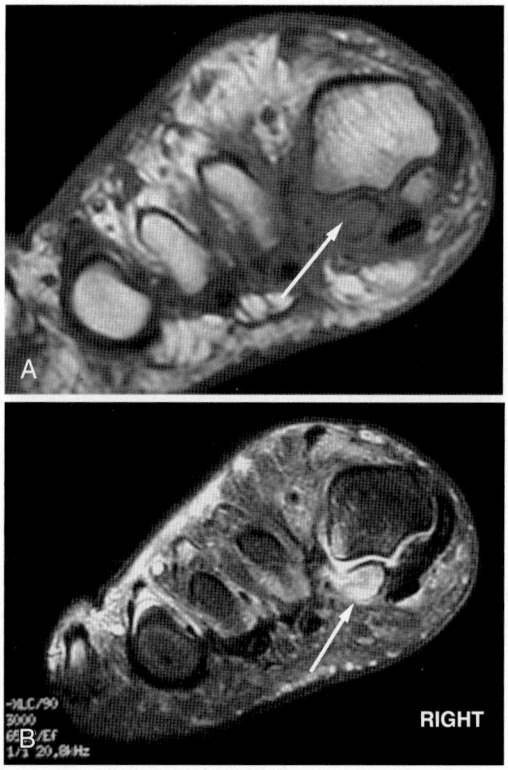

FIG. 12.22 **Osteomyelitis.** Axial T1 (A) and T2 (B) weighted images through the forefoot in this diabetic shows low T1 signal (*arrow*, A) and high T2 signal (*arrow*, B) in the lateral sesamoid. Cortical disruption is present which is diagnostic for osteomyelitis.

TABLE 12.1 Common Causes of Chronic Lateral Ankle Pain
Anterior talofibular ligament disruption or scarring
Sinus tarsi syndrome
Longitudinal split tears of the peroneus brevis
Anterolateral impingement

exactly where the pathology is, which then allows the surgeon to direct his therapy more precisely.[8]

Injury to the anterior talofibular ligament from an inversion ankle sprain is the common thread running through all of these diagnoses, being associated in around 80% in each entity. These four entities should be looked for in every ankle MR, as they are commonly found even in only minimally symptomatic patients.

Isolated chronic injury to the anterior talofibular ligament may be a cause of chronic lateral ankle pain, or it may be only one part of the problem. An 80% association with sinus tarsi syndrome and longitudinal split tears (both of which were discussed earlier in this chapter) has been reported, either of which can be a cause of chronic lateral ankle pain by themselves.

Another cause of chronic lateral ankle pain, which has a high association with chronic disruption of the anterior talofibular ligament, is anterolateral impingement or lateral gutter syndrome. The lateral gutter is

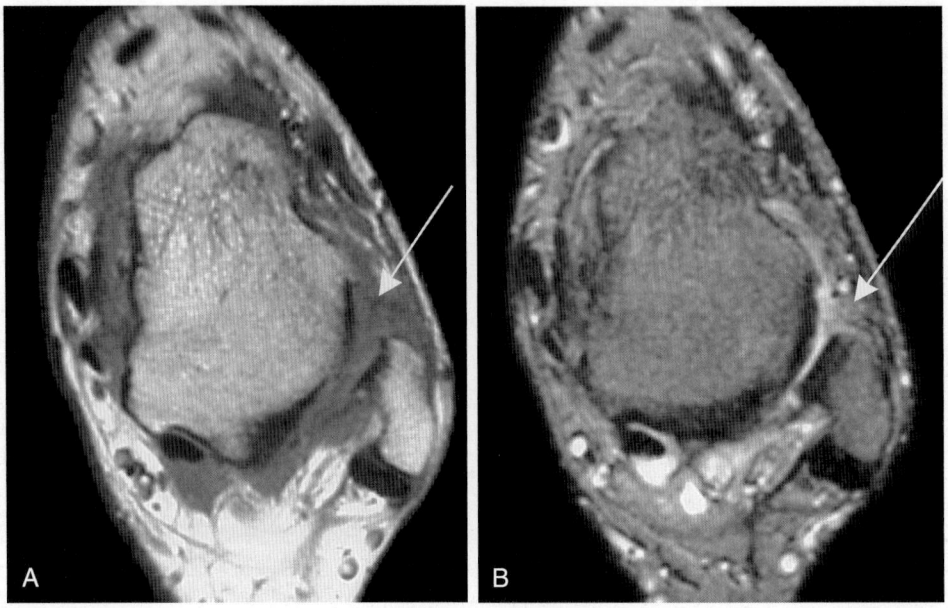

FIG. 12.23 **Anterolateral Impingement.** This axial T1-weighted image through the ankle (A) reveals absence of the anterior talofibular ligament *(arrow)*. The corresponding T2-weighted image (B) shows low signal scar tissue deep to the expected location of the anterior talofibular ligament *(arrow)*, which indicates anterolateral impingement syndrome.

simply the lateral joint space between the distal tibia and talus medially and the fibula and lateral collateral ligaments laterally. The synovium gets thickened and scarred from an inversion ankle injury and causes a painful, mechanical block to dorsiflexion. It is easily identified with MRI by noting low-signal scar tissue in the joint just deep to the anterior talofibular ligament where one should see joint fluid (Fig. 12.23). It is treated by arthroscopically debriding the scar tissue and, if necessary, reconstructing the lateral collateral ligaments.

REFERENCES

1. Kneeland J, Macrandar S, Middleton W, Cates J, Jesmanowicz A, Hyde J. MR imaging of the normal ankle: correlation with anatomic sections. *AJR*. 1988;151:117–126.
2. Balen PF, Helms CA. Association of posterior tibial tendon injury with spring ligament injury, sinus tarsi abnormality, and plantar fasciitis on MR imaging. *AJR*. 2001;176:1137–1143.
3. Rosenberg Z, Cheung Y, Jahss M, Noto A, Norman A, Leeds N. Rupture of posterior tibial tendons: CT and MR imaging with surgical correlation. *Radiology*. 1988;169:229–236.
4. Keigley B, Haggar A, Gaba A, Ellis B, Froelich J, Wu K. Primary tumors of the foot: MR imaging. *Radiology*. 1989;171:755–759.
5. Erickson S, Quinn S, Kneeland J, et al. MR imaging of the tarsal tunnel and related spaces: normal and abnormal findings with anatomic correlation. *AJR*. 1990;155:323–328.
6. Erickson S, Smith J, Ruiz M, et al. MR imaging of the lateral collateral ligament of the ankle. *AJR*. 1991;156:131–136.
7. Klein M, Spreitzer A. MR imaging of the tarsal sinus and canal: normal anatomy, pathologic findings, and features of the sinus tarsi syndrome. *Radiology*. 1993;186:233–240.
8. Anzilotti K, Schweitzer ME, et al. Effect of foot and ankle MR imaging on clinical decision making. *Radiology*. 1996;201:515–517.

CHAPTER 13

Miscellaneous Magnetic Resonance Imaging

There are several additional areas in which magnetic resonance (MR) imaging is useful but should be covered in detail in texts devoted to musculoskeletal (MSK) MRI. They will be only superficially mentioned here. Included in this group are MR of the wrist, hip, elbow, and bone marrow.

WRIST

MR imaging of the wrist has been slower to develop than that of other joints. Similarly, wrist arthrography has not enjoyed the same popularity as that of the knee or shoulder. Nevertheless, MR imaging of the wrist has some definite utility. It is useful in evaluating the carpal bones for fractures and avascular necrosis (AVN). It seems to have some use for evaluating the triangular fibrocartilage (TFC) and the intercarpal ligaments.[1]

Imaging Techniques

Thin-section (2 to 3 mm) T1- and T2-weighted images in both an axial and a coronal plane are usually employed with a dedicated wrist coil or a small surface coil. Some recommend sagittal images as well. A small field of view (FOV) (5 to 8 cm) should be used for maximal resolution. Three-dimensional volumetric coronal images with thin (1 to 2 mm) slices are used in many centers to replace the T2-weighted images. These are especially useful for examining the TFC and the intercarpal ligaments.[2]

Pathology

Triangular Fibrocartilage

The TFC lies between the distal ulna and the carpal bones and is thought to have some shock-absorbing function. It can tear or become detached and cause significant wrist pain and dysfunction. Tears of the TFC can be diagnosed with arthrography or with MR imaging, although it is somewhat controversial as to the significance of a torn TFC. That is because torn TFCs (and torn intercarpal ligaments, for that matter) are found with a high frequency in older patients who do not have wrist pain or dysfunction. Nevertheless, in a young patient with a painful, torn TFC, most hand surgeons would surgically intervene if conservative care was ineffective. For this reason, imaging may play a role.

The normal TFC is predominantly low signal on all imaging sequences and seen to be triangular in shape with the base attaching to the ulna and the apex attaching onto the radius (Fig. 13.1). A detached or torn TFC is best seen in the coronal plane with T2 or gradient-echo sequences and is usually accompanied by joint fluid in both the distal radioulnar and the proximal carpal joints (Fig. 13.2).

Avascular Necrosis

The wrist has several bones that have a propensity to undergo AVN. The lunate is commonly affected and is known as Kienböck malacia. It is seen as uniform low signal on T1- and T2-weighted images (Fig. 13.3). As is found with AVN in other joints, MR imaging can be useful in showing AVN when plain films are normal.

The proximal pole of the scaphoid often undergoes AVN following a fracture. MR can demonstrate the AVN earlier than plain films, allowing earlier treatment (Fig. 13.4). Subtle or occult fractures of the scaphoid (or any other carpal bone) can be identified with MR. MR should be considered when clinical suspicion of a fracture is high and plain films are negative, since a missed fracture of the scaphoid can lead to AVN. We have found it cost-effective to perform an MR of the wrist to rule out a fracture in a patient with trauma, pain in the snuff box, and a negative plain film, as opposed to casting the patient for a week and having them return for a follow-up x-ray.[3]

Intercarpal Ligaments

The intercarpal ligaments can tear and cause pain and instability in the wrist. The scapholunate ligament is the most commonly torn intercarpal ligament. It should be identified at the proximal part of the scapholunate joint in every MRI of the wrist unless it is torn (Fig. 13.5). A torn scapholunate ligament will have linear disruption of the normal triangular or band-like configuration (Fig. 13.6). The next most common intercarpal ligament to tear is the lunatotriquetral ligament, which is found at the proximal portion of the

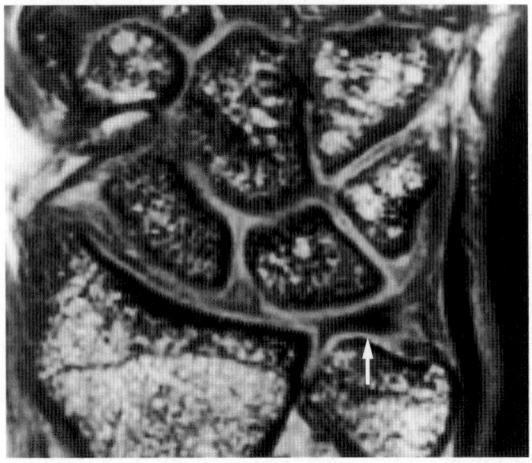

FIG. 13.1 **Normal Triangular Fibrocartilage (TFC).** A coronal gradient-echo 3D-volume thin-section image of a normal wrist shows the TFC *(arrow)* with its attachment to the radius separated by a thin layer of cartilage.

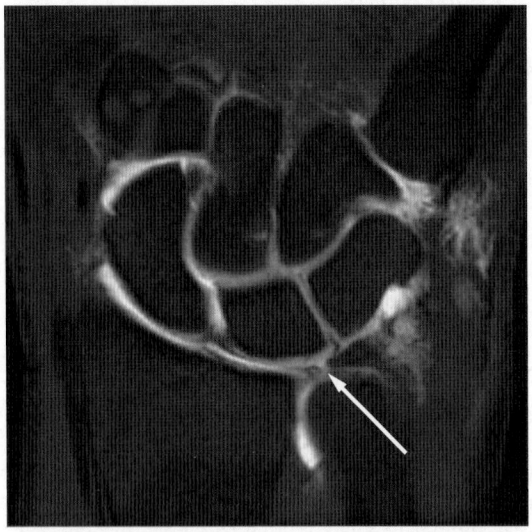

FIG. 13.2 **Torn Triangular Fibrocartilage (TFC).** A coronal T1WI of a wrist arthrogram in a patient with ulnar-sided wrist pain shows the TFC to be torn in its midsubstance *(arrow)*. Note the gadolinium/fluid that has extended into the distal radioulnar joint, which would only be present with a torn TFC.

joint. Unfortunately, it is not always visualized, even with excellent images; hence, it is difficult to diagnose a torn lunatotriquetral ligament with any certainty.

Further complicating the diagnosis of torn intercarpal ligaments is the fact that they can be torn as a

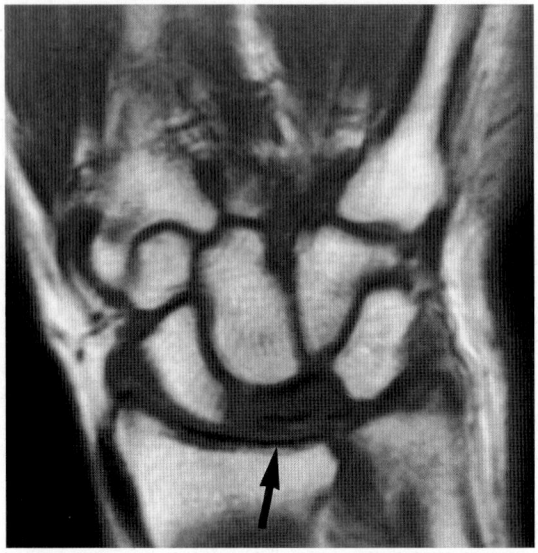

FIG. 13.3 **Kienböck Malacia.** A coronal T1-weighted image shows the lunate *(arrow)* to be devoid of the normal high signal from fatty marrow. This is diagnostic of avascular necrosis (AVN), called Kienböck malacia when it occurs in the lunate.

matter of aging and wear and tear without being symptomatic. Hence, diagnosing a torn ligament may have no clinical significance whatsoever. Cadaver studies have reported torn intercarpal ligaments in up to 80% of older people.

Carpal Tunnel Syndrome

The median nerve can become impinged in the carpal tunnel by a variety of processes and result in paresthesia in the hand and fingers. Surgical removal of the offending agent (if any—it is most often idiopathic or due to overuse of the hands in stressful positions, such as typing) and excision of the flexor retinaculum is usually curative if conservative treatment fails. Although MR imaging is useful in identifying tumors, ganglia, swollen flexor tendon sheaths, or other masses in the carpal tunnel, MRI has little role in carpal tunnel syndrome because of the ease with which the diagnosis of carpal tunnel syndrome is made clinically. If surgery is performed, it is easy to inspect the entire carpal tunnel, making preoperative imaging unnecessary.

Tendons

MRI plays a valuable role in identifying tendon abnormalities in the wrist. The extensor tendons seem to have more pathology associated with them than the flexor tendons. The most commonly affected extensor tendon

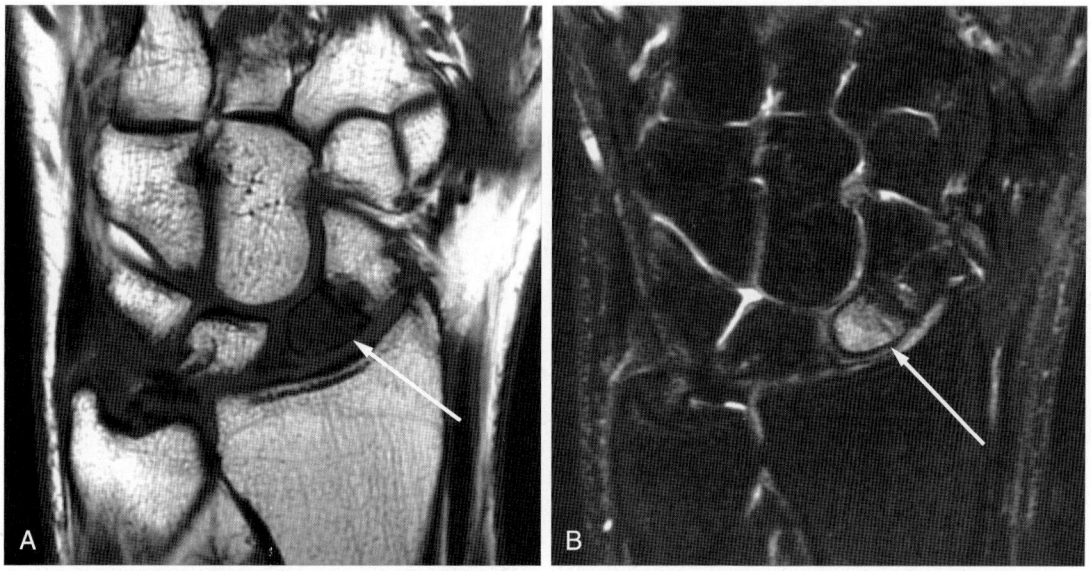

FIG. 13.4 **Scaphoid Avascular Necrosis (AVN).** Coronal images in a patient who suffered a fracture of his scaphoid several months prior shows low signal in the proximal pole on the T1WIs (A), which is high in signal on the T2WIs (B). This is worrisome but not diagnostic of AVN. If the T2WIs were low in signal, it would indicate AVN, but with high T2 signal, the proximal pole might still be viable.

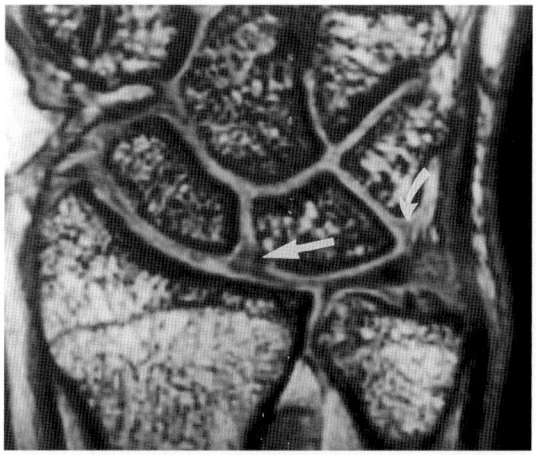

FIG. 13.5 **Scapholunate Ligament.** A coronal 3D-volume thin-section image of a normal wrist shows the appearance of the scapholunate ligament *(arrow)*. A normal lunatotriquetral ligament *(curved arrow)* can also be seen, although it is not always identified.

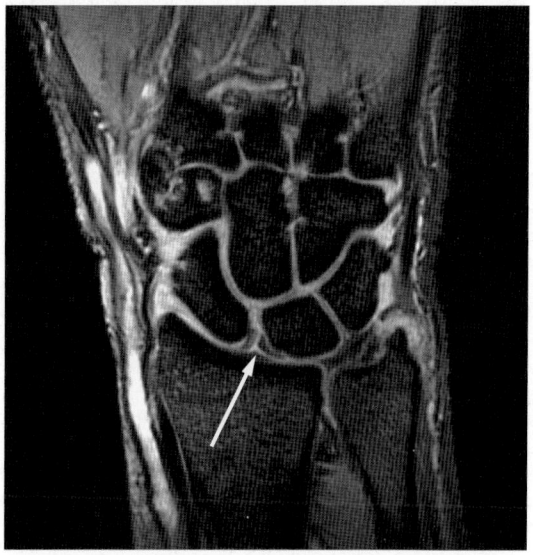

FIG. 13.6 **Torn Scapholunate Ligament.** This coronal T2WI demonstrates a torn scapholunate ligament *(arrow)* with linear disruption of the ligament. The body of the triangular fibrocartilage (TFC) is also torn.

is the extensor carpi ulnaris. It commonly has tendinosis with swelling and increased signal intensity, which is easily identified on the axial images. Longitudinal split tears (Fig. 13.7), as in tendons in the ankle, may have the same significance as complete tears. The abductor pollicis longus and extensor pollicis brevis tendons have a common tendon sheath on the radial aspect of the wrist and often have tenosynovitis and/or tendinosis, which can result in a "trigger thumb." This is where the thumb catches on attempted flexion and then suddenly gives way. This is

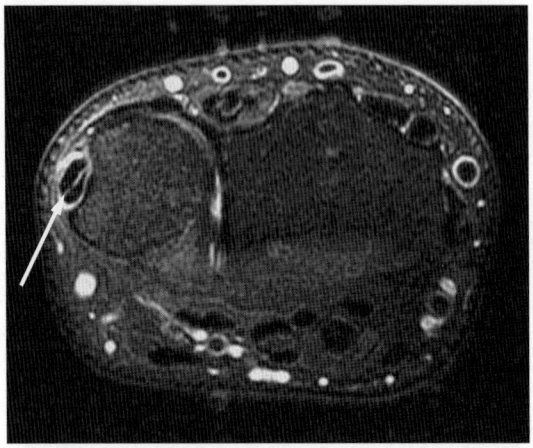

FIG. 13.7 **Longitudinal Split Tear of the Extensor Carpi ulnaris (ECU).** The ECU tendon has a split tear seen on this axial T2WI *(arrow)*.

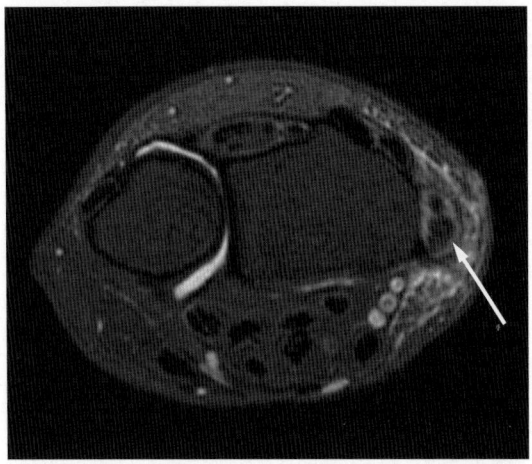

FIG. 13.8 **De Quervain.** This axial T2WI through the wrist at the distal radius in a patient complaining of a trigger thumb shows distension of the common tendon sheath surrounding the abductor pollicis longus and the extensor pollicis brevis tendons *(arrow)*. The fluid is not very T2 bright, suggesting synovitis. The abductor pollicis longus is somewhat thickened with some increased signal, indicative of tendinosis.

called De Quervain syndrome. MRI shows the fluid distending the tendon sheath (tenosynovitis) and will show the tendinosis, if present (Fig. 13.8).

Septic tenosynovitis in any of the flexor tendons (Fig. 13.9) is considered a surgical emergency by most hand surgeons, and when seen on MRI deserves a phone call to the surgeon. An infection in a flexor tendon sheath can easily spread to the common flexors in the wrist and lead to a terrible outcome for the patient.

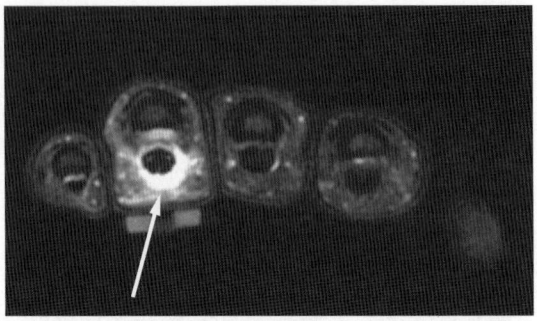

FIG. 13.9 **Flexor Tenosynovitis.** An axial T2WI through the fingers in a patient with painful swelling of the fourth digit shows tenosynovitis of the fourth flexor tendon *(arrow)*, which is worrisome for a septic tenosynovitis. Septic tenosynovitis is considered a surgical emergency, although magnetic resonance imaging (MRI) cannot tell if it is septic or aseptic.

MRI cannot differentiate a sterile tenosynovitis from an infectious tenosynovitis, but can alert the surgeon to the possibility of septic tenosynovitis.

HIP

MRI has proved to be useful in a number of abnormalities of the hip, including AVN, fractures (see Chapter 5), idiopathic transient osteoporosis of the hip (ITOH; see Chapter 8), torn acetabular labra, and femoroacetabular impingement (FAI).

Osteonecrosis (AVN)

AVN can be diagnosed with great sensitivity with MR imaging. It has a characteristic appearance with involvement of the anterosuperior portion of the femoral head. The area of AVN typically is surrounded by a low-signal serpiginous border (Fig. 13.10). AVN can be diagnosed earlier and more reliably using MR imaging than with plain films or nuclear medicine.

Acetabular Labrum

The acetabular labrum is analogous to the glenoid labrum of the shoulder. It can tear or detach, resulting in a painful, snapping hip. The labrum can be arthroscopically debrided or repaired, with a good clinical outcome reported by multiple surgeons.

The acetabular labrum is best visualized with an MR arthrogram.[4] Imaging should be done with a small FOV and only one hip studied. Bilateral exams with a large FOV and nonarthrogram studies have an extremely low sensitivity for labral tears. When the labrum tears or detaches, it most commonly is abnormal in the anterosuperior quadrant (Fig. 13.11).

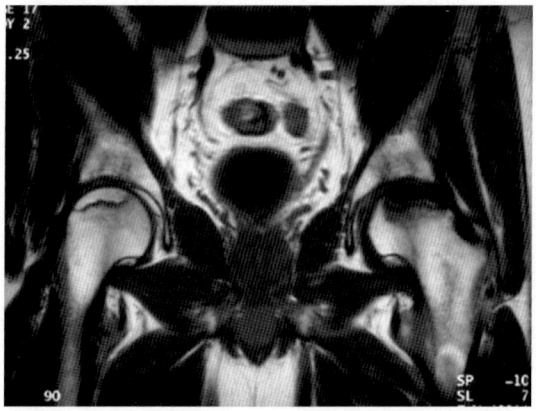

FIG. 13.10 **Avascular Necrosis (AVN) of the Femoral Heads.** A T1-weighted coronal image shows marked low signal in the left femoral head, which indicates advanced hip AVN. The right hip has AVN demonstrated by high signal surrounded by a low-signal serpiginous border. This is characteristic for AVN.

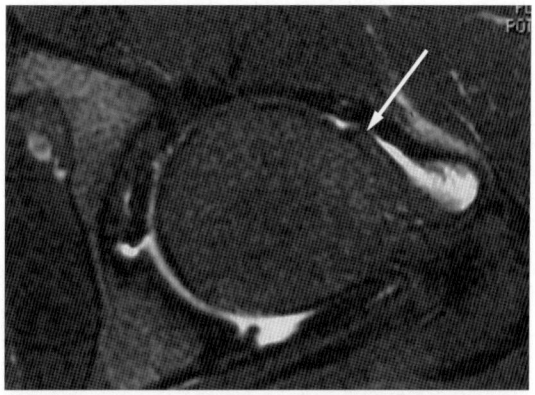

FIG. 13.12 **Femoroacetabular Impingement (FAI).** An axial T2WI in an athlete with hip pain shows a bony prominence in the subcapital portion of the femoral neck *(arrow)*. He had marked pain relief and increased range of motion following surgical excision of the bony prominence.

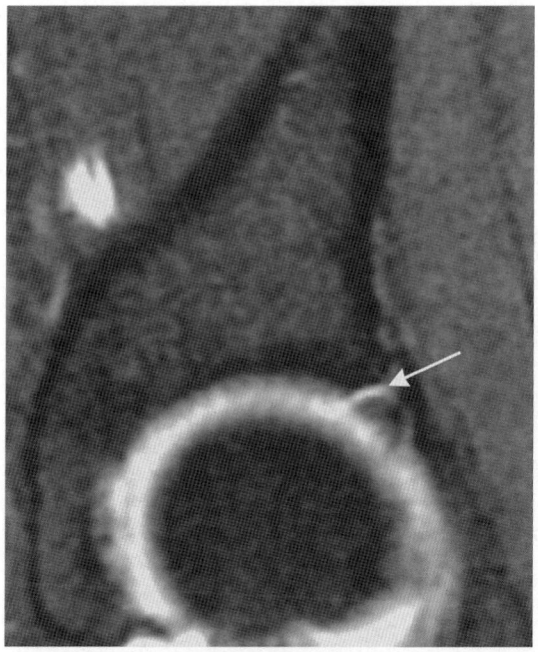

FIG. 13.11 **Torn Acetabular Labrum.** This coronal T1-weighted, fat-suppressed arthrogram of the hip shows fluid between the bony acetabulum and the labrum *(arrow)*, indicating a detached labrum.

Femoroacetabular Impingement

The labrum is often torn or macerated due to FAI. This is a relatively recently described entity that is a result of bony prominence or even a protuberance at the lateral subcapital region of the femoral neck (Fig. 13.12) and/or from overcoverage of the femoral head by the acetabulum. Abduction of the hip causes the bony prominence on the femur to abut the acetabulum (which may also be prominent), squeezing the labrum, and often tearing it. If the main problem is a bony prominence on the femur, it is termed "cam" impingement, whereas if the acetabulum is prominent, it is termed "pincer" impingement. Cam impingement is more common in males, while pincer impingement is said to be more common in females. In fact, the vast majority of patients with impingement have a combination of the two types. Multiple measurements about the hip have been described to diagnose FAI; however, they do not seem to be reliably reproduced, and many asymptomatic individuals have abnormal measurements. Therefore I do not report any measurements. I simply evaluate for a subcapital bony prominence or for overextension of the acetabulum and let the surgeon decide if the patient has clinical signs of FAI.

ELBOW

MRI of the elbow has been shown to be useful in diagnosing collateral ligament tears, biceps tendon tears, and for loose bodies. It can show high T1 signal in the flexor tendons as they insert on the medial epicondyle and in the extensor tendons on the lateral epicondyle in so-called golfer's and tennis elbow. Tendinosis of the flexor and extensor tendons is the most common abnormality seen on elbow MRI. Partial tears of the flexor or extensor tendons show high T2 signal (Fig. 13.13). Bony and cartilaginous abnormalities can also be seen with MRI.

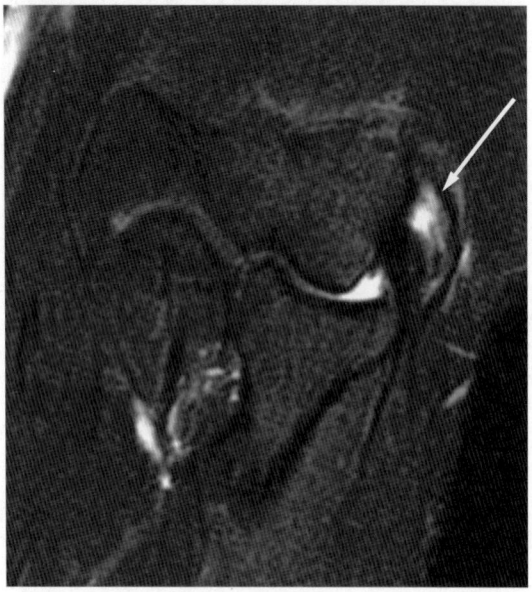

FIG. 13.13 **Partial Tear of the Common Extensors.** A coronal T2WI of the elbow shows fluid signal at the insertion of the common extensor tendons onto the lateral epicondyle *(arrow)*. This indicates a partial tear of the tendons.

The imaging protocol typically includes axial and coronal T1- and T2-weighted images. Sagittal images are optional in some centers; however, we have found them to be useful and routinely obtain them. MR arthrography is utilized when a partial tear of the ulnar collateral ligament or loose bodies are clinical considerations.

The ulnar collateral ligament is reliably identified on coronal T2 images. If it is torn, it will show discontinuity and high T2-weighted signal (Fig. 13.14).

BONE MARROW

MRI readily shows the bone marrow throughout the skeleton. Its appearance varies with age and location within the skeleton. For instance, a young person's skeleton has more red (hematopoietic) marrow, while an elderly person has more fatty marrow. The axial skeleton (spine and pelvis) have more red marrow than the peripheral skeleton.

One of the best tips for differentiating red marrow from an infiltrative process is that red marrow is *always* higher in signal on T1WI than adjacent muscle, or, in the lumbar spine, higher on signal than the discs (Fig. 13.15). An infiltrative process, such as tumor or infection, only rarely is higher in signal than muscle or disc on a T1 sequence. Even the most severe anemia with marked red marrow hyperplasia will obey this rule

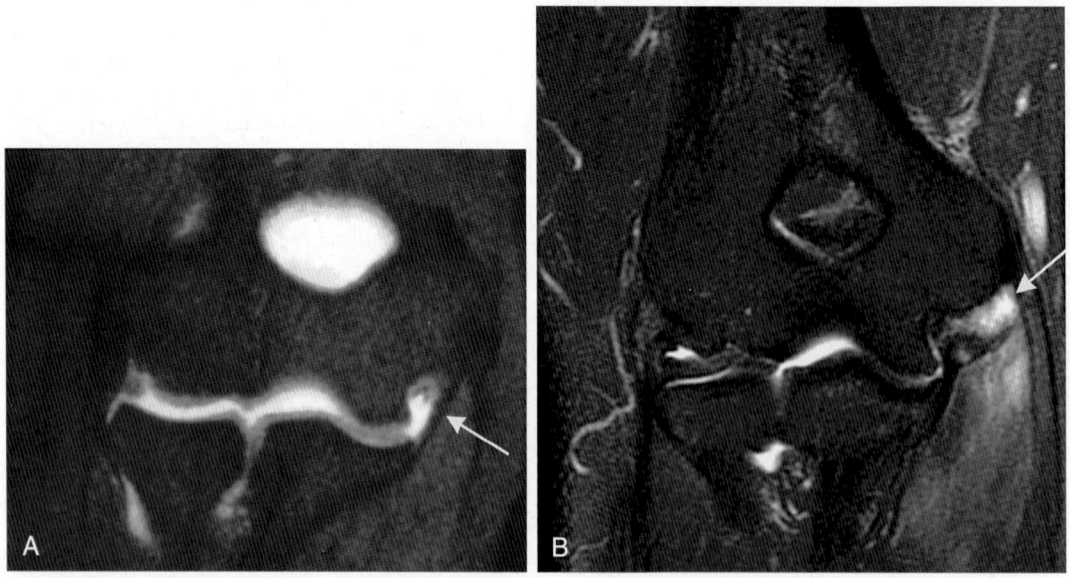

FIG. 13.14 **Ulnar Collateral Ligament.** Coronal T1-weighted, fat-suppressed arthrograms of the elbow show the normal ulnar collateral ligament (A) *(arrow)* and one that is torn off of the attachment to the medial epicondyle *(arrow)*.

unless there is iron overload, as in hemochromatosis. Care must be taken not to confuse diffuse increased bone density with abnormal marrow, since both may have marked low signal on T1WIs.

When I see red marrow hyperplasia, it is usually in a 30- to 40-year-old obese woman who smokes. Those factors often rev up the red marrow. My residents and fellows routinely mention these as an etiology for the increased red marrow, and most times they are probably right. However, it's important to suggest anemia as a cause (Fig. 13.16) because anemia is easily diagnosed with a simple blood test and easily treated with iron supplements, usually with a noticeable difference for the patient. Obesity and smoking are unlikely to be cured, so I usually mention only anemia as a cause for the increased red marrow.

The epiphyses should always have fatty marrow seen as high signal on T1 sequences. If red marrow is seen in the epiphyses, anemia should be suggested (Fig. 13.17). Fatty marrow will be present in a geographic pattern following radiation treatment as the hematopoietic marrow is obliterated.

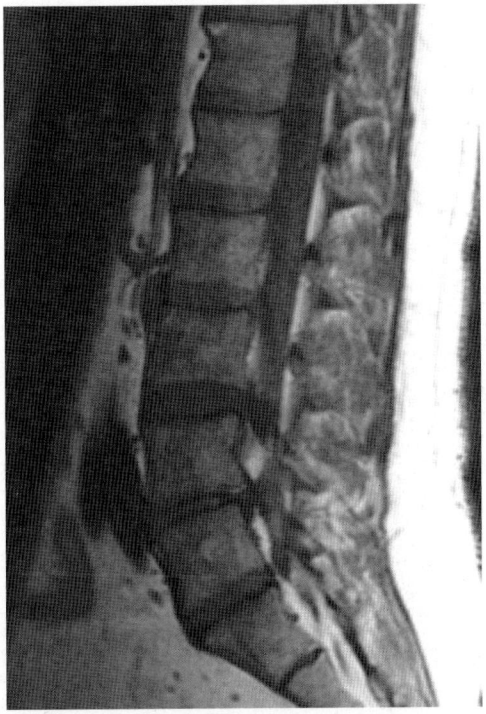

FIG. 13.15 **Normal Red Marrow.** This sagittal T1WI of the lumbar spine in a 25-year-old shows the appearance of normal red marrow in the vertebral bodies. Note that the low signal in the marrow is higher in signal than the discs.

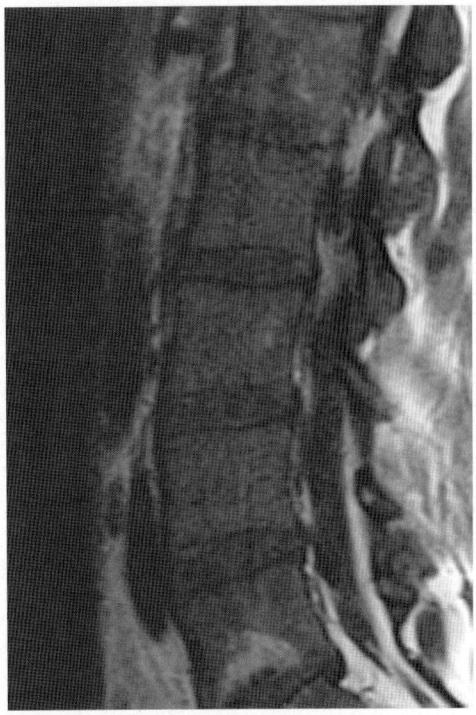

FIG. 13.16 **Increased Red Marrow in Anemia.** A sagittal T1WI through the lumbar spine in a 40-year-old woman with anemia shows a marked increase in the red marrow. Note that it remains higher in signal than the discs.

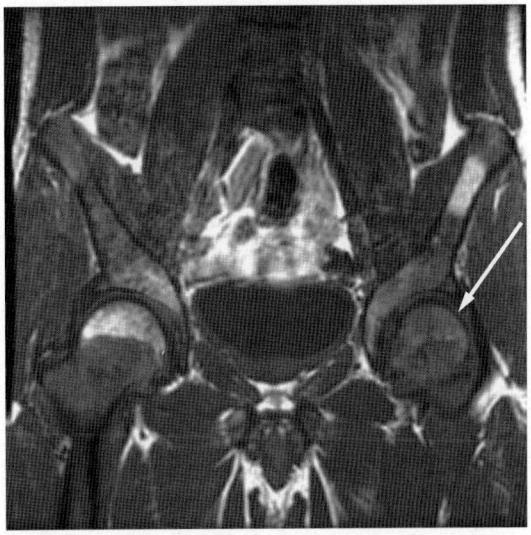

FIG. 13.17 **Sickle Cell Anemia.** A coronal T1WI of the pelvis in a patient with sickle cell anemia shows low signal in the left femoral head epiphysis *(arrow)*, indicative of red marrow hyperplasia. The right femoral head shows the normal appearance with fatty marrow.

REFERENCES

1. Kang H, Kindynis P, Brahme S, et al. Triangular fibrocartilage and intercarpal ligaments of the wrist: MR imaging. Cadaveric study with gross pathologic and histologic correlation. *Radiology*. 1991;181:401–404.
2. Totterman S, Miller R, Wasserman B, Blebea J, Rubens D. Intrinsic and extrinsic carpal ligaments: evaluation by three-dimensional Fourier transform MR imaging. *AJR*. 1993;160:117–123.
3. Dorsay TA, Major NM, et al. Cost-effectiveness of immediate MR imaging versus traditional follow-up for revealing radiographically occult scaphoid fractures. *AJR*. 2001;177:1257–1263.
4. Petersilge CA. MR arthrography for evaluation of the acetabular labrum. *Skeletal Radiol*. 2001;30:423–430.

Index

A
ABCs. *See* Aneurysmal bone cysts (ABCs)
Abrams, Herbert, 1
Acetabular labrum, 242, 243f
Achilles tendon, MRI for, 225–226, 226f
Achondroplasia, 167, 167f
ACL (anterior cruciate ligament), MRI for, 187–188, 189f–190f
Acromegaly, 132
Adamantinoma, 11f
Age
  malignant tumors and, 40t
  nonossifying fibroma and, 17–19
Aggressive osteoporosis, 152, 154f
Anemia, 245, 245f
Aneurysmal bone cysts (ABCs), 20–24, 23f
  cortical destruction and, 35, 37f
  MRI for, 23f
  osteoblastoma and, 19–20
  primary type of, 22–24
  secondary type of, 22–24
Ankle
  MRI for, 225–238
    anatomy of, 225, 227f
    anterolateral impingement, 238f
    chronic lateral ankle pain, 235–238, 237t
    osteomyelitis, 237f
    stress fracture, 237f
  Ottawa Rules, 3–4
  unnecessary examinations in, 3–4, 4f
Ankylosing spondylitis, 91–92, 125, 127f–128f
  spine fracture in, 93f
Annular tear, of disc, 214f
Anterior cruciate ligament (ACL), MRI for, 187–188, 189f–190f
Anterior inferior iliac spine, avulsion from, 108f
Anterior talofibular ligament, 232–234, 234f
Anterior wedge compression fracture, 89–91, 91f
Anterolateral impingement, 238f
Arm, trauma to
  displaced fat pads, 102f–103f
  fractures, 98–105
    Colles, 98–99, 99f
    Galeazzi, 100, 101f
    glenoid, 105f
Arm, trauma to *(Continued)*
    Monteggia, 99, 101f
    plastic bowing deformity of forearm, 98–99, 100f
  shoulder
    dislocations, 102, 103f
    Hill-Sachs deformity, 102–103
    normal anteroposterior view of, 104f
    pseudodislocation of, 63, 68f–69f
Arthritis, 119–150
  anatomical distribution of, 119
    in hands and wrists, 120t
  avascular necrosis in, 144–149
    Freiberg's infraction, 146–149, 149f
    geodes, 146, 148f
    of hip, 145f–146f
    Kienböck's malacia, 146–149, 149f
    Köhler disease, 146–149, 149f
    Legg-Perthes disease, 146–149
    MRI in, 146
    Osgood-Schlatter disease, 146–149
    osteochondral lesion, 146, 147f–148f
    Scheuermann's disease, 146–149, 150f
    of shoulder, 147f
  collagen-vascular diseases, 132
  crystal-induced, 129–132
    gout, 129–130, 131f–132f
    pseudogout (calcium pyrophosphate crystal deposition disease), 130–132
  differential diagnoses of, 119
  hemophilia, 134, 140f
  HLA-B27 spondyloarthropathies, 124–129
    ankylosing spondylitis, 125, 127f–128f
    Reiter syndrome, 125–129, 130f
    syndesmophytes, 125, 126f–127f
    variants, 124
  joint effusions, 137–144
    knee, 144, 145f
    teardrop measurements of, 138–144, 144f–145f
  large joint involvement, 120t
  osteoarthritis, 120–121
    DISH, 120–121, 121f
    geodes, 121, 123f, 123t
Arthritis *(Continued)*
    hallmarks of, 120b
    joint space narrowing, 120
    letter joints with, 121, 123t
    primary, 121, 122f
    secondary, 121
    in shoulder, 120f
    SI joints, 109f, 123f
    subchondral cysts, 121, 123f, 123t
  paralysis, 134
  psoriatic, 126–128, 128f–129f
    CT of, 128f
  PVNS, 136, 142f–143f
  rheumatoid, 121–123, 123t, 124f
    CPPD, 123
    of hip, 125f
    juvenile, 134, 139f
    migration routes of, 124f
    secondary degenerative disease and, 126f
    in shoulder, 125t
  sarcoidosis, 132, 137f
  in SI joints, 119, 120t
    osteoarthritis, 109f
  side-to-side symmetry of, 119
    bilateral, 120b
  synovial osteochondromatosis, 134–136, 141f
    MRI in, 136
    muscular dystrophy, 140f
    without calcification, 142f
  systemic lupus erythematosus, 132, 135f
Athletes, osteosclerosis in, 160
Atypical synovial cyst, 55f
"Automatics", 30, 30b
Avascular necrosis (AVN), 167, 168f, 168t, 239, 243f
  arthritis and, 144–149
    Freiberg's infraction, 146–149, 149f
    geodes, 146, 148f
    of hip, 145f–146f
    Kienböck's malacia, 146–149, 149f
    Köhler disease, 146–149, 149f
    Legg-Perthes disease, 146–149
    MRI in, 146
    Osgood-Schlatter disease, 146–149
    osteochondral lesion, 146, 147f–148f

Note: Page numbers followed by "f" indicate figures and "t" indicate tables.

Avascular necrosis (AVN) *(Continued)*
Scheuermann's disease, 146–149, 150f
of shoulder, 147f
causes of, 168t
etiology of, 167
MRI for, 167
of scaphoid, hand and wrist trauma, 98f
in tendon, 229–230, 230f
osteochondritis dissecans, 229–230, 230f
Avulsion injuries, 59, 62f
pelvic fractures, 105–106

B

Baker's cysts, 54
Baseball finger. *See* Mallet finger
Benign lytic lesions, 7–34
additional points for, 29–30
aneurysmal bone cyst, 20–24, 23f
MRI for, 23f
osteoblastoma and, 19–20
primary type of, 22–24
secondary type of, 22–24
automatics, 30, 30b
chondroblastoma, 28, 28f
chondromyxoid fibroma, 29, 29f
cystic angiomatosis, 26f
enchondroma, 11–12, 12f
bone infarcts, 12, 13f
chondrosarcoma, 12
Maffucci syndrome, 12, 14f
MRI, 12
multiple, 12
Ollier disease, 12, 14f
periostitis, 12
eosinophilic granuloma, 12–14, 15f
appearances of, 12–13
bony sequestrum of, 14, 16f, 16t
monostotic, 13
FEGNOMASHIC, 7–8, 9t
definition of, 7–8
discriminators, 8
giant cell tumor, 8
unicameral bone cyst, 8
fibrous dysplasia, 8–11, 9f–10f
adamantinoma and, 11f
assessment, 8
chondrosarcoma and, 11
classic description of, 10
differential diagnosis, 8
McCune-Albright syndrome and, 11
monostotic, 10, 10f
periostitis and, 8
polyostotic, 10
giant bone island, 30–31, 31f
giant cell tumor, 14–16, 16f–17f
criteria for, 14–16
eccentric locations of, 15
FEGNOMASHIC, 8
nonossifying fibromas and, 15–16
Benign lytic lesions *(Continued)*
hemangiomas, 25–26
hyperparathyroidism, 25
brown tumors of, 25, 25f
subperiosteal bone resorption and, 25
infection, 26
metastatic disease, 20, 22f
renal cell carcinoma, 23f
myeloma, 20
nonossifying fibroma, 17–19, 17f
age and, 17–19
CT of, 17–19, 19f
giant cell tumor and, 15–16
healing, 18f
large, 20f
MRI for, 19, 21f
resolving, 32f
osteoblastoma, 19–20, 22f, 22t
aneurysmal bone cysts and, 19–20
osteomyelitis with pyoarthritis, 27f
plasmacytoma, 22f
sclerotic lesion, differential diagnosis of, 30–31
solitary bone cyst, 24–25, 24f–25f
Benign tumors, malignant *versus*, 35–36
Bennett fracture, 92, 93f
Boehler's angle, in normal calcaneus, 117f
Bone infarcts
as benign lesions, 69–75, 79f–80f
enchondroma and, 12, 13f
Bone islands, 67, 77f
Bone marrow
edema, painful, 176–177, 177f–178f
MRI for, 244–245, 245f
Bowtie sign, 184–185, 186t
Brodie abscess, 26f
Brower, Anne, 119
Brown tumors, 25, 25f
Bucket handle tear, 183–184, 184f–185f
Buford complex, 205, 206f
Bursitis, 194, 196f–197f

C

Calcaneal stress fractures, 109–110, 113f, 237f
Calcaneus
fracture, 117f
pseudocyst of, 78f
Calcium pyrophosphate crystal deposition disease (CPPD), 130–132
arthropathy, 133f–134f
gout and, 129–130
hemochromatosis and, 133
in knee, 132f
pseudo-Charcot joint in, 134, 135f
in wrist, 133f
Carpal tunnel syndrome, 240
Central canal stenosis, 217–218, 217f
Cervical spine (C-spine)
ligamentous disruption in, 5
normal, 85f–86f
unnecessary examinations for, 5
Chance fracture, 88
Charcot joint, 133–134, 138f–139f
Chondroblastoma, 28, 28f
as "don't touch" lesions, 64–65, 73f
Chondromalacia, 194, 196f
Chondromyxoid fibroma, 29, 29f
Chondrosarcoma, 11–12, 43, 47f
Chronic lateral ankle pain, 235–238, 237t
Clay-shoveler fracture, 87, 87f
Coccyx, unnecessary examinations of, 2
Collagen-vascular diseases, 132
Colles fracture, 98–99, 99f
Computed tomography (CT)
of fractured hook of hamate, 97f
of lumbar spine, 212f
for nonossifying fibroma, 17–19, 19f
for osteoid osteoma, 172
for osteoporosis, 151
of posttraumatic lesions, 59
of psoriatic arthritis, 128f
skull, 1–2
Contusions, 194, 198f
Cortical desmoid, as posttraumatic lesions, 59, 62f–64f
Cortical destruction, 35
aneurysmal bone cysts, 35, 37f
giant cell tumor and, 37f
Cortical holes, in osteoporosis, 152, 154f–155f
Costochondritis, 63, 69f
Crystal-induced arthritis, 129–132. *See also* Calcium pyrophosphate crystal deposition disease
gout, 129–130, 131f–132f
Cystic angiomatosis, 26f
Cysts. *See specific cysts*

D

De Quervain syndrome, 240–242, 242f
Desmoid, 45, 45f, 49f
Diaphyseal dysplasia, 167, 169f
Diffuse idiopathic skeletal hyperostosis (DISH), 91–92
osteoarthritis and, 120–121, 121f
Disc disease, 211–216, 212f, 222f
mimics, 221–223
renal cell carcinoma, 223f
sacroiliitis, 223f
Disc protrusions, 213, 213f
Discitis, 161f
Discogenic vertebral disease, 59–63, 67f
Discoid meniscus, 186, 186f
lateral, 187f
DISH (diffuse idiopathic skeletal hyperostosis), 91–92

Dislocations
anterior, transscapular view of, 104f
examples of, 87–92
of hip, 106f
lunate, 96f
posterior, transscapular view of, 105f
Disuse osteoporosis, 152
"Don't touch" lesions, 59–82
benign, 66–75
bone infarcts, 69–75, 79f–80f
bone islands, 67, 77f
lipidization, 67–69
nonossifying fibroma, 66–67, 75f–77f
Pitt's pit, 75, 80f
pseudocyst of calcaneus, 78f
unicameral bone cysts, 67–69, 78f
chondroblastoma, 64–65, 73f
dorsal defect of patella, 63–64, 71f
MRI scans of, 71f
normal variants, 63–66
osteopoikilosis, 66, 74f–75f
posttraumatic, 59–63
avulsion injury, 59, 62f
cortical desmoid, 59, 62f–64f
CT of, 59
fracture, 63, 68f
geodes, 59, 65f–66f
MRI for, 59
myositis ossificans, 59, 60f–61f
os odontoideum, 65–66, 73f–74f
osteogenic sarcoma, 61f
osteophytosis, 59–63
pseudocyst of humerus, 64–65, 72f
pseudodislocation of shoulder, 63, 68f–69f
from trauma, 59
Dorsal defect, of patella, 63–64, 71f
MRI scans of, 71f

E
Elbow
fat pad of, normal anterior, 103f
MRI for, 243–244
Enchondroma, 11–12, 12f
bone infarcts and, 12, 13f
chondrosarcoma and, 12
Maffucci syndrome and, 12, 14f
MRI, 12
multiple, 12
Ollier disease and, 12, 14f
periostitis and, 12
Engelmann disease, 167, 169f
Eosinophilic granuloma, 12–14, 15f
appearances of, 12–13
bony sequestrum of, 14, 16f, 16t
monostotic, 13
Ewing sarcoma, 42–43, 46f–47f
Examinations. *See* Unnecessary examinations
Exostoses, multiple hereditary, 170–172, 171f–172f
Extensors, partial tear of, 244f

F
Facet hypertrophy, causing stenosis, 217f
Fast spin-echo (FSE) T2-weighted sequence, 181, 199
FEGNOMASHIC, 7–8, 9t
Femoral stress fracture, 110f–111f
Femoroacetabular impingement, 243, 243f
Ferris, Hall, 1
FHL (flexor hallucis longus), 226–227, 227f
Fibrous dysplasia, 8–11, 9f–10f
adamantinoma and, 11f
assessment in, 8
chondrosarcoma and, 11
classic description of, 10
differential diagnosis, 8
McCune-Albright syndrome and, 11
monostotic, 10, 10f
periostitis and, 8
polyostotic, 10
Fibular stress fractures, 109, 113f
Flexion teardrop fracture, 88, 89f
Flexor hallucis longus, 226–227, 227f
Fluorosis, 160
Foot
fracture, 117
Lisfranc, 134
MRI for, 225–238
Forrester, Debbie, 119
Fractures, 83, 87–92
anterior wedge compression, 89–91, 91f
arm, 98–105
Colles, 98–99, 99f
Galeazzi, 100, 101f
glenoid, 105f
Monteggia, 99, 101f
plastic bowing deformity of forearm, 98–99, 100f
of base of fifth metatarsal, 117, 117f–118f
calcaneal, 117f
chance, 88
clay-shoveler, 87, 87f
flexion teardrop, 88, 89f
foot, 117
Lisfranc, 134
hand and wrist, 92–98
Bennett, 92, 93f
hook of the hamate, 96–97, 96f
pseudo-Bennett, 92
Rolando, 92, 93f
of scaphoid, 97, 98f
transscaphoid, 96
triquetral, 98, 99f
hangman's, 88, 88f
of hip, 115f
Jefferson, 87, 87f
leg, 109–118
calcaneal stress, 109–110, 113f
with completion, 111f–112f
Fractures *(Continued)*
femoral, 153f
femoral stress, 109, 110f
fibular stress, 109, 113f
tibial plateau, 110–117, 116f
Looser's, 153
metabolic bone survey for, 3
pelvic, 105–109
avulsion injuries, 105–106
"Honda sign", 105, 107f
sacral, 105
as posttraumatic lesions, 63, 68f
sacral insufficiency, 63, 70f
of sacrum, 106f
seat belt, 88, 90f
Smith, 88, 98–99, 100f
supra-acetabular insufficiency, 63, 70f
unilateral locked facets, 88, 89f
Freiberg's infraction, 146–149, 149f
FSE (fast spin-echo) T2-weighted sequence, 181, 199

G
Galeazzi fracture, 100, 101f
Gamekeeper's thumb, 92–94, 94f
Geodes
in avascular necrosis, 146, 148f
in osteoarthritis, 121, 123f, 123t
as posttraumatic lesions, 59, 65f–66f
Giant bone island, 30–31, 31f
Giant cell tumor, 8, 14–16, 16f–17f
criteria for, 14–16
eccentric locations of, 15
FEGNOMASHIC, 8
malignant, 37f, 43–44
nonossifying fibromas and, 15–16
in tendon, 230, 231f
Glenoid fracture, 105f
Gonadal radiation, lumbar spine, 3
Gout, 129–130, 131f–132f

H
Hall, Ferris, 1
Hand and wrist
fractures, 92–98
Bennett, 92, 93f
pseudo-Bennett, 92
Rolando, 92, 93f
of scaphoid, 97, 98f
transscaphoid, 96
triquetral, 98, 99f
lunate dislocation, 94–95, 95f
lunate/perilunate dislocation, 94–95, 95f
normal lateral radiograph, 94f
schematic depiction of, 95f
trauma to
arthritis, 120t
calcium pyrophosphate crystal deposition disease, 133f
Kienböck's malacia, 98, 98f
rotatory subluxation of scaphoid, 97, 97f

Hangman's fracture, 88, 88f
Harris, Jack, 83
Harris, William, 83
Healing nonossifying fibroma, 18f
Hemangioma, 25–26
  in osteoporosis, 152, 156f
  soft tissue tumors, 52–54, 54f
Hematoma, 54, 56f
Hemochromatosis, 133, 137f
Hemophilia, 134, 140f
Hemorrhagic cyst, 57f
Hill-Sachs deformity, 102–103
  in shoulders, 202, 203f
Hip
  dislocation of, 106f
  MRI for, 242–243
HLA-B27 spondyloarthropathies, 124–129
  ankylosing spondylitis, 125, 127f–128f
  Reiter syndrome, 125–129, 130f
  syndesmophytes, 125, 127f
  variants, 124
"Honda sign", 105, 107f
HPO (hypertrophic pulmonary osteoarthropathy), 169, 169f, 169t
Humerus, pseudocyst of, 64–65, 72f
Hunter syndrome, 169–170
Hurler syndrome, 169–170, 170f–171f
Hyperparathyroidism (HPT), 25, 153–155, 158f–159f
  calcium pyrophosphate crystal deposition disease and, 132
  causes of, 153
  discitis, 161f
  metabolic bone surveys for, 3
  primary, 153
  with sacroiliac joint subperiosteal erosion, 159f
  subperiosteal bone resorption in, 153–154
Hypertrophic pulmonary osteoarthropathy (HPO), 169, 169f, 169t
Hypophosphatasia, 132

I

Idiopathic transient osteoporosis, of hip, 177f
Impingement, 200
Infection, in benign cystic lesion, 26, 26f–27f
Intercarpal ligaments, 239–240, 241f
Intraosseous lipoma, 67–69
Ischium, avulsion of, 108f

J

Jefferson fracture, 87, 87f
Joint effusions, 137–144
  knee, 144, 145f
  teardrop measurements of, 138–144, 144f–145f
Juvenile rheumatoid arthritis, 134, 139f

K

Kienböck malacia, 240f
  AVN and, 146–149, 149f
  wrist, 98, 98f
Knee
  calcium pyrophosphate crystal deposition disease in, 132f
  joint effusions, 144, 145f
  MRI of, 181–198
    ACL, 187–188, 189f–190f
    axial images of, 182
    bony abnormalities, 194
    bowtie sign, 184–185, 186t
    bucket handle tear, 183–184, 184f–185f
    bursitis, 194, 196f–197f
    chondromalacia, 194
    collateral ligaments, 192–193, 192f–194f
    contusions, 194, 198f
    coronal images, 181
    cruciate ligaments, 187–192, 189f–190f
    discoid meniscus, 186, 186f–187f
    imaging protocol for, 181–182, 182t
    ligament of Wrisberg, 190–191, 191f
    loose body, 190–191, 191f
    MCL, 192, 192f–193f
    meniscal cysts, 186, 188f
    meniscal tears, 182, 183f–184f
    menisci, 182–186, 182f–183f
    meniscocapsular separation, 192–193, 193f
    parrot beak tear, 184, 185f
    patella and cartilage, 194
    PCL, 188–190, 190f
    plica, 194, 196f
    posterolateral corner, 193, 195f
Köhler disease, 146–149, 149f
Kummell disease, 89–91, 92f

L

Large nonossifying fibroma, 20f
Lateral collateral ligament, 193, 194f, 232–234, 233f
Lateral recess stenosis, 219, 219f
Legg-Perthes disease, 146–149
Lesions. *See* "Don't touch" lesions; Malignant tumors
Ligament of Humphrey, 191–192, 192f
Ligament of Wrisberg, 190–191, 191f
Ligaments, MRI for, 232–234, 233f, 235f
Ligamentum flavum hypertrophy, 217–218, 218f
Lipidization, 67–69
Lisfranc fracture, 116f, 117, 134
Looser's fractures
  metabolic bone survey for, 3
  in osteomalacia, 153, 157f
Lumbar myelograms, 4–5, 4f
Lumbar spine
  annular tear in, 214f
  conjoined root in, 215, 215f
  CT of, 212f
  desiccated disc in, 212f
  disc bulges in, 212f
  disc disease, 211–216, 212f, 222f
    mimics, 221–223
    renal cell carcinoma, 223f
    sacroiliitis, 223f
  disc protrusions, 213, 213f
  end-plate changes in, 220–221
  free fragments in, 214–215, 214f–215f
  gonadal radiation dose in, 3
  imaging protocols for, 211
  lateral discs in, 216, 216f
  marrow changes in, 220–221, 221f–222f
  MRI for, 212f, 213–214
  postoperative scars in, 219, 220f
  spondylolisthesis in, 2–3, 219–220
  spondylolysis in, 219–220, 221f
  stenosis, 217–219
    central canal, 217–218, 217f
    facet hypertrophy causing, 217f
    lateral recess, 219, 219f
    ligamentum flavum hypertrophy, 217–218, 218f
    neuroforaminal, 218–219, 218f
  unnecessary examinations of, 2–3
    with MRI, 4–5, 5f
Lunate dislocation, 96f
Lytic osteosarcoma, 43f

M

Maffucci syndrome, enchondroma and, 12, 14f
Magnetic resonance imaging (MRI)
  of aneurysmal bone cyst, 23f
  of avascular necrosis, 146, 167
    in tendons, 229–230, 230f
  of bone marrow, 244–245, 245f
    anemia, 245, 245f
    sickle cell anemia, 245, 245f
  of bony abnormalities, 234–235
  of calcaneal stress fracture, 114f, 237f
  of dorsal defect of patella, 71f
  of elbow, 243–244
    partial tear, of extensors, 244f
    ulnar collateral ligament, 244f
  for enchondroma, 12
  of foot and ankle, 225–238
    anatomy of, 225, 227f
    anterolateral impingement, 238f
    chronic lateral ankle pain, 235–238, 237t
    osteomyelitis, 237f
  of hip, 242–243
    acetabular labrum, 242, 243f
    avascular necrosis, 243f
    femoroacetabular impingement, 243, 243f
    osteonecrosis, 242–243

Magnetic resonance imaging (MRI) *(Continued)*
of hip fracture, 115f
of knee, 181–198
ACL, 187–188, 189f–190f
axial images of, 182
bowtie sign, 184–185, 186t
bucket handle tear, 183–184, 184f–185f
bursitis, 194, 196f–197f
chondromalacia, 194
collateral ligaments, 192–193, 192f–194f
contusions, 194, 198f
coronal images of, 181
cruciate ligaments, 187–192, 189f–190f
discoid meniscus, 186, 186f–187f
imaging protocol for, 181–182, 182t
ligament of Humphrey, 191–192, 192f
ligament of Wrisberg, 190–191, 191f
loose body in, 190–191, 191f
MCL, 192, 192f–193f
meniscal cysts, 186, 188f
meniscal tears, 182, 183f–184f
menisci, 182–186, 182f–183f
parrot beak tear, 184, 185f
patella and cartilage, 194
PCL, 188–190, 190f
plica, 194, 196f
posterolateral corner, 193, 195f
of ligaments, 232–234, 233f, 235f
sinus tarsi syndrome, 234, 235f–236f
of lumbar spine, 4–5, 4f–5f, 212f, 213–214
malignant tumors, zone of transition, 40f
for nonossifying fibroma, 19, 21f
of posttraumatic lesions, 59
of sacral insufficiency fracture, 107f
of shoulders, 199–210
acromion, 200, 202
anatomy, 199, 200f
biceps tendon, 205–206, 206f–207f
bony abnormalities, 202
Buford complex, 205, 206f
coronal images, 199, 200f
FSE, 199
glenoid labrum, 202–205, 204f–205f
Hill-Sachs lesion, 202, 203f
imaging protocol, 199–200
impingement, 200
os acromiale, 202, 203f
Parsonage-Turner syndrome, 208–209, 208f
partial tears, 202, 203f–204f

Magnetic resonance imaging (MRI) *(Continued)*
quadrilateral space syndrome, 208, 208f
rotator cuff, 200–202, 201f–202f
suprascapular nerve entrapment, 206–208, 207f
supraspinatus tendon, 200, 201f–202f, 202
tendinosis, 201f
of skull, 1–2
of synovial osteochondromatosis, 136
of wrist, 239–242
avascular necrosis, 239
carpal tunnel syndrome, 240
De Quervain syndrome, 240–242, 242f
imaging techniques, 239
intercarpal ligaments, 239–240, 241f
Kienböck malacia, 240f
pathology of, 239–242
septic tenosynovitis, 242, 242f
tendons, 240–242, 242f
triangular fibrocartilage, 239, 240f
Malignant fibrous histiocytoma (MFH), 44–45, 48f
Malignant tumors, 35–58. *See also* Soft tissue tumors
appearance, 46
benign *versus*, 35–36
chondrosarcoma, 43, 47f
cortical destruction, 35, 36f
aneurysmal bone cyst, 35, 37f
giant cell tumor and, 37f
desmoid, 45, 49f
differentiating types of, 36–55, 40t
enchondroma, 43
Ewing sarcoma, 42–43
fibrous histiocytoma, 44–45, 48f
giant cell tumor, 43–44
metastatic disease, 46
prostate carcinoma, 50f
myeloma, 46–51
multiple, 50f–51f
plasmacytoma, 51
orientation/axis of, 35–36, 39f–40f
osteosarcoma, 40–41, 41f–42f
lytic, 43f
Paget's disease and, 41
parosteal, 41
parosteal osteogenic sarcoma, 44f
patient age and, 40t
periostitis, 35
benign, 38f
primary lymphoma of bone, 45, 49f
zone of transition, 36, 39f
on MRI, 40f
narrow, 36, 39f
permeative, 36, 39f
wide, 36, 39f
Mallet finger, 92, 94f
Marked osteoporosis, 152f

Mastocytosis, 159, 164f
McCune-Albright syndrome, 11
Medial collateral ligament (MCL), MRI for, 192, 192f–193f
Melorheostosis, 169, 170f
Meniscal tears, 182, 183f–184f
Menisci, 182–186, 182f–183f
Meniscocapsular separation, 192–193, 193f
Metabolic bone disease, 151–166. *See also* Hyperparathyroidism
osteomalacia, 153
Looser fractures in, 153, 157f
rickets, 153, 157f
osteoporosis, 151–153
aggressive, 152, 154f
causes of, 151
cortical holes in, 152, 154f–155f
CT for, 151
disuse, 152
femoral fracture in, 153f
hemangioma in, 152, 156f
marked, 152f
mild, 152f
normal mineralization in, 153f
permeative process in, 152, 155f
primary, 151
secondary, 151
osteosclerosis, 155–160
in athletes, 160
differential diagnosis for, 155–156
fluorosis, 160
mastocytosis, 159, 164f
metastatic carcinoma and, 159
myelofibrosis, 157, 162f
osteopetrosis, 157, 162f–163f
Paget's disease, 159–160, 164f–166f
pyknodysostosis, 157–159, 164f
renal osteodystrophy, 156–157
sickle cell disease, 157, 162f
thalassemia, 160, 166f
Metabolic bone survey, 3
Metastatic bone survey, 3
Metastatic carcinoma, 159
Metastatic disease, 20, 22f, 46, 50f
renal cell carcinoma, 23f
MFH (malignant fibrous histiocytoma), 44–45, 48f
Mild osteoporosis, 152f
Mineralization, normal, in osteoporosis, 153f
Monostotic fibrous dysplasia, 10, 10f–11f
Monteggia fracture, 99, 101f
Morquio syndrome, 169–170, 170f
MRI. *See* Magnetic resonance imaging
Mucopolysaccharidoses, 169–170, 170f–171f
Hunter syndrome, 169–170
Hurler syndrome, 169–170, 170f–171f
Morquio syndrome, 169–170, 170f

Multiple enchondroma, 12
Multiple hereditary exostoses, 170–172, 171f–172f
Multiple myeloma, 50f–51f
Muscular dystrophy, 140f
Myelofibrosis, 157, 162f
Myelograms, lumbar, 4–5, 4f
Myeloma, 20, 46–51
  multiple, 50f–51f
  plasmacytoma, 51, 52f
Myositis ossificans
  parosteal osteosarcoma and, 41, 45f
  as posttraumatic lesions, 59, 60f–61f

N

Nasal bone, unnecessary examinations of, 2
Neuroforamen, 218f
Neuroforaminal stenosis, 218–219, 218f
New England Journal of Medicine, 1
Nonossifying fibroma (NOF), 17–19, 17f–18f
  age and, 17–19
  as benign lesions, 66–67, 75f–77f
  CT of, 17–19, 19f
  giant cell tumor and, 15–16
  healing, 18f, 30f
  large, 20f
  MRI for, 19, 21f
  resolving, 32f

O

Occult lesions, metastatic bone surveys, 3
OCL (osteochondral lesion), 146, 147f–148f
Ollier disease, enchondroma and, 12, 14f
Os acromiale, 202, 203f
Os odontoideum, 65–66, 73f–74f
Osgood-Schlatter disease, 146–149
Osteoarthritis, 120–121
  causing geodes, 121, 123f, 123t
  causing subchondral cysts, 121, 123f, 123t
  DISH, 120–121, 121f
  hallmarks of, 120b
  joint space narrowing in, 120
  letter joints with, 121, 123t
  primary, 121, 122f
  secondary, 121
  of shoulder, 120f
  in SI joints, 109f, 123f
Osteoblastoma, 19–20, 22f, 22t
Osteochondral lesion (OCL), 146, 147f–148f
Osteochondritis dissecans, 229–230, 230f
Osteogenic sarcoma, 61f
Osteoid osteoma, 172, 173f–175f
  CT scan for, 172
  double density sign of, 172
  etiology of, 172
Osteomalacia, 153
  Looser fractures in, 153, 157f
  rickets, 153, 157f
Osteomyelitis
  of foot and ankle, 237f
  with pyoarthritis, 27f
Osteonecrosis, 242–243
  secondary to radiation, 152–153, 156f
Osteopathia striata, 172, 176f
Osteopetrosis, 157, 162f–163f
Osteophytosis, 59–63
Osteopoikilosis, 66, 74f–75f, 176, 176f
Osteoporosis, 151–153
  aggressive, 152, 154f
  causes of, 151
  cortical holes in, 152, 154f–155f
  CT for, 151
  disuse, 152
  femoral fracture in, 153f
  hemangioma in, 152, 156f
  marked, 152f
  mild, 152f
  normal mineralization in, 153f
  permeative process in, 152, 155f
  primary, 151
  secondary, 151
Osteosarcoma, 40–41, 41f–42f
  lytic, 43f
  parosteal, 41, 44f, 46f
    cortical desmoid, 45f
    location of, 41
    myositis ossificans, 41, 45f
Osteosclerosis, 155–160
  in athletes, 160
  differential diagnosis for, 155–156
  fluorosis, 160
  mastocytosis, 159, 164f
  metastatic carcinoma and, 159
  myelofibrosis, 157, 162f
  osteopetrosis, 157, 162f–163f
  Paget's disease, 159–160, 164f–166f
  pyknodysostosis, 157–159, 164f
  renal osteodystrophy, 156–157
  sickle cell disease, 157, 162f
  thalassemia, 160, 166f
Ottawa Rules, for ankle, 3–4

P

Pachydermoperiostosis, 176, 176f
Paget's disease
  osteosarcoma and, 41
  osteosclerosis and, 159–160, 164f–166f
Painful bone marrow edema, 176–177, 177f–178f
Paralysis, 134
Parathyroid hormone (PTH) discitis, 161f
Parosteal osteosarcoma, 41, 44f, 46f
  cortical desmoid, 45f
  location of, 41
  myositis ossificans, 41, 45f
Parrot beak tear, 184, 185f
Parsonage-Turner syndrome, 208–209, 208f
Partial tear, of extensors, 244f
Patella, MRI of, 194
  with dorsal defect, 63–64, 71f
PCL (posterior cruciate ligament), MRI of, 188–190, 190f
Periosteal osteogenic sarcoma, 46f
Periostitis, 8, 169, 169t
  benign, 35, 38f
  enchondroma and, 12
  fibrous dysplasia and, 8
  malignant tumors, 35
Permeative process, in osteoporosis, 152, 155f
Peroneal tendons, 227–229, 229f
Pigmented villonodular synovitis (PVNS), 51–52, 52f, 54f
  arthritis and, 136, 142f–143f
Pitt, Michael, 75
Pitt's pit, as benign lesions, 75, 80f
Plasmacytoma, 22f, 51, 52f
Plastic bowing deformity of forearm, 98–99, 100f
Plica, 194, 196f
Polyostotic fibrous dysplasia, 10
Posterior cruciate ligament (PCL), MRI of, 188–190, 190f
Posterior tibial tendons, 226, 228f
Posttraumatic lesions, 59–63
  avulsion injury, 62f
  cortical desmoid, 62f–64f
  CT of, 59
  fracture, 63, 68f
  geodes, 59, 65f–66f
  MRI for, 59
  myositis ossificans, 59, 60f–61f
  os odontoideum, 65–66, 73f–74f
  osteogenic sarcoma, 61f
  osteophytosis, 59–63
  pseudocyst of humerus, 64–65, 72f
  pseudodislocation of shoulder, 63, 68f–69f
  from trauma, 59
Primary lymphoma of bone (reticulum cell sarcoma), 45, 49f
Primary osteoarthritis, 121, 122f
Primary osteoporosis, 151
Pseudo-Bennett fracture, 92
Pseudocyst
  of calcaneus, 78f
  of humerus, 64–65, 72f
Pseudodislocation, of shoulder, 63, 68f–69f
Psoriatic arthritis, 126–128, 128f–129f
  CT of, 128f
PVNS. *See* Pigmented villonodular synovitis
Pyknodysostosis, 157–159, 164f
Pyoarthritis, osteomyelitis with, 27f

Q

Quadrilateral space syndrome, 208, 208f

R

Radial tear, 184, 186f
Radiation, osteonecrosis secondary to, 152–153, 156f
Radiology, 1
The Radiology of Emergency Medicine (Jack and William Harris), 83
Radiology of Skeletal Trauma (Rogers), 83
Radionuclide scans, metastatic bone surveys, 3
Reiter syndrome, 125–129, 130f
Renal cell carcinoma, 23f
  disc disease, 223f
Renal osteodystrophy, 156–157
Resnick, Don, 119
Rheumatoid arthritis, 121–123, 123t, 124f
  CPPD, 123
  of hip, 125f
  juvenile, 134, 139f
  migration routes of, 124f
  secondary degenerative disease and, 126f
  in shoulder, 125t
Rib, unnecessary examinations of, 2
Rickets, 153, 157f
Rogers, Lee, 83, 99
Rolando fracture, 92, 93f
Rotator cuff, 200–202, 201f–202f
Rotatory subluxation of scaphoid, 97, 97f

S

Sacral insufficiency fractures, 63, 70f
Sacroiliac (SI) joints
  arthritis in, 119, 120t
  osteoarthritis in, 109f, 123f
  subperiosteal erosion, hyperparathyroidism with, 159f
Sacroiliac osteophytosis, 110f
Sacroiliitis, disc disease, 223f
Sacrum, fractures of, 106f
  insufficiency, 107f
Sarcoid, 177, 178f
Sarcoidosis, 132, 137f
Sarcoma, osteogenic, 61f
Scheuermann disease, 146–149, 150f
Schwannoma, 56f
Scleroderma, 132, 136f
Sclerotic lesion, differential diagnosis of, 30–31
Seat belt fracture, 88, 90f
Secondary osteoarthritis, 121
Secondary osteoporosis, 151
Septic tenosynovitis, 242, 242f
Shoulders
  avascular necrosis of, 147f
  MRI of, 199–210
Shoulders *(Continued)*
  acromion, 200, 202
  anatomy, 199, 200f
  biceps tendon, 205–206, 206f–207f
  bony abnormalities, 202
  Buford complex, 205, 206f
  coronal images, 199, 200f
  FSE, 199
  glenoid labrum, 202–205, 204f–205f
  Hill-Sachs lesion, 202, 203f
  imaging protocol, 199–200
  impingement, 200
  os acromiale, 202, 203f
  Parsonage-Turner syndrome, 208–209, 208f
  partial tears, 202, 203f–204f
  quadrilateral space syndrome, 208, 208f
  rotator cuff, 200–202, 201f–202f
  suprascapular nerve entrapment, 206–208, 207f
  supraspinatus tendon, 200, 201f–202f, 202
  tendinosis, 201f
  osteoarthritis of, 120f
  posterior dislocation of, 104f
  pseudodislocation of, 63, 68f–69f
  rheumatoid arthritis in, 125t
SI joints. *See* Sacroiliac (SI) joints
Sickle cell anemia, 245, 245f
Sickle cell disease, 157, 162f
Sinus tarsi syndrome, 234, 235f–236f
Sinus, unnecessary examinations in, 1–2, 2f
Sinusitis, 1–2
Skull, unnecessary examinations in, 1, 2f
SLE (systemic lupus erythematosus), 132
Slipped capital femoral epiphysis, 177, 179f
Smith fracture, 88, 98–99, 100f
Soft tissue tumors, 51–55
  Baker's cysts, 54
  hemangioma, 52–54, 54f
  hemorrhagic cyst, 57f
  misdiagnosis, 54–55
  PVNS, 52, 54f
  synovial osteochondromatosis, 51–52, 52f
  tumefactive synovial osteochondromatosis, 53f
Solitary bone cyst, 24–25, 24f–25f
Spine. *See also* Fractures
  C-spine
    ligamentous disruption in, 5
    normal, 85f–86f
    unnecessary examinations for, 5
  trauma, 83–92
    C1-2 dislocation, 86f
    C-7, 83, 84f
Spine *(Continued)*
    C-spine examination of, 83–87
    CT, 83
    disc spaces, 85
    prevertebral soft tissue, 83
    spinolaminal line, 84
Spondylolisthesis, 89, 91f
  in lumbar spine, 2–3, 219–220
Spondylolysis, 88–89, 90f
  in lumbar spine, 219–220, 221f
Stenosis, 217–219
  central canal, 217–218, 217f
  facet hypertrophy causing, 217f
  lateral recess, 219, 219f
  ligamentum flavum hypertrophy, 217–218, 218f
  neuroforaminal, 218–219, 218f
Stress fractures
  calcaneal, 109–110, 113f, 237f
  femoral, 109, 110f
  fibular, 109, 113f
  tibial, 112f
Subchondral cysts, 121, 123f, 123t
Subperiosteal bone resorption, 25
  in hyperparathyroidism, 153–154
  metabolic bone survey for, 3, 3f
Sudeck atrophy, 137, 143f
Supra-acetabular insufficiency fracture, 63, 70f
Suprascapular nerve entrapment, 206–208, 207f
Supraspinatus tendon, tear, 200, 201f–202f, 202
Swischuk, Leonard, 138–144
Symphysis pubis, 106
  osteoarthritis of, 108f–109f
Syndesmophytes, 125, 126f–127f
Synovial osteochondromatosis, 52f, 134–136, 141f
  MRI in, 136
  muscular dystrophy, 140f
  without calcification, 142f
Synovial sarcomas, 51–52
Systemic lupus erythematosus (SLE), 132, 135f

T

Tarsal coalition, 236f
Tarsal tunnel syndrome, 232, 232f
Tendinosis, 201f, 225
Tendons, 225–229
  Achilles, 225–226, 226f
  avascular necrosis, 229–230, 230f
    osteochondritis dissecans, 229–230, 230f
  flexor hallucis longus, 226–227, 227f
  MRI for, in wrist, 240–242, 242f
  peroneal, 227–229, 229f
  posterior tibial, 226, 228f
  spring ligament, 229f
  supraspinatus, 200, 201f–202f, 202
  tendinosis, 201f, 225

Tendons *(Continued)*
tumors, 230–232
anomalous muscles, 232, 233f
bone cyst, 231f
giant cell, 231f
tarsal tunnel syndrome, 232, 232f
Tenosynovitis, 225
Thalassemia, 160, 166f
Tibia
plateau fracture of, 110–117, 116f
stress fracture of, 112f
Tietze syndrome, 63
Toulouse-Lautrec syndrome, 157–159
Transscaphoid fracture, 96
Transverse ligament, pseudotear from, 186, 188f
Trauma, 83–118. *See also* Arm; trauma to; Fractures; Hand and wrist; trauma to
DISH, 91–92
Kummell disease, 89–91, 92f
mallet finger, 92, 94f
posttraumatic lesions from, 59
rotatory subluxation of scaphoid, 97, 97f
spine, 83–92
C1-2 dislocation, 86f
Trauma *(Continued)*
C-7, 83, 84f
C-spine examination of, 83–87
CT, 83
disc spaces, 85
prevertebral soft tissue, 83
spinolaminal line, 84
spondylolisthesis, 89, 91f
spondylolysis, 88–89, 90f
Triangular fibrocartilage, 239, 240f
Triquetral fracture, 98, 99f
Tumefactive synovial osteochondromatosis, 53f
Tumors. *See also* Benign tumors; Malignant tumors
tendons, MRI for, 230–232
anomalous muscles, 232, 233f
bone cyst, 231f
giant cell, 231f
tarsal tunnel syndrome, 232, 232f

U

Ulnar collateral ligament, 244f
Unicameral bone cysts, 8, 67–69, 78f
Unilateral locked facets fracture, 88, 89f
Unnecessary examinations, 1–6
ankle, 3–4, 4f
of cervical spine, 5
of coccyx, 2
lumbar myelograms as, 4–5
of lumbar spine, 2–3
medicolegal considerations in, 1
metastatic bone survey as, 3
of nasal bone, 2
rib, 2
sinus, 1–2, 2f
skull, 1, 2f
technical considerations for, 5–6

W

Wilson disease, 132
Wrist, MRI for, 239–242
avascular necrosis, 239
carpal tunnel syndrome, 240
De Quervain syndrome, 240–242, 242f
imaging techniques, 239
intercarpal ligaments, 239–240, 241f
Kienböck malacia, 240f
pathology of, 239–242
septic tenosynovitis, 242, 242f
tendons, 240–242, 242f
triangular fibrocartilage, 239, 240f

BMA LIBRARY
BRITISH MEDICAL ASSOCIATION
WITHDRAWN
FROM LIBRARY